ADVANCES IN
Cardiac Surgery®

VOLUME 10

ADVANCES IN Cardiac Surgery®

VOLUMES 1 THROUGH 6 AND 8 (OUT OF PRINT)

VOLUME 7

VOLUME 9

Surgical Approach to Vascular Rings, *by Carl L. Backer and Constantine Mavroudis*

Double-Switch Operation for Congenitally Corrected Transposition, *by Yasuharu Imai*

Volume Reduction Surgery in the Treatment of End-stage Heart Diseases, *by Tomas A. Salerno and Joginder Bhayana*

Video-assisted Coronary Surgery, *by Guido Sani, Gianfranco Lisi, Massimo A. Mariani, Massimo Maccherini, Patrick Nataf, Federico J. Benetti, and Michele Toscano*

Postoperative Atrial Fibrillation, *by Kenneth A. Ellenbogen, Mina K. Chung, Craig R. Asher, and Mark A. Wood*

Left Ventricular Assist, *by O.H. Frazier*

Pediatric Cardiac Transplantation, *by David C. McGiffin, James K. Kirklin, and F. Bennett Pearce*

Surgery for Kawasaki Disease, *by Soichiro Kitamura, Yoichi Kameda, and Yasunaru Kawashima*

Arterial Grafts for Coronary Artery Bypass, *by Noel L. Mills*

Revision of the Traditional Atriopulmonary Fontan Connection, *by Frank G. Scholl, Juan C. Alejos, and Hillel Laks*

ADVANCES IN
Cardiac Surgery®

VOLUME 10

Mosby

St. Louis Baltimore Boston Carlsbad Naples New York Philadelphia Portland
London Madrid Mexico City Singapore Sydney Tokyo Toronto Wiesbaden

Mosby
Dedicated to Publishing Excellence

A Times Mirror Company

Associate Publisher: Cynthia Baudendistel
Developmental Editor: Gary O'Brien
Manager, Periodical Editing: Kirk Swearingen
Production Editor: Stephanie M. Geels
Project Supervisor, Production: Joy Moore
Production Assistant: Laura Bayless

Printed in the United States of America
Composition by The Clarinda Company
Printing/binding by The Maple-Vail Book Manufacturing Group

Editorial Office:
Mosby, Inc.
11830 Westline Industrial Drive
St. Louis, Missouri 63146

International Standard Serial Number: 0889–5074
International Standard Book Number: 0–8151–9804–3

Contributors

Kit V. Arom, M.D., Ph.D.
Cardiovascular Surgeon, Cardiac Surgical Associates, Minneapolis Heart Institute, St. Paul Heart and Lung Institute, St. Paul, Minnesota

John H. Artrip, M.D.
Research Fellow, Columbia University; Research Fellow, Department of Surgery, Columbia Presbyterian Medical Center, New York, New York

Miguel L. Barbero-Marcial, M.D.
Associate Professor, Chief of Pediatric Cardiac Surgery, Heart Institute, University of São Paulo Medical School, São Paulo, Brazil

Vincent Dor, M.D.
Professor of Thoracic and Cardiovascular Surgery, Marseille and Nice University; Head of Surgical Department, Cardio-Thoracic Center of Monaco, Monte Carlo, Monaco

Donald B. Doty, M.D.
Clinical Professor of Surgery, University of Utah School of Medicine; Chief, Department of Surgery, LDS Hospital, Salt Lake City, Utah

John R. Doty, M.D.
Resident, Division of Cardiac Surgery, The Johns Hopkins Hospital, Baltimore, Maryland

Ann M. Emery, R.N.
Cardiac Surgical Associate Research Foundation, Minneapolis–St. Paul, Minnesota

Robert W. Emery, M.D.
Director of Cardiothoracic Transplantation and Cardiovascular and Thoracic Surgeon, Minneapolis Heart Institute, St. Paul Heart and Lung Institute; President, International Society for Minimally Invasive Surgery; Cardiac Surgical Associates, Minneapolis–St. Paul, Minnesota

Richard N. Gates, M.D.
Assistant Clinical Professor of Surgery, Division of Cardiothoracic Surgery, UCLA School of Medicine, UCLA Medical Center, Los Angeles, California; Children's Hospital of Orange County, Orange, California

Peter Hanrath, M.D.
Professor and Chief of Cardiology, Medicine Clinic I, University Hospital Aachen, Aachen, Germany

Keith A. Horvath, M.D.
Assistant Professor of Surgery, Division of Cardiothoracic Surgery, Northwestern University Medical School, Chicago, Illinois

Ranjit John, M.D.
Research Fellow, Columbia University; Research Fellow, Department of Surgery, Columbia Presbyterian Medical Center, New York, New York

Heinrich G. Klues, M.D.
Associate Professor, Department of Cardiology, Medicine Clinic I, University Hospital Aachen, Aachen, Germany

Jon A. Kobashigawa, M.D.
Associate Clinical Professor of Medicine, UCLA School of Medicine; Medical Director, UCLA Heart Transplant Program, University of California, Los Angeles, California

Hillel Laks, M.D.
Professor and Chief, Division of Cardiothoracic Surgery; Director, Heart and Heart–Lung Transplant Program, UCLA Medical Center, Los Angeles, California

Kenneth L. Mattox, M.D.
Professor and Vice Chair of Surgery, Baylor College of Medicine; Chief of Staff and Chief of Surgery, Ben Taub General Hospital, Houston, Texas

Bruno J. Messmer, M.D.
Professor and Chief of Thoracic and Cardiovascular Surgery, University Hospital Aachen, Aachen, Germany

Robert E. Michler, M.D.
Karl P. Klassen Professor of Surgery, Ohio State University; Chief, Cardiothoracic Surgery, Ohio State University Medical Center, Columbus, Ohio

Noel L. Mills, M.D.
Clinical Professor, Department of Surgery, Tulane University School of Medicine, New Orleans, Louisiana

John M. Murkin, M.D., F.R.C.P.C.
Professor of Anesthesia; Director, Cardiac Anesthesia, University Campus, London Health Sciences Center, University of Western Ontario, London, Ontario, Canada

Sebastian Reith, M.D.
Junior Fellow, Department of Cardiology, Medicine Clinic I, University Hospital Aachen, Aachen, Germany

Friedrich A. Schoendube, M.D., Ph.D.
Associate Professor, Department of Thoracic and Cardiovascular Surgery, University Hospital Aachen, Aachen, Germany

Carla Tanamati, M.D.
Fellow, Cardiac Surgery, Heart Institute, University of São Paulo Medical School, São Paulo, Brazil

Contents

CHAPTER 1

Minimally Invasive Coronary Artery Bypass Surgery: State of the Art

Robert W. Emery, M.D.
Director of Cardiothoracic Transplantation and Cardiovascular and Thoracic Surgeon, Minneapolis Heart Institute, St. Paul Heart and Lung Institute; President, International Society for Minimally Invasive Surgery; Cardiac Surgical Associates, Minneapolis–St. Paul, Minnesota

Kit V. Arom, M.D., Ph.D.
Cardiovascular Surgeon, Cardiac Surgical Associates, Minneapolis Heart Institute, St. Paul Heart and Lung Institute, St. Paul, Minnesota

Ann M. Emery, R.N.
Cardiac Surgical Associate Research Foundation, Minneapolis–St. Paul, Minnesota

Minimally invasive cardiac surgery may be a misnomer in that these procedures are still major surgical interventions.[1] Nevertheless, the concept of less tissue disruption, shortened patient recovery, and cost-effective delivery of myocardial revascularization was thrust upon the profession in surprisingly rapid fashion beginning in early 1995 and was readily accepted by the patient population and media. The implicit success of minimally invasive coronary bypass surgery (MICAB), however, lay in many previous initiatives. Laparoscopic surgery developed by the obstetric and gynecologic practitioners was extended to the field of general surgery. General surgeons did not readily accept laparoscopic procedures, but with the accumulation of data and experience, procedures such as laparoscopic cholecystectomy and herniorrhaphy became well-accepted alternatives to standard approaches. These procedures demonstrated that operations previously performed through larger incisions could be performed by alternative means with similar results and proven patient well-being. The logical extension was video-assisted thoracoscopic surgery. Thoracic and cardiovascular surgeons were thus introduced to procedures involving smaller incisions and the necessity of learning new skills to deal with surgery at a "distance." The introduction of MICAB procedures is the latest and most visible initiative. A detailed history of MICAB development has been published.[2]

Work published by Buffolo, Benetti, and their associates indicated that coronary bypass surgery without the use of cardiopulmonary bypass (CPB) on the beating heart could be safely performed in large populations of patients.[3,4] These reports demonstrated that surgery on the beating heart obviated the morbid side effects of CPB. In addition, cost containment was realized in emerging countries that had the capability of performing open-heart surgery but had fewer resources available. Robinson et al. reported the first MICAB performed through a small anterior thoracotomy incision with support from CPB.[5] It soon became apparent that circulatory support was not necessary and early presentations by Subramanian et al. and Calafiore and colleagues further evolved the field.[6,7] Port-access MICAB developed in parallel and allows myocardial revascularization via a minimal incision with the use of CPB and myocardial arrest.[8,9] Thorascopic assistance to harvest necessary conduit and to assist with the procedure itself has subsequently been introduced.[10–12] Over this time, of course, the internal mammary artery became recognized as the conduit of choice for bypass of the left anterior descending (LAD) coronary artery and lent itself readily to MICAB.[13,14]

The definition of minimally invasive surgery is still unclear, however. At a recent meeting the participating audience was asked to define minimally invasive surgery. Eighty-one percent believed that absence of the use of CBP was the defining factor, whereas 19% believed that the size of the incision was a more important component.[15] A definition of minimally invasive surgery remains difficult because the field is so fluid and changes are ongoing at a rapid pace.[16] Over the past 2½ years, evolution into the current state of three methods of revascularization has occurred. Although some of the indications and contraindications for each overlap, each of these surgical methods of revascularization allows an opportunity for the cardiovascular surgeon to offer alternatives to the standard means of performing coronary bypass surgery to patients with specific disease conditions or contraindications to routine bypass surgery because of significant co-morbid risk factors.[17] Currently used techniques include coronary bypass surgery performed via complete sternotomy without the use of CPB, minimally invasive coronary artery bypass surgery performed via a small incision under direct visualization of the beating heart, and port-access surgery using small incisions, CPB with cardiac standstill, and endovascular instrumentation. Each plays an important role in the further development of MICAB. The ultimate goal is to provide complete, multiconduit revascularization with minimal invasion while maximizing the safety and minimizing the risk and recovery time for patients requiring such surgical procedures.

OFF-PUMP CORONARY BYPASS VIA COMPLETE STERNOTOMY

Although the first coronary artery bypasses were performed without CPB and Ankenny in 1975 presented a series of patients on whom CPB was not used, developmental milestones were achieved by using CPB with myocardial standstill.[2, 18] Subsequently, large series of patients on whom multivessel coronary bypass surgery was performed without CPB have been published.[3, 4] The necessity of providing cardiovascular care in environments with limited economic means was the primary thrust for developing off-pump techniques. This impetus did not gain popularity in industrialized countries because of the ready availability of equipment and resources for CPB. However, with the introduction of off-pump surgery via small incisions, interest was rekindled. Arom et al. indicated that through a small skin incision with adequate tissue mobilization a complete sternotomy and multivessel procedure could be accomplished.[19] Access to the lateral circulation is somewhat more difficult, but the anterior descending and right coronary systems are easily approached.

The performance of revascularization via complete sternotomy without CPB is a reconfiguration of accepted surgical techniques. The development of stabilization devices has allowed more accurate surgery on the beating heart with traditional suture techniques.[20–22] Although many stabilizing devices are useful for the anterior wall of the heart, a stabilizing device such as the Medtronic "Octopus" (Fig 1), with its suction cups, allows adherence to and retraction of the heart into the operative field with less packing and manipulation of the ventricle.[22] Hemodynamic compromise is less likely to occur.[23] Other pressure plate–type stabilizing devices have no means of adherence to the epicardium and do not seem to serve the dual purpose of being a retractor as well as a stabilizer, but they function well in many circumstances. The advantages of off-pump bypass surgery via sternotomy are shown in Table 1. Avoiding CPB is an important aspect in expanding surgical indications in that multivessel coronary bypass surgery can be completed in patients

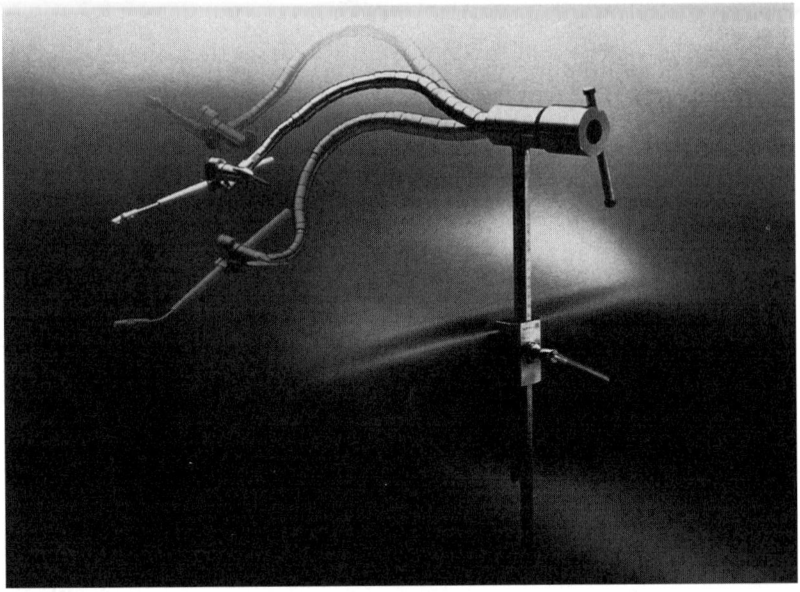

FIGURE 1.
Medtronic Octopus is demonstrated with its articulated arms and suction cups. This device not only permits stabilization of the myocardial surface for the placement of precise sutures but also acts as a retractor for drawing the heart into the operative field. (Courtesy of Medtronic, Inc.)

who have contraindications to the use of standard techniques.[24] Examples might include patients with calcific or severe exophytic disease of the ascending aorta, patients with severe depression of their ejection fraction, or patients in whom significant co-morbid factors such as disease of the kidneys, CNS, or lungs may be substantially worsened by the use of CPB.[17, 25, 26] This application may be especially valid for elderly patients or those at risk for neurologic injury.[27] Gundry and associates and Pagni et al. have reported a greater incidence of disease recurrence in the vessels of patients treated off as opposed to on CPB and have related this to the use of vascular snares.[28, 29] Others have disagreed.[30, 31] Experience with full sternotomy off-pump coronary bypass surgery continues to develop. The ongoing development of new technology is easing the burden on the surgeon for completing such procedures. Excellent midterm outcomes from such procedures have recently been reported, but more information is necessary.[30] Aside from serving as an accepted procedure, operating in such a manner also serves as a learning tool for developing techniques to operate on the beat-

TABLE 1.
Off-Pump Sternotomy Coronary Bypass

Advantages
1. Obviates morbidity of cardiopulmonary bypass
2. Cost-effective
3. Extends indications for surgery to patients who are not candidates for routine approaches
4. Capability of multivessel, multiconduit coronary bypass
5. Utilization of standard operative techniques
6. No aortic manipulation
7. Familiar exposure
Disadvantages
1. Complete sternotomy necessary
2. Surgery technically more difficult
3. Approach to the posterior ventricular wall difficult

ing heart inasmuch as the exposure is familiar to all cardiovascular surgeons.

MINIMALLY INVASIVE OFF-PUMP APPROACHES

The original approach to minimally invasive bypass grafting was reported by Robinson et al. in 1995 and included anterior descending artery grafting with the mammary artery through a small anterior thoracotomy.[5] In this report, CPB was performed via a small groin incision with arterial and venous cannulation of the common femoral artery and vein. This operation was subsequently modified by Calafiore et al. and Subramanian and colleagues and defined by Calafiore et al. as the LAST operation—left anterior small thoracotomy.[6, 7] A variety of approaches to minimally invasive, beating-heart surgery have been developed, including right anterior small thoracotomy for bypass grafting of the right coronary artery, an abdominal approach for utilization of the gastroepiploic vessel in bypassing the posterior descending or distal right coronary artery, and partial sternotomy and combination incisions for bilateral or multivessel bypass in all successful multiple centers worldwide.[17, 19, 32–35] Video-assisted harvesting of the internal mammary artery also allows greater variability in the small thoracotomy incision.[12] The incision does not have to abut the sternum to allow direct retrieval of the mammary artery. The incision may be moved to the third inner space and more laterally where the

TABLE 2.
Minimally Invasive Direct Beating-Heart Coronary Bypass

Advantages	
	1. Limited tissue disruption
	2. Improved patient recovery
	3. Extended indications to patients with contraindications to standard techniques
	4. Cost-effective
	5. Improved cosmesis
	6. No aortic manipulation
	7. No cardiopulmonary bypass
	8. Multiple approaches available
	9. Reconfiguration of accepted surgical techniques
Disadvantages	
	1. Limited access to the anterior and anterolateral ventricular wall
	2. Technically difficult
	3. Pedicled conduits necessary
	4. No proven long-term results
	5. Applicable to a minority of patients
	6. Questions of anastomotic graft patency

first diagonal and ramus intermedius or high obtuse marginal branches can be approached, thereby allowing for multivessel bypass grafting through these small incisions.

Currently, this original approach to minimally invasive surgery has application to only a minority of patients.[15] The advantages and disadvantages of this process are shown in Table 2. Indications include single- or double-vessel disease that may be bypassed by using pedicled conduits. Additional grafts may be accomplished by using alternative conduits such as the saphenous vein or radial artery, with the proximal anastomosis being constructed to the versatile internal mammary artery. Access to the aorta is not possible through these incisions. The development of myocardial stabilizing devices has improved the technical performance of this operation.[29] Three prototype stabilizing devices are shown in Figures 2, 3, and 4. All use a pressure plate to compress the myocardium surrounding the vessel to be bypassed, thereby stabilizing the vessel and allowing fine suturing in a stationery field. These devices are designed to be conveniently placed through small incisions. The experience gained by surgeons has allowed excellent confidence in performing the anastomosis.[35] Most reports would indicate that internal mammary patency has improved with the use of stabiliz-

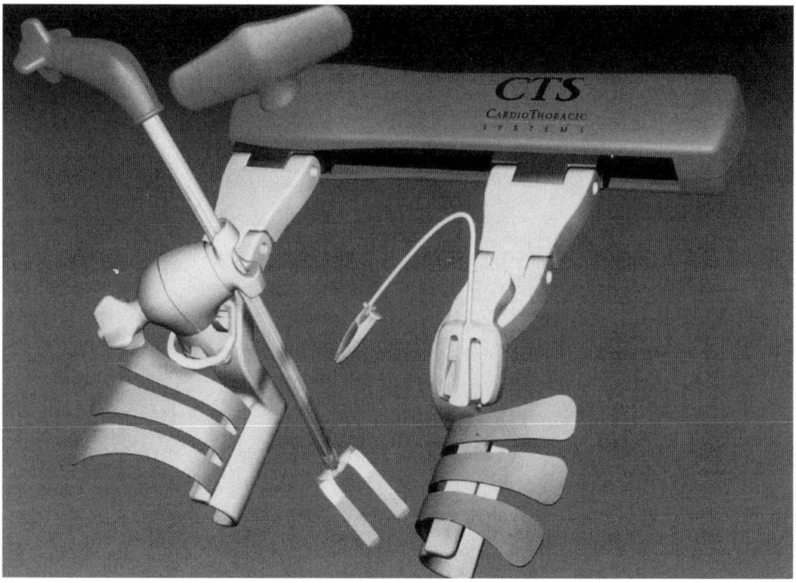

FIGURE 2.

A pressure plate stabilizer developed by CTS, Inc. This latest-generation device is adapted to multivessel bypass and may be used on many areas of the heart. Incorporated into the base of the retractor are sites for a blowing device and a light. This retractor system is disposable and modifications are ongoing. (Courtesy of CTS, Inc.)

ing devices.[7, 21, 29] It must be remembered that three components account for the patency of anastomoses, only one of which is the technical skill of the surgeon. The other two are the quality of the artery being grafted and the quality of the conduit used. Each of these may vary according to patient-related factors.

Substantial worldwide experience has been gained and reports are accruing on the benefits of this operation in terms of patient acceptance, graft patency, and economic savings.[17, 36, 37] Intermediate-term improvement in outcomes of type C LAD lesions as compared with angioplasty has also been demonstrated.[38] Long-term follow-up is not yet available.

The application of minimally invasive techniques to the beating heart, such as the LAST procedure, carries important implications for expanding the indications for coronary artery surgery to patients who in the past have not been considered candidates for routine techniques. Additionally, patients who have significant comorbid risk factors such as advanced age and cerebrovascular disease may have internal mammary–LAD bypass grafting and then

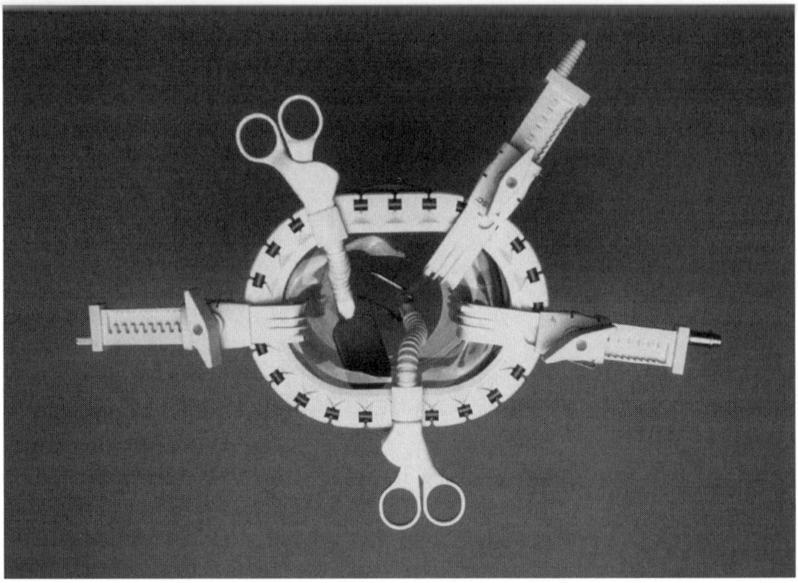

FIGURE 3.
A stabilizing retractor developed by U.S. Surgical Corporation. This device has a very low profile and a gooseneck footplate stabilizing device that attaches to the retractor base. Different sizes of chest retractors are available for use depending on the thickness of the chest wall, as well as different lengths of stabilization devices. This device has also been adapted to a larger size for use in sternotomy and multivessel bypass procedures. The low-profile design keeps all material clear of the operative field. (Courtesy of U.S. Surgical Corporation.)

be treated with angioplasty or stenting of other diseased vessels, so-called hybrid procedures.[25, 39–41] As patients advance in age and illness, the use of minimally invasive techniques coupled with hybrid procedures or culprit lesion grafting to the LAD, the dominant vessel in patients with otherwise moderate coronary artery disease, may be a logical choice, particularly in those at neurologic risk from CPB.[27] These approaches may be especially valuable in reoperative surgery, where dense scaring of the mediastinum may be avoided.[17, 42, 43] Other applications of such minimally invasive techniques continue to be developed. Recently, William B. Cohn, M.D., presented an H-graft technique wherein the mammary artery is left in situ and a separate conduit such as saphenous vein, inferior epigastric artery, or radial artery is sewn to the side of the mammary artery and then to the LAD or diagonal branches (Advanced Laparoscopy Training Center Course, Atlanta, November 1997).

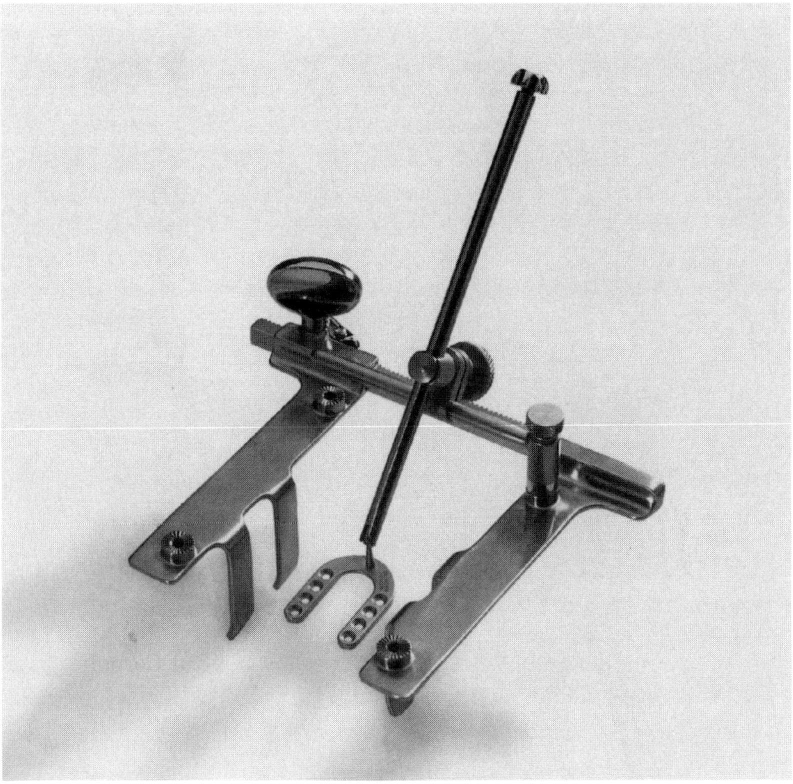

FIGURE 4.
A prototype retractor designed by Genzyme Surgical Products also uses footplate technology. This retractor, however, is nondisposable. The footplate stabilizer may be placed on any of the mobile bars, which permits use for multivessel revascularization. (Courtesy of Genzyme Surgical Products.)

This procedure allows for a smaller operative incision and no disruption of the chest wall during internal mammary artery harvest. The anterior descending coronary artery is fed in similar fashion to the renal artery, which exits at right angles from the aorta. Such innovative approaches will further extend the ability of surgeons to apply such minimally invasive techniques to an expanded patient population.

PORT-ACCESS TECHNIQUES

The development of endovascular technology has allowed coronary artery bypass grafting and valve replacement to be completed

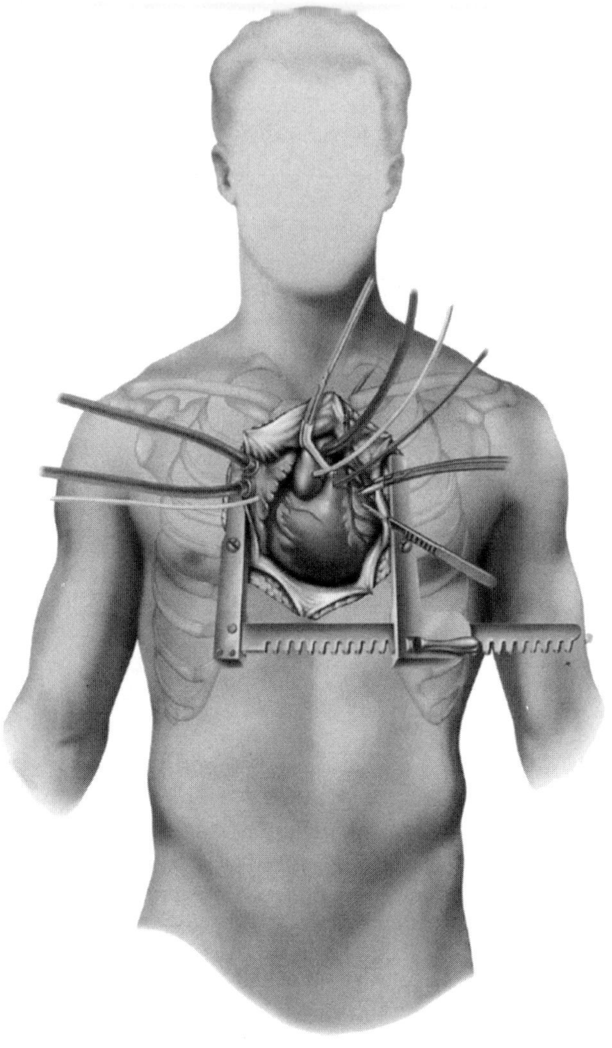

CONVENTIONAL
OPEN-CHEST
HEART SURGERY

FIGURE 5.

Port-access coronary bypass surgery as opposed to conventional open-chest surgery is shown in this figure. Complete coronary bypass grafting may be completed through a small incision with the heart decompressed and stopped via femorally accessed pulmonary bypass. (Courtesy of Heartport, Inc.)

(continued)

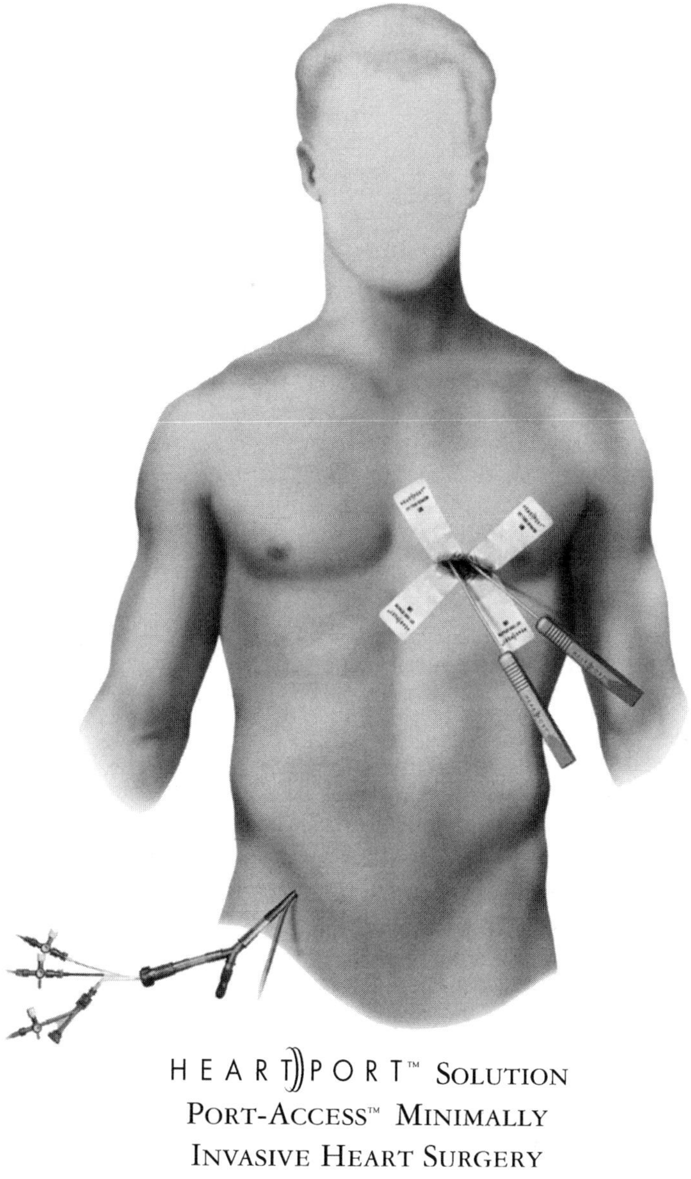

FIGURE 5. (continued)

TABLE 3.
Port-Access On-Pump Coronary Bypass

Advantages
1. Less tissue disruption
2. Improved recovery
3. Tool for the development of thorascopic-only surgery
4. Complete multivessel, multiconduit bypass can be accomplished
5. Improved cosmesis

Disadvantages
1. Morbidity of cardiopulmonary bypass maintained
2. Peripheral and central vascular disease must be absent
3. Cost-ineffective
4. Technology dependent
5. Surgical technique difficult (steep learning curve)
6. Small incidence of endovascular complications
7. May be time consuming

via small incisions with the patient on CPB.[8] Heartport, Inc., has led the field (Fig 5). Mitral valve repair/replacement and tricuspid valve procedures have been accomplished with femoral-femoral bypass and endo-aortic technology as described by Fann et al. or with videoscopic assistance and transthoracic aortic occlusion as described by Chitwood et al.[9, 44] Additionally, multivessel bypass grafting using multiple conduits with access to all areas of the heart has recently been accomplished, thus extending the use of small-incision complete myocardial revascularization surgery.[45] Even through a LAST incision with the heart decompressed on CPB, the ascending aorta can be accessed to perform proximal anastomoses, thereby obviating the need for pedicled conduits only. The advantages and disadvantages of such surgery are shown in Table 3. Experience continues to accumulate, although reports are limited. Importantly, the technology of allowing minimal access with still-heart surgery will advance the development of techniques and instrumentation for complete port-access, multivessel, multiconduit bypass grafting. Feasibility studies have already been undertaken.[46, 47]

TECHNOLOGY

Minimally invasive coronary bypass surgery is technology dependent, and technological advances occur virtually weekly. Areas of technology that will allow advancement in this field include vessel stabilization, control of blood flow within the lumen of the vessel, the development of visual (video) modalities to allow intrathoracic visualization adequate to perform fine surgical procedures, and specialized instrumentation for anastomotic construction.

Initially, stabilization devices were simply handheld tools designed along the lines of a fork with the middle tines removed (J.D. Hill, personal communication). Right-angle clamps or C-shaped clamps were handheld devices used to depress the myocardium on either side of the vessel to be sutured.[48] Advances in these devices allowed retractors to be developed with footplate stabilizers that were static and attached to the chest wall retractor. Multiple variants have been developed (see Figs 2, 3, and 4). Use of these stabilizing devices improved the confidence of the surgeon in performing the anastomosis and has also improved the patency rate (Subramanian VC, presented at Society of Thoracic Surgeons, San Diego, January 1997). Beating-heart surgery appears to be the ultimate target for revascularization, and further development of stabilizing devices and refinement of current models, including those using suction stabilization (i.e., the Octopus device, see Fig 1), will be ongoing to allow multivessel stabilization through port access.[49]

Control of blood flow in arteries to be bypassed is a twofold problem. Blood flow has to be controlled or eliminated to visualize the vessel edges for suturing. This leads to a secondary problem of distal ischemia. In the early stages of minimally invasive bypass surgery, distal ischemia was believed to be a significant problem and a variety of safety net devices were developed.[50] As experience was gained, distal ischemic problems and myocardial arrhythmias or hypotension when operating on the LAD or the circumflex system were found to be rare events. On the other hand, surgery on the right coronary artery was associated with frequent and severe problems with radical arrhythmias and hypotension. Subsequently, two different methods of control have been developed. Vessel occlusion is the simplest and most common means of controlling blood flow. It can be accomplished with virtual impunity on the left side of the heart because of extensive collateral flow. Occlusion devices, including suture, vessel loops (Quest Medical, Inc.), and low-profile clips (U.S. Surgical Corp), that can be applied to the vessel are available, although anastomotic complications may be an issue with external occluding devices.[29] Suction or a blowing apparatus is used to keep the lumen free of collateral blood flow so that the anastomosis can be constructed. A variety of shunts have also been developed to maintain intraluminal blood flow yet keep the field dry to allow for suture placement. These are generally bulb-tipped, longitudinal devices that are inserted into the lumen of the vessel when the anastomosis is nearly completed and the shunt is removed. Shunts maintain blood flow and are available in a variety of sizes. Originally, the shunts were offshoots of carotid shunt prototypes; however, miniaturized developments with new biomaterials such as the Rivetti-Levinson shunt have allowed the devices greater flexibility and side port accessibility.[51] Problems with insertion of a shunt include disruption of the endothelium and potential endothelial damage from foreign body insertion. Difficulty in insertion can also be a factor. Newer strides in the control of intraluminal blood flow have been undertaken in Utrecht, The Netherlands, by Gründeman, Borst, Jansen, and their colleagues.[52] A polyurethane contact lens–shaped device with a keel much akin to an upside-down surfboard has been developed. This is inserted inside an arteriotomy to cap the arteriotomy site. This device does not substantially extend into the lumen or touch the inferior half of the lumen of the vessel. This clear device allows the surgeon to visualize the presence of blood flow through the lumen and maintain distal perfusion without intraluminal invasion. The device is flexible, and suture placement can be accomplished by depressing the device slightly with a needle as the suture is placed. Before completion of the anastomosis, the flexible device is removed easily by retracting on the "keel" portion of the device; the last few stitches of the anastomosis are then completed. Ongoing development of such ingenious devices to control blood flow and obviate ischemia will be important in the development of distal anastomotic construction as thorascopic approaches develop in parallel.

Visual equipment that can produce three-dimensional views of the intrathoracic cavity and the heart to allow precise construction of anastomoses is being developed. Innovative and new equipment by several manufacturers allows brilliant light to be placed inside the thoracic cavity, and three-dimensional views can be seen either on a cross-table full-screen television set or in mounted headset cameras such as that manufactured by Vista Medical, Inc. (Fig 6). This allows the surgeon multiple views of the anastomosis through digital video reproduction as the anastomosis is being constructed. Fine thorascopic instruments with 3- and 5-mm points (Genzyme, Inc.) are available and provide excellent visualization and access through tiny incisions. Coupling of these devices with robotic assistance to direct a camera or instruments as required by

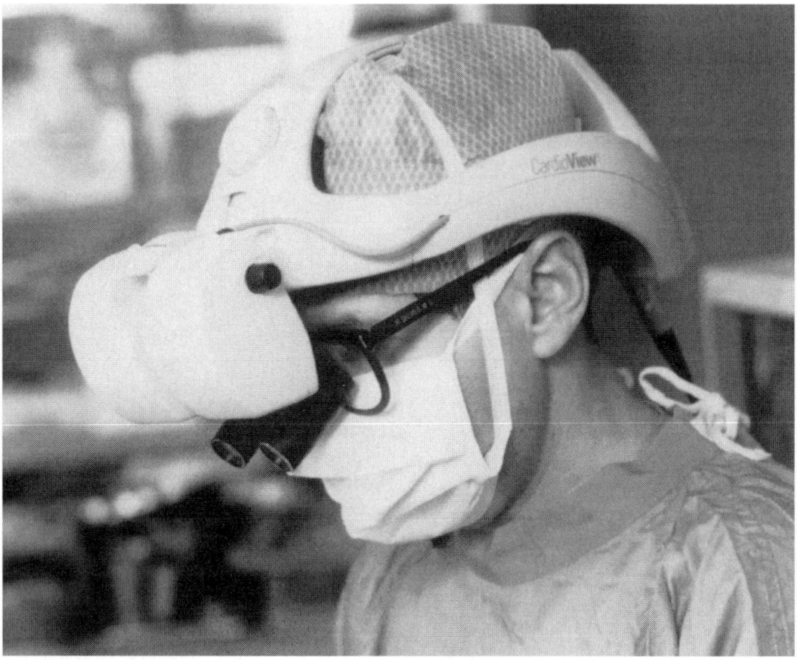

FIGURE 6.
This three-dimensional video system developed by Vista Medical, Inc., allows the transmission of images to television screens located on a head-mounted device. The surgeon may either use his own direct vision via small incisions or, by altering his gaze upward, view internal or other views of anatomy depending on placement of the camera. (Courtesy of Vista Medical, Inc.)

the surgeon, particularly those that are voice controlled (Computer Motion, Inc.), will further abet anastomotic construction by enhancing the view the surgeon can achieve for precise placement of sutures (Fig 7).

The development of instrumentation to complete an anastomosis through a thoracoscope in a reasonable time frame is also being explored. Alternatives for anastomotic construction include sutures, stapling devices, and biological glue.[53] All three are under development along with devices to facilitate the placement of sutures through small vessels at a distance. Development of this portion of the process, which will allow the construction of patulous vessel-to-vessel anastomoses at a distance in a reasonable time frame, probably represents the key missing piece in the process of total thorascopic coronary bypass surgery.

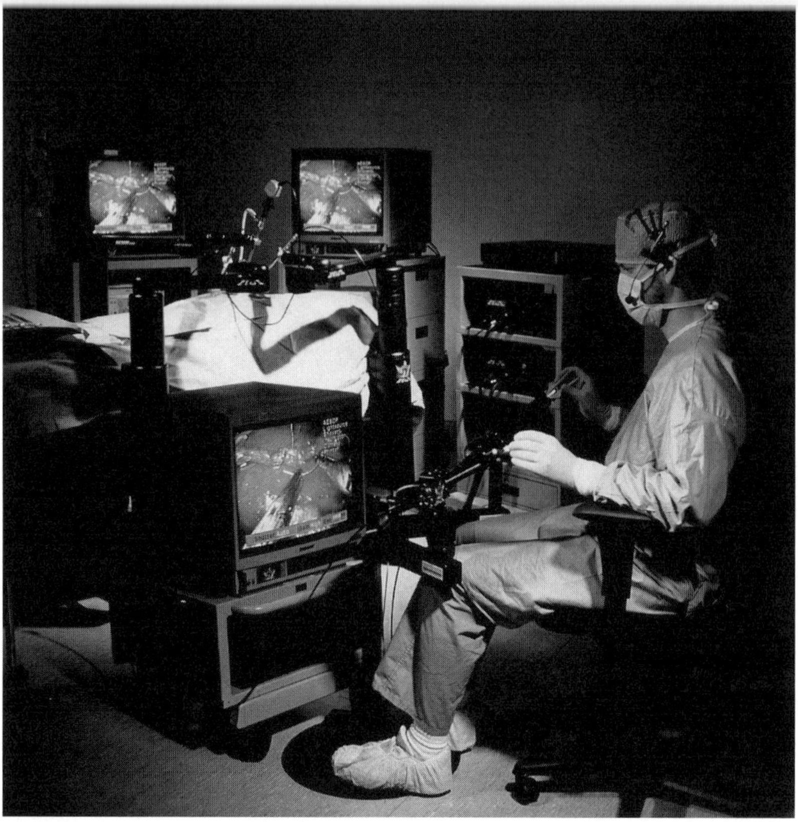

FIGURE 7.
The operating room of the future may allow the surgeon to operate at a distance. Robotic systems and excellent visualization will allow steady suture placement with finely controlled movements via robotic arms, as well as voice-activated camera placement and surgical assistance. Systems such as this are currently being developed. (Courtesy of Computer Motion, Inc.)

The sine qua non of the aforementioned procedures is to obtain a patent anastomosis. Currently, the gold standard for evaluation of patency remains angiography; however, this can be cumbersome and difficult. Originally, Doppler US was used to assess gross patency; however, this proved inadequate. A flow-measuring US probe (Transsonic, Inc.) has been used with success to quantitate levels of flow, but correlates with patency are not currently available.[48] Transthoracic Doppler evaluation has been used but has not proved specific enough.[48, 54] Thermal angiography may be used to assess graft patency, but it is not quantitative and the equipment is expensive.[20, 55] Contrast cineangiography after the surgical procedure is believed to provide the most important indication of graft patency and quality; however, this often requires the patient to return to the catheterization laboratory, which can be time consuming and expensive and subjects the patient to a further interventional procedure. In addition, should there be a problem with the graft, reoperation may prove to be more difficult. Currently, on-table evaluation of bypass grafts with ease of use has been reported and, importantly, determination of the state of the anastomosis at the time of surgery so that operative correction can be undertaken if necessary.[12, 56, 57] Some angiographically acute abnormalities in the anastomosis may prove to be resolvable over time, but this is not well defined.[58] Therefore, angiography in and of itself may not prove to be the answer to anastomotic quality. Because of the difficulties in appreciating angiographic narrowings within bypassed vessels, the use of a functionally significant anatomical determinate of an anastomosis is inadequate. There are no current data to indicate the importance of angiographic abnormalities within the first 24 hours of left internal mammary artery (LIMA) implantation, and thus the angiographic data available have no comparable information to suggest that an angiographic abnormality may be functionally significant. Physiologic assessment of the LIMA anastomosis has been proposed as a method to assure the operator that adequate patency has been maintained at the conclusion of the procedure. Intravascular Doppler-guided wire measurements have been performed in a limited number of patients in the operating room and have demonstrated that proximal inflow from the native LAD through the anastomosis contributes to volumetric flow through the LIMA anastomosis. Assessment of LIMA flow then depends on minimizing native LAD inflow and assessing the waveform and hyperemic response of distal LAD flow during occlusion and release of the LIMA (personal communication, Morton J. Kern, St. Louis). An anastomosis that is unrestrictive to increases in flow is a physiologically satisfactory anastomosis regardless of the angiographic appearance. Currently, the use of intravascular Doppler probes is beyond the scope of operative use. Future evaluations of anastomotic patency will involve translesional pressure as well as flow velocity techniques. A surface Doppler probe would facilitate the surgeon's appreciation of distal LAD flow through a patent anastomosis. Intraoperative angiography may have value in determining functional significance when coupled with the physiologic measurements just mentioned. Currently, intraoperative angiography would be warranted in cases of beating-heart surgery. Determination of anastomotic patency by angiographic methods has not become routine, but it is the preferred method by the majority of surgeons.

EDUCATION

The rapid changes in the field of coronary bypass surgery have dramatically altered the preparation and choices the surgeon has to make for revascularization. There are a multiplicity of conduits and approaches such that "designer surgery" can be selected for the needs and co-morbidities of an individual patient. With the patient population requiring coronary bypass becoming older and sicker, these approaches are warranted.[59] Because technology is rapidly evolving, educational processes become even more essential in keeping surgeons current in the state of the art and establishing a format for teaching the skills necessary for performing minimally invasive coronary artery bypass surgery. Although many of these procedures apply standard techniques, there are applications of new, complex technology that require subspecialty training. Guidelines have yet to be established for the qualification and credentialing of surgeons performing minimally invasive bypass surgery and for the use of specific technologies. This is important to consider for the future because a strong background education and ongoing continuing medical education are required for surgical competency. Unlike the case with standard procedures, volume alone may not be adequate.[60] The forums for such educational processes have yet to be established. A multiplicity of programs are touting education in minimally invasive cardiac surgery; however, the caliber and content of the programs vary and they are not critically peer reviewed. A new society, the International Society for Minimally Invasive Cardiac Surgery, has been formed and, one hopes, will create a platform for the scientific scrutiny and investigation of minimally invasive techniques and instrumentation coupled with comprehensive peer review. The official peer-reviewed journal is *The Heart Surgery Forum,* an on-line multimedia publication. This society's first meeting is in June 1998. The intention is to provide a dais for a broad base of information exchange and critique conducted between the medical profession and industry for the development of this technologically dependent field. This effort will provide an ongoing forum for critical review as has been suggested by others.[61, 62] The New Technology Assessment Committee of the Society of Thoracic Surgeons is also working toward approving courses and creating guidelines for credentialing surgeons in minimally invasive cardiac surgery as well as being proactive in assessing new technologically dependent procedures, of which the minimally invasive arena is only one. It behooves surgeons and institutions to be assured that appropriate preparation is accomplished before embarking on programs of minimally invasive cardiac surgery.

COMMENT

Minimally invasive coronary artery bypass surgery continues to evolve. The pace is rapid, and as in the computer world, equipment and techniques rapidly become outmoded. The trend of progress is to develop methods to perform multivessel, multiconduit, complete myocardial revascularization via port access on the beating heart without the use of CPB—basically, same-day myocardial revascularization surgery. Many technical steps and innovations are required, but a great deal of effort is being expended toward the development of such technologies. Furthermore, with appropriate education, the techniques are becoming more manageable so that they are applicable across the broad spectrum of the skills of cardiovascular surgeons and not the privilege of a few talented individuals. The procedures described for minimally invasive surgery currently belong in the armamentarium of modern cardiovascular surgeons and enable the creation of "designer" myocardial revascularization. Dr. Denton A. Cooley noted that we must tailor the operation to the patient and not the patient to the operation.[63] With the developing expertise, cardiovascular surgeons will be able to better conform to this ideal. Rather than taking one specific procedure (i.e., coronary artery bypass grafting on CPB via sternotomy) and applying this to all patients regardless of confounding risk factors, revascularization can be designed directly for the needs of the patients, thereby reducing risk, lessening morbidity, and improving patient recovery. These advances and efforts are truly global inasmuch as cardiovascular surgeons and their colleagues from all of the world's continents are contributing.

REFERENCES

1. Ancalmo N, Busby JR: Minimally invasive coronary artery bypass surgery: Really minimal. *Ann Thorac Surg* 64:928–929, 1997.
2. Westaby S: Coronary surgery without cardiopulmonary bypass: Rationale and evolution of technique, in Emery RW, Arom KV, Fonger JD, et al (eds): *Techniques for Minimally Invasive Direct Coronary Artery Bypass (MIDCAB) Surgery.* Philadelphia, Hanley & Belfus, 1997, pp 3–8.

3. Buffolo E, Andrade JCS, Succi J, et al: Direct myocardial revascularization without cardiopulmonary bypass. *J Thorac Cardiovasc Surg* 33:26–29, 1985.
4. Bennetti FJ, Naselli G, Wood M, et al: Direct myocardial revascularization without extra corporeal circulation. *Chest* 100:312–316, 1991.
5. Robinson MC, Gross DR, Zeman W, et al: Minimally invasive coronary artery bypass grafting: A new method using an anterior mediastinotomy. *J Cardiac Surg* 10:529–536, 1995.
6. Subramanian VA, Sani G, Benetti FJ, et al: Minimally invasive coronary bypass surgery: A multi-center report of preliminary clinical experience. *Circulation* 92:645A, 1995.
7. Calafiore AM, Di Giammarco G, Teodori G, et al: Left anterior descending coronary artery grafting via left anterior small thoracotomy without cardiopulmonary bypass. *Ann Thorac Surg* 61:1658–1665, 1996.
8. Stevens JH, Burdon TA, Peters WS, et al: Port-access coronary artery bypass grafting: A proposed surgical method. *J Thorac Cardiovasc Surg* 111:567–573, 1996.
9. Fann JI, Pompili MF, Stevens JH, et al: Port-access operations with cardioplegic arrest. *Ann Thorac Surg* 63:535–539, 1997.
10. Benetti FJ, Balleston C, Sani G, et al: Video-assisted coronary artery bypass surgery. *J Card Surg* 10:620–625, 1995.
11. Nataf P, Lima L, Regan M, et al: Minimally invasive coronary surgery with thorascopic internal mammary artery dissection: Surgical technique. *J Card Surg* 11:288–292, 1996.
12. Ohtsuka T, Wolf RK, Hiratzka LF, et al: Thorascopic internal mammary artery harvest for MICAB using the Harmonic scalpel. *Ann Thorac Surg* 63:107–109, 1997.
13. Loop FD, Lytle BW, Cosgrove DW, et al: Influence of the internal mammary artery graft on 10-year survival and other cardiac events. *N Engl J Med* 314:1–6, 1986.
14. Loop FD: Internal thoracic artery grafts—biologically superior coronary arteries. *N Engl J Med* 334:263–265, 1996.
15. Shennib H, Mack MJ, Lee AGL: A survey on minimally invasive coronary artery bypass grafting. *Ann Thorac Surg* 64:110–115, 1997.
16. Oz MC, Argenziano M, Rose EA: What is "minimally invasive" coronary artery bypass surgery: Experience with a variety of surgical revascularization procedures for single vessel disease. *Chest* 112:1409–1416, 1997.
17. Arom KV, Emery RW, Nicoloff DM, et al: Minimally invasive direct coronary artery bypass grafting: Experimental and clinical experiences. *Ann Thorac Surg* 63:548–552, 1997.
18. Ankeney JL: To use or not use the pump oxygenator in coronary bypass operations. *Ann Thorac Surg* 19:108–109, 1975.
19. Arom KV, Emery RW, Nicoloff DM: Mini-sternotomy for coronary artery bypass grafting. *Ann Thorac Surg* 62:1271–1272, 1996.
20. Emery RW, Arom KV, Lillehei TJ, et al: Suture techniques of MIDCAB

surgery, in Emery RW, Arom KV, Fonger JD, et al (eds): *Techniques for Minimally Invasive Bypass (MIDCAB) Surgery.* Philadelphia, Hanley & Belfus, 1997, pp 87–93.

21. Boonstra PW, Grandjean JG, Mariani MA: Local immobilization of the left anterior descending coronary artery for minimally invasive coronary bypass grafting. *Ann Thorac Surg* 63:576, 1997.
22. Borst C, Jansen WL, Tulleken CA, et al: Coronary artery bypass grafting without cardiopulmonary bypass and without interruption of native coronary flow using a novel anastomosis site restraining device (Octopus). *J Am Clin Cardiol* 27:1356–1364, 1996.
23. Gründeman PF, Borst C, van Herwaarden JA, et al: Hemodynamic changes during displacement of the beating heart by the Utrecht Octopus method. *Ann Thorac Surg* 63:88S–93S, 1997.
24. Corso PG: Cardiopulmonary bypass and coronary artery bypass graft: Are the risks necessary? *Chest* 100:298–299, 1991.
25. Gaudino M, Santarelli P, Bruno P, et al: Palliative coronary artery surgery in patients with severe non-cardiac disease. *Am J Cardiol* 80:135, 1997.
26. Tashiro T, Todo K, Haruta Y, et al: Coronary artery bypass grafting without cardiopulmonary bypass for high-risk patients. *Cardiovasc Surg* 4:207–211, 1996.
27. Roach GW, Kanchuger M, Mangano CW, et al: Adverse cerebral outcomes after coronary artery bypass surgery. *N Engl J Med* 335:1857–1863, 1996.
28. Gundry SR, Rozzouk AJ, Bailey LL: Coronary artery bypass with and without the heart-lung machine: A case-matched 6-year follow-up. *Circulation* 94:52S, 1996.
29. Pagni S, Paqish NK, Senior DG, et al: Anastomotic complications in minimally invasive coronary bypass surgery. *Ann Thorac Surg* 63:564–567, 1997.
30. Moshkovite Y, Lusky A, Mohr R: Coronary artery bypass without cardiopulmonary bypass: Analysis of short-term and mid-term outcome in 220 patients. *J Thorac Cardiovasc Surg* 110:979–987, 1995.
31. Perrault LP, Menashe P, Biodouard JP, et al: Suturing of the target vessels in less invasive bypass operations does not cause endothelial dysfunction. *Ann Thorac Surg* 63:751–755, 1997.
32. Hau MH, Vatsia SK: Successful minimally invasive triple coronary artery bypass through bilateral parasternal incisions. *Ann Thorac Surg* 64:1484–1486, 1997.
33. Svensson LG: Minimal-access "J" or "j" sternotomy for valvular, aortic and coronary operations or reoperations. *Ann Thorac Surg* 64:1501–1503, 1997.
34. Watanabe G, Misaki T, Kotuh K, et al: Bilateral minimally invasive direct coronary artery bypass grafting with the use of two anterior grafts. *J Thorac Cardiovasc Surg* 113:949–951, 1997.
35. Borst C, Santamore WP, Smedira NG, et al: Minimally invasive coro-

nary artery bypass grafting: On the beating heart and via limited access. *Ann Thorac Surg* 63:1S–5S, 1997.

36. King RC, Reece B, Hurst JL, et al: Minimally invasive coronary artery bypass grafting decreases hospital stay and costs. *Ann Thorac Surg* 225:805–811, 1997.
37. Zenati M, Domit TM, Saul M, et al: Resource utilization for minimally invasive direct and standard coronary artery bypass grafting. *Ann Thorac Surg* 63:84S–87S, 1997.
38. Mariani M, Boonstra PW, Grandjean JG, et al: Minimally invasive coronary artery bypass grafting versus angioplasty for isolated type C stenosis of the left anterior descending coronary artery. *J Thorac Cardiovasc Surg* 114:434–439, 1997.
39. Emery RW, Emery AM, Flavin TF, et al: Revascularization using angioplasty and minimally invasive technique documented by thermal imaging. *Ann Thorac Surg* 62:591–593, 1996.
40. Mooney MR, Mooney J: MIDCAB: An interventionalist's view, in Emery RW, Arom KV, Fonger JD, et al (eds): *Techniques for Minimally Invasive Direct Coronary Artery Bypass (MIDCAB) Surgery.* Philadelphia, Hanley & Belfus, 1997, pp 107–112.
41. Liekweg WG, Misra R: Minimally invasive direct coronary artery bypass, percutaneous transluminal coronary angioplasty and stent placement for left main stenosis. *J Thorac Cardiovasc Surg* 113:411–412, 1997.
42. Allen KB, Matheny RG, Robison RJ, et al: Minimally invasive versus conventional reoperative coronary artery bypass. *Ann Thorac Surg* 64:616–622, 1997.
43. Boonstra PW, Grandjean JG, Mariani MA: Reoperative coronary bypass grafting without cardiopulmonary bypass through a small thoracotomy. *Ann Thorac Surg* 63:405–407, 1997.
44. Chitwood WR, Elbeery JR, Chopman WH, et al: Video-assisted minimally invasive valve surgery: The "micro-mitral." *J Thorac Cardiovasc Surg* 113:413–414, 1997.
45. Schwartz DS, Ribakov GH, Grossi EA, et al: Single and multivessel port-access grafting with cardioplegic arrest: Technique and reproducibility. *J Thorac Cardiovasc Surg* 114:46–52, 1997.
46. Peters WS, Burdon TA, Siegel LC, et al: Port-access bilateral internal mammary artery grafting for left main coronary artery disease: Canine feasibility study. *J Card Surg* 12:1–7, 1997.
47. Soulez G, Gagner M, Therasse E, et al: Catheter-assisted totally thorascopic coronary artery bypass grafting: A feasibility study. *Ann Thorac Surg* 64:1036–1040, 1997.
48. Fonger JD: Monitoring MIDCAB grafting, in Emery RW, Arom KV, Fonger JD, et al (eds): *Techniques for Minimally Invasive Direct Coronary Artery Bypass (MIDCAB) Surgery.* Philadelphia, Hanley & Belfus, 1997, pp 93–106.
49. Takahashi M, Yamamoto S, Tabata S: Immobilized instrument for

minimally invasive direct coronary artery bypass: MIDCAB doughnut. *J Thorac Cardiovasc Surg* 114:680–681, 1997.
50. Robinson MC: Identification and management of coronary arteries: Immobilization and control, in Emery RW, Arom KV, Fonger JD, et al: *Techniques for Minimally Invasive Direct Coronary Artery Bypass (MIDCAB) Surgery.* Philadelphia, Hanley & Belfus, 1997, pp 79–88.
51. Rivetti LA, Gandra SMA: Initial experience using an intraluminal shunt during revascularization of the beating heart. *Ann Thorac Surg* 63:1742–1747, 1997.
52. Heijmen RH, Borst C, van Daten R, et al: Temporary intravascular anteriotomy seal (IVAS) during end-to-side anastomosis suturing. *Circulation* 96:248S, 1997.
53. Werker PMN, Kon M: Review of facilitated approaches to vascular anastomosis surgery. *Ann Thorac Surg* 63:5122–5127, 1997.
54. Takemura H, Kawasuji M, Sakakibara N, et al: Internal thoracic artery graft function during exercise assessed by transthoracic Doppler echocardiography. *Ann Thorac Surg* 61:914–919, 1996.
55. Falk V, Diegeler A, Walther T, et al: Intraoperative patency control of arterial grafts in minimally invasive coronary artery bypass graft operations by means of endoscopic thermal coronary angiography. *J Thorac Cardiovasc Surg* 114:507–509, 1997.
56. Gill I, Fitzgibbon GM, Higginson LA, et al: Minimally invasive coronary artery bypass: A series with early qualitative angiographic follow-up. *Ann Thorac Surg* 64:710–714, 1997.
57. Elbeery J, Chitwood WR: Intraoperative catherization of the left internal mammary artery via the left radial artery. *Ann Thorac Surg,* in press.
58. Calafiore AM, Di Giammarco G, Teodori G, et al: Midterm results after minimally invasive coronary surgery (LAST operation). *J Thorac Cardiovasc Surg,* in press.
59. Blanche C, Matloff JM, Denton TA, et al: Cardiac operations in patients 90 years of age and older. *Ann Thorac Surg* 63:1685–1690, 1997.
60. Crawford FA Jr, Anderson RP, Clark RE, et al: Volume requirement for cardiac surgery credentialing: A critical review. *Ann Thorac Surg* 61:12–16, 1996.
61. Ullyot DJ: Look ma, no hands. *Ann Thorac Surg* 61:10–11, 1996.
62. Lytle BE: Minimally invasive cardiac surgery. *J Thorac Cardiovasc Surg* 111:554–555, 1997.
63. Westaby S: Invited commentary of Ott et al. *Ann Thorac Surg* 64:478–481, 1997.

CHAPTER 2

Repair of Ventricular Aneurysm

Vincent Dor, M.D.
Professor of Thoracic and Cardiovascular Surgery, Marseille and Nice University; Head of Surgical Department, Cardio-Thoracic Center of Monaco, Monte Carlo, Monaco

Since the first resection of a left ventricular aneurysm under extracorporeal circulation in 1958 by Cooley and associates,[1] this technique of surgery for ventricular wall ischemia quickly expanded and improved. However, even though most left ventricular ectatic lesions are treated by resection of the exteriorized dyskinetic area and longitudinal suturing of the opening, this classic technique is considered by cardiologists like Froelich et al.[2] to not lead to improvement in left ventricular morphology and performance. For this reason, some technical modifications have been adopted, such as septal plicature by Cooley[3] and circular suturing of the opening by Jatene.[4] Since 1984 we have thought that the use of an endoventricular patch sutured in the contractile area and excluding the akinetic areas leads to significant and measurable improvement in left ventricular function. Gradually the technique of left ventricular reconstruction by endoventricular circular patch–plasty with exclusion of the akinetic septum was established. This technique had already been presented in 1985 at the 17th Congress of the International Society of Cardiovascular Surgeons.[5] Our team's experience over the last 12 years is based on 781 cases (120 patients who underwent surgery at Nice Hospital and 661 at the Cardio-Thoracic Center of Monaco between May 1987 and July 1997).

By examining these cases we are able to answer the following questions:

- In what circumstances does an ischemic condition of the left ventricular wall lead to surgery?

TABLE 1.
Nice University Series

Indications	CHF	37%
	Angina	47%
	S.V.A.	8%
	(emergency)	10%
Results	Hospital Mortality	10%
	1st control on 90 patients	
	delayed control on 45 patients	

Abbreviations: CHF, congestive heart failure; *SVA,* spontaneous sustained ventricular arrhythmia.
(Courtesy of Georg Thieme Verlag, from Dor V, Saab M, Coste P, et al: Left ventricular aneurysm: A new surgical approach. *J Thorac Cardiovasc Surg* 37:11–19, 1989.)

- What type of lesions are encountered?
- Which technique should be used?
- What clinical and hemodynamic results can one expect?
- What should the indications for surgery be?

These questions have already been partially answered, especially questions pertaining to the first series of 120 patients (Nice Hospital) (Table 1). To obtain the maximum amount of data, a standardized study was performed on the most recent series of 661 patients (Table 2) who underwent surgery at the Cardio-Thoracic Center of Monaco; in addition to clinical and mechanographic data, each case included a complete preoperative hemodynamic and angiographic study, right catheterization with measurement of cardiac output and pulmonary artery pressure, and if there were no contraindication, programmed ventricular stimulation to search for any inducible ventricular tachycardia. During left heart catheterization, the morphology of the left ventricle was studied on right and left anterior oblique projections, and the left ventricular ejection fraction was checked globally, as well in the contractile portion after exclusion of the akinetic area. After surgery, a hemodynamic study in conjunction with programmed ventricular stimulation was performed during the first postoperative month, provided that there was no contraindication related to renal insufficiency or patient refusal. After 1 year, the same hemodynamic study involving coronary angiography in conjunction with programmed ven-

TABLE 2.
Cardio-Thoracic Center of Monaco Series

Age	
Mean, yr	60.4 ± 9.1 yr (32–81)
+ 65 yr	150
Patients (*n* = 661)	
M	572
F	89
Main Indications	
Angina	397
CHF	257
Spontaneous VT	89 (______)
Location	
ASA	562
Posterior and Posterolateral	32
Bifocal	27
Delay from MI (mean)	51.43 ± 63.69 mo (1 wk–312 mo)
Emergencies	116
NYHA	
Class I & II	290
Class III & IV	371 (56.12%)
LVEF	
< 20%	110 (44.47%)
21% to 30%	184
31% to 40%	144
> 40%	223
Mean PAP above 25 mm Hg (systemic PAP 54 mm Hg [30–90])	145 (22%)

Abbreviatons: CHF, congestive heart failure; *VT,* ventricular tachycardia; *ASA,* anteroseptoapical; *MI,* myocardial infarction; *NYHA,* New York Heart Association; *LVEF,* left ventricular ejection fraction; *PAP,* pulmonary artery pressure.

tricular stimulation was proposed to the patients and accepted by more than half of them. The details of this series of patients are shown in Table 2.

MAIN INDICATIONS

In 397 patients (60%), angina led to coronary bypass surgery, the particulars of which were determined by the scar lesions of the left ventricle. In 257 patients (39%), recurring or refractory cardiac failure led to surgery for wall motion abnormalities. In 89 patients (13.4%), spontaneous ventricular arrhythmias (sustained ventricular tachycardia, 82 patients; ventricular fibrillation, 7 patients) were the primary indications for surgery, but if the 175 other patients with inducible spontaneous ventricular tachycardia are included, a total of 264 patients (39.9%) underwent surgery for ventricular arrhythmias. In 116 cases (17.5%), indications for surgery were deemed emergencies because of mechanical complications stemming from recent myocardial infarction (parietal rupture, septal rupture, acute mitral insufficiency), refractory ventricular arrhythmia, or permanent cardiac failure that previously required intra-aortic balloon pumping.

TYPE AND LOCATION OF LESIONS

The scars resulting from myocardial infarction and wall motion abnormalities appear either as an actual dyskinesia with paradoxical contraction during systole—ventricular aneurysm—or as an akinesia with outlines and limits that are more difficult to evaluate on angiography, particularly on the septum. In the series of patients who underwent surgery at the Cardio-Thoracic Center of Monaco (661 cases), 339 dyskinetic aneurysms and 223 akinesias were noted. In the remaining patients it was difficult to isolate either akinesia or dyskinesia. The location of the lesions was mainly anterior, anteroapical, or anteroseptal (562 cases); posterior or posterolateral lesions were found in 34 patients (Table 3). In 27 patients the lesion was considered bifocal, i.e., anterior and posterior; however, there were more patients with an old posterior scar in addition to a recent anteroseptal lesion. Finally, 13 patients in this series who underwent resection for an anteroseptal aneurysmal scar had persistent extensive septal akinesia and dyskinesia.

TECHNICAL METHODS

All operations are performed under aortic cross-clamping with crystalloid or blood cardioplegia when the ejection fraction is below 30%,[7] in addition to local irrigation with frozen serum. Coronary revascularization of the contractile areas as well as the diseased area is conducted first, with the internal mammary artery used in more than 80% of the cases.

ANTEROSEPTOAPICAL LESIONS

The technique, depicted in Figure 1, involves gaining access to the fibrous endocardium through a ventricular anteroapical incision

TABLE 3.
Type and Location of Wall Motion Abnormalities ($n = 661$)

Location	Akinesia	Dyskinesia (Aneurysm)
Anteroseptoapical	223	339
Posterior and posterolateral	13	21
Bifocal		27

and evaluating the contractile area inside the ventricle. The endocardium is mobilized and resected if calcified or covered with mural thrombi, particularly in the case of ventricular arrhythmia. In the presence of ventricular arrhythmia, cryotherapy at −60° _ is directed at the edge of the resection for 2 minutes. If there is no indication for endocardiectomy, the patch can be inserted directly into the left ventricle in the contractile area. To measure the dimensions of the patch, 2-0 Monofilament suture is passed into the muscular edge at the border of the fibrous lesions (Fontan maneuver[8]) and tightened. The Dacron or pericardium patch is fixed on this guiding line with the same suture. When the septal endocardium is fibrous and resistant, a hemicircular patch of material is cut to the size of the remaining opening after tightening the suture (Fig 2, A).

After hemostasis, the fibrous epicardial or myocardial edges excluded are either sutured directly above the patch or simply folded or glued on the septum and the patch to avoid restraint on the right ventricle and occlusion of the left anterior descending artery and its branches in the interventricular groove. This endoventricular patch can be used in the case of septal rupture to exclude the diseased septum from the left ventricular cavity (Fig 2, B).

POSTERIOR AND POSTEROLATERAL LESIONS

An opening in the left ventricle is cut in a fibrous area after locating the mitral papillary muscle, and endocardiectomy is performed on the posterior and postero-inferior side of the septum (Fig 3). If the posterior papillary muscle is completely involved, it is resected with the endocardium and a mitral prosthesis is inserted through the ventricle (13 cases). The ventricle is reconstructed with a triangular patch sutured in a contractile area of the left ventricle; the mitral annulus serves as the base of the triangle and the apex is fixed at the root of the posterior or lateral papillary muscle. The edges excluded are sutured above the patch.

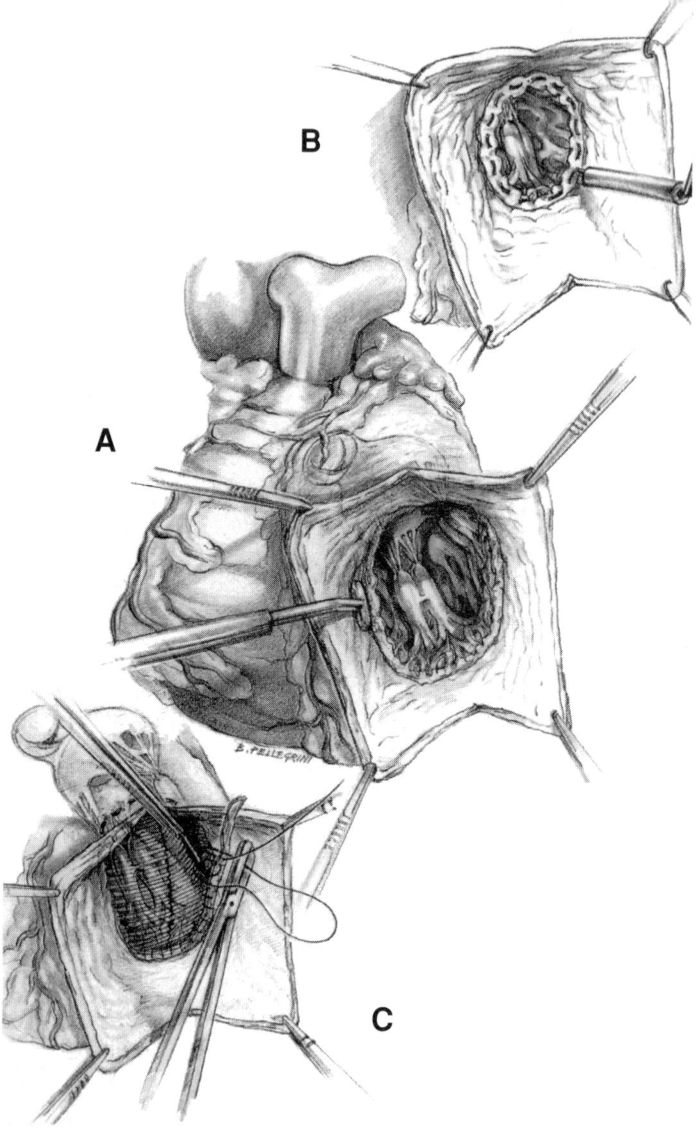

FIGURE 1.
Left ventricular reconstruction for anteroseptoapical aneurysm. **A,** appearance of the left ventricular cavity after endocardial resection. The cryotherapy probe is applied to the edges of the resection. **B,** endoventricular continuous suture to shorten the opening. **C,** Dacron patch fixed with 2-0 Monofilament with or without pericardial strips.

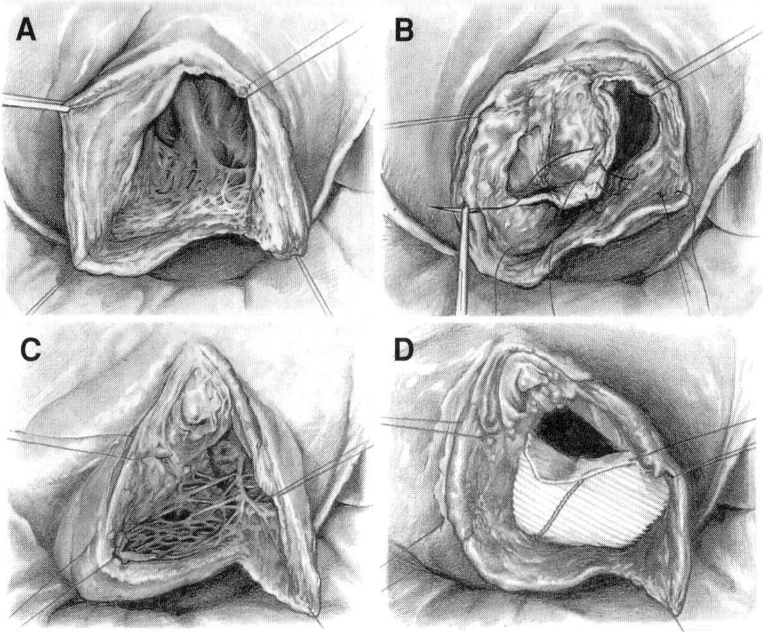

FIGURE 2.

Endoventricular patch reconstruction. **A,** utilization of the septal scar as an autologous patch. A semicircular portion of the scar mobilized from the septum with a septal hinge is sutured on contractile muscle inside the left ventricle. **B,** septal rupture. The patch is anchored above the dehiscence, which is excluded from the left ventricular cavity.

BIFOCAL LESIONS

Through the anterior opening, the posterior fibrosis is treated by cryotherapy in case of arrhythmia. In only two patients was resection followed by direct suture performed, the anterior part being treated by a patch with exclusion of the apicoseptal scar.

REMAINING APICOSEPTAL SCARS

The lesions that were not treated by the classic linear suture method are excluded by an endoventricular circular patch; in these cases the left anterior descending artery, very often involved in the first operative suture, cannot be revascularized.

MITRAL INSUFFICIENCY

Mitral insufficiency requires specific care. In the case of posterior lesions, either valvular replacement or mitral reconstruction can be performed through the posterior ventricular opening, and the

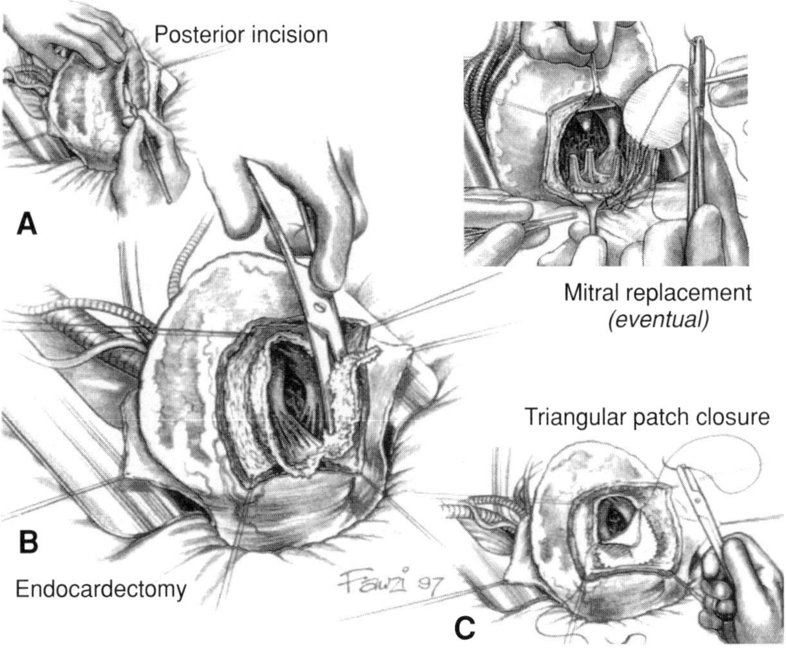

FIGURE 3.
A, posterior incision. **B**, endocardiectomy. **C**, triangular patch closure. **C′**, the same triangular patch after mitral replacement.

morphology of the annulus and the left ventricular cavity can be reconstructed with a triangular Dacron patch as mentioned earlier.

In the case of anteroseptal lesions, mitral insufficiency has to be estimated by a transatrial approach, and simple annular dilatations without valvular prolapse are treated by annuloplasty. However, associated degenerative lesions (posterior and anterior leaflets, chordae rupture) must be corrected by quadrangular resection with annuloplasty for the posterior leaflet and shortening and new chordae for the anterior valve, this being done through the ventricle. Of 23 mitral valvuloplasties performed in this series, the posterior leaflet was involved in 8 cases and the anterior leaflet in 4.

Perioperative transesophageal echocardiography was performed in all cases. The technical methods used in this series are summarized in Table 4.

RESULTS

MORTALITY

The series of 120 patients who underwent surgery at Nice University from 1984 to April 1987 has been analyzed previously in 1989.

TABLE 4.
Surgery Data

Patch	
Dacron	417 (63%)
Autologous (and pericardium)	211 (32%)
Coronary revascularization	643 (97%)
IMA	595 (90%)
Endocardectomy	359 (54%)
Associated procedures	
Mitral valve	56
Repair	41
Replacement	15
Aortic valve replacement	4

Abbreviation: IMA, internal mammary artery.

Hospital Mortality

Global hospital mortality in the series of 661 patients who underwent surgery at the Cardio-Thoracic Center of Monaco was 8.01% (53 cases), but specific mortality varied according to the surgical condition. Nineteen of the 116 patients who received emergency surgery died (16.38%), as opposed to only 34 of 545 who were scheduled for surgery (6.24%). In addition, the mortality rate was 17.27% (19/110) in patients with an ejection fraction below 20%, whereas it was only 1.43% (3/210) in patients with an ejection fraction above 40%. Twenty-two of the 145 patients (15.17%) with mean pulmonary hypertension greater than 25 mm Hg died.

Late Mortality

All surviving patients were checked clinically or contacted by telephone. Forty-two (6.35%) died between the 2nd and 100th postoperative month.

Differences in mortality according to age group, ventricular function, and pulmonary hypertension are shown in Table 5.

POSTOPERATIVE COMPLICATIONS

Postoperative low cardiac output necessitated the use of intraaortic balloon pumping in 87 cases (13.2%) (Table 6). Hemorrhagic complications requiring re-entry for hemostasis occurred in 30 patients (4.5%), and 125 patients needed transfusions (18.9% of the series). Renal insufficiency (31 cases) was treated medically without a need for hemodialysis or hemofiltration. The only infections

TABLE 5.
Post Operative and Late Mortality Related to Patient Categories (N = 536)

Category	Postoperative Mortality	Late Mortality
Age		
32–55 yr (*n* = 56)	3 (5.3)*	2 (3.7)
55–65 yr (*n* = 190)	9 (4.5)	11 (5.7)
> 65 yr (*n* = 104)	16 (15.3)	5 (5.6)
Ejection fraction		
≤ 20% (*n* = 39)	7 (17.9)	3 (9.3)
20% to 40% (*n* = 190)	17 (8.9)	11 (6.3)
≥ 40% (*n* = 131)	2 (1.5)	4 (3.1)
Pulmonary artery pressure		
25 mm Hg (*n* = 208)	13 ____	9 (4.6)
≥ 25 mm Hg (*n* = 62)	11 (17.7)	5 (9.8)

*Values in parentheses are percentages.

reported affected the lungs in patients who were ventilated for longer than 3 days. Finally, 4 patients had to receive heart transplants between 1 week and 6 months after left ventricular reconstruction for persistent, nonreversible cardiac failure.

HEMODYNAMIC RESULTS

Among the 607 survivors, 495 had at least one postoperative hemodynamic and angiographic control examination[9] (Table 7). A return to a more normal ventricular shape resulted in an improved ejection fraction that exceeded all theoretical values of the ejection fraction in the contractile area[10] (Fig 4).

The angiographic controls demonstrated disappearance of the dyskinetic areas and recovery of normal septal contraction (Fig 5). For coronary bypass, revascularization was checked more precisely. Bypasses of the infarcted area were patent in 94% of a series of 114 left internal mammary arteries implanted on diseased left anterior descending arteries.

The mean preoperative global ejection fraction of 32.62% (range, 6% to 79%) rose to 50.19% at the first postoperative checkup and was 46.24% at the delayed checkup. The end-diastolic volume index decreased from 112.78 to 76.58 mL/m^2 at the early checkup but then increased to 89.77 at the delayed

TABLE 6.
Postoperative Complications and Mortality

LCO with IABP	87
Re-entry (bleeding)	30
Blood transfusion	125
Renal insufficiency	31
Pulmonary infection (long respiratory support)	29
Neurologic disorder (transient in 15)	31
Gastrointestinal bleeding	11
Heart Transplantation	4
Hospital mortality	53 (8%)

Abbreviations: LCO, low cardiac output; *IABP,* intra-aortic balloon pumping.

TABLE 7.
Hemodynamic Results

	Preoperative	First Month	First Year
EF (%)	32.62 ± 13.52	50.19 ± 12.98	46.24 ± 13.25
EDVI	112.78 ± 48	76.58 ± 24.10	89.77 ± 28.26
PAP (mm Hg)	21.83 ± 9.45	18.27 ± 6.82	25.76 ± 13.61
CI (mL/min/m^2)	2.74 ± 1.19	2.70 ± 0.61	2.64 ± 0.61

Note: Patients not improved, 73 (11%).
Abbreviations: EF, ejection fraction; *EDVI,* end-diastolic volume index; *PAP,* pulmonary artery pressure; *CI,* cardiac index.

checkup. The cardiac index and cardiac output did not vary significantly, but this could be a problem with measurement.

Finally, two important facts should be mentioned:

1. The mean pulmonary pressure, which decreased from 21.83 mm Hg preoperatively to 18.27 mm Hg at the first checkup, rose to 25.76 mm Hg at the delayed checkup; this indicated a tendency to secondary deterioration of the remaining ventricle.
2. Seventy-three patients (11%) were not improved hemodynamically at the first checkup because of persistent deterioration of the remaining contractile area. Clinical[11] as well as hemody-

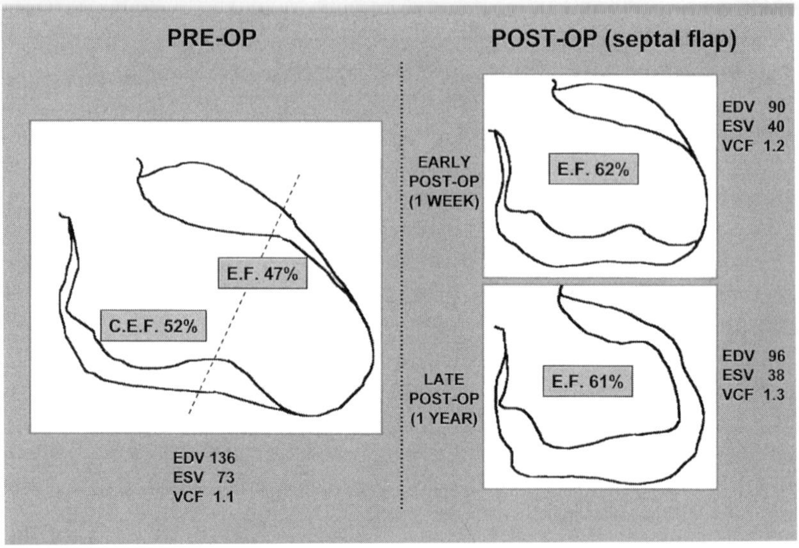

FIGURE 4.
Preoperative and postoperative left ventricular ejection fraction. The postoperative ejection fraction at 1 week and 1 year exceeds the preoperative theoretical contractile ejection fraction *(CEF). Abbreviations: E.F.*, ejection fraction; *EDV*, end-diastolic volume; *ESV*, end-systolic ventricular volume; *VCF*, velocity of circumferential fibers.

namic[12] study of systolic and diastolic function of the remaining contractile area is of great interest to cardiologists searching for angiographic, hemodynamic, or pathologic preoperative criteria that could anticipate this problem.

VENTRICULAR ARRHYTHMIAS

Results on ventricular arrhythmias (Table 8) have already been analyzed in a recent publication in the *Journal of Thoracic and Cardiovascular Surgery*. The mortality rate in this group was 6.4% (17 of 264). Of 89 spontaneous ventricular tachycardias, 7 reappeared in the immediate postoperative course and 4 were inducible by medical treatment without requiring the use of a defibrillator; after 1 year, only 1 of these 4 patients was inducible.

Of 175 cases of inducible ventricular tachycardia (147 inducible only and 28 spontaneous and inducible), 4 patients remained inducible in the early postoperative course, and 2 again become negative at the delayed checkup. Therefore, almost 91% of the cases of spontaneous ventricular tachycardia and 97% of the cases of inducible ventricular tachycardia were controlled by ventricular resection with endocardiectomy. These results are comparable with those obtained by mapped guide endocardiectomy.[12, 13]

It is interesting to note that of the 450 programmed ventricular stimulations performed postoperatively in this series, besides the 19 inducible tachycardias already mentioned there were also 10 inducible tachycardias in patients with a negative preoperative test and 5 inducible tachycardias found in patients whose stimulation test had been considered to be contraindicated preoperatively (ejection fraction less than 20% or thrombus in the left ventricle); this raises the problem of extension of endocardiectomy during surgery or induction of an arrhythmogenic area through the surgical scar.[15]

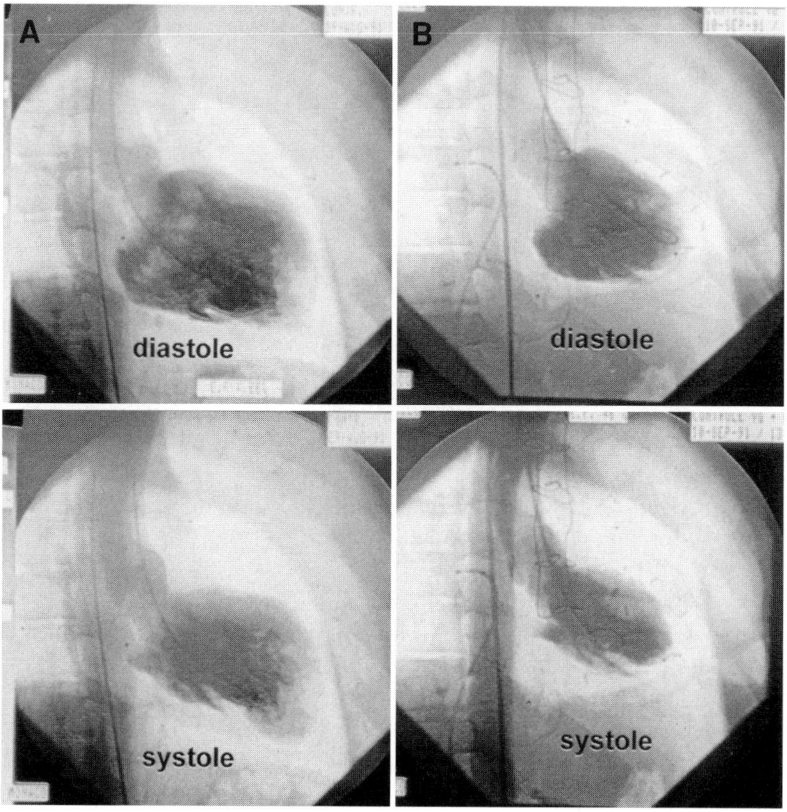

FIGURE 5.

Left ventricular angiograms in a patient with anteroseptoapical dyskinesia. **A,** preoperative diastole and systole in a right anterior oblique projection (left ventricular ejection fraction [LVEF], 28%). **B,** postoperative views of **A** (LVEF, 46%). *(continued)*

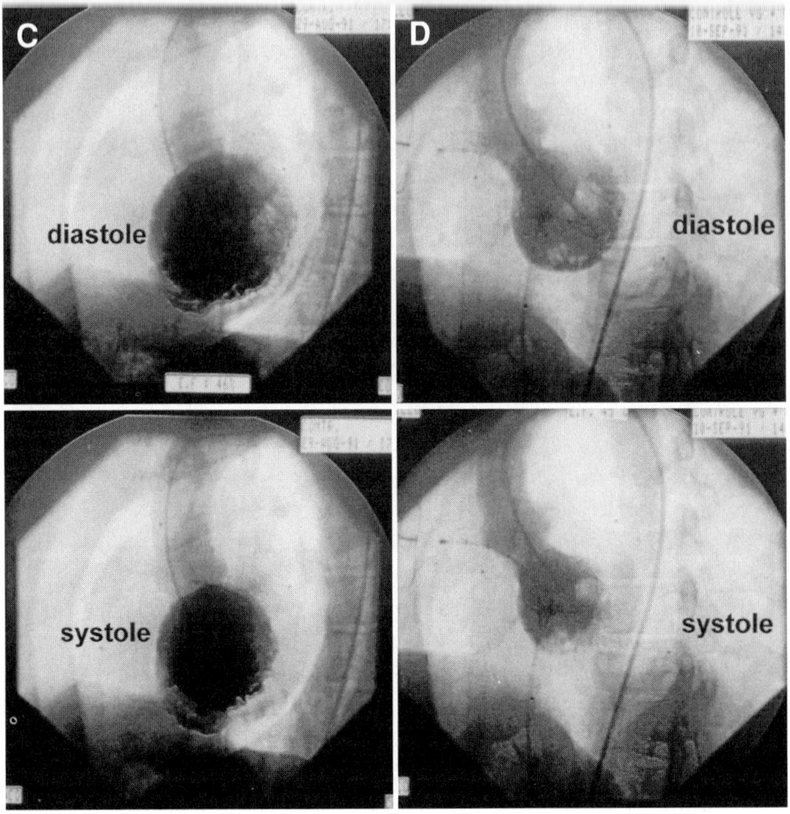

FIGURE 5. (continued)
C, preoperative diastole and systole in a left anterior oblique projection. **D,** postoperative views of **C.**

DELAYED CONTROL

After the first postoperative year, of 211 patients treated by autologous endoventricular patches, 123 (58%) were in New York Heart Association class I, 71 (33%) were in class II, 13 (6%) were in class III, and 5 (2%) were in class IV. There were thus 18 (8.5%) nonimproved patients and more than 90% in satisfactory clinical condition.[15]

INDICATIONS

These results, which are clinically satisfactory in more than 90% of our cases (8.5% of those in New York Heart Association classes III and IV) and in more than 90% of those with ventricular arrhyth-

TABLE 8.
Ventricular Arrhythmias

	Preoperative	Died in Hospital	Postoperative
SVT	89	9	7/80 (8.75%)
IVT	175	8 (4.57%)	4/167 (2.39%)
IVT + SVT	28	1	2/27 (7.4%)

Note: Postoperative PVS was performed 450 times and stimulated IVTs in 19 patients, 4 of whom were PVS-postive preoperatively, 10 of whom were PVS-negative preoperatively, and in 5 of whom PVS was contraindicated or not done. *Abbreviations: SVT,* spontaneous sustained ventricular tachycardia; *IVT,* inducible ventricular tachycardia; *PVS,* programmed ventricular stimulation.

mias and an ejection fraction at 1 year persistently superior to the contractile ejection fraction evaluated preoperatively, led us to propose the following indications:

- This ventricular reconstruction can be proposed without hesitation to all patients with ventricular aneurysms or akinesia with angina, arrhythmias, or attacks of cardiac insufficiency when the global ejection fraction is greater than 30% and the contractile ejection fraction is greater than 40%. In this category of patients, the operative mortality rate varied from 1.5% to 3%, these results clearly being better than allowing the pathology to evolve naturally. This is an elective indication.
- In emergencies when safe immediate circulatory assistance or a cardiac transplant is not available, left ventricular reconstruction can give hope of survival to more than 80% of these patients; on the other hand, there is no hope with natural evolution of the aneurysm.
- These mandatory indications must therefore be taken into consideration.

Finally, the indication for surgical reconstruction is questionable in two opposing circumstances:

- In asymptomatic patients when hemodynamic and angiographic evaluation after myocardial infarction shows left ventricular dyskinesia, the classic cardiologic attitude is abstention from surgery.
- It then seems advisable to propose tests for adaptation to exer-

else to such patients (stress ECG, isotopic ventriculography, and oxygen consumption measurement) to be sure that there are no symptoms; in particular, it is important to note that deterioration of the remaining contractile area can appear around the 40th month after myocardial infarction. Consequently, if the global ejection fraction of such patients is below 40% and the contractile ejection fraction is below 50%, it seems wise to propose left ventricular reconstruction to prevent an unfavorable evolution of the condition.

- On the contrary, in the category of end-stage ischemic cardiomyopathies when the ejection fraction is below 20%, the contractile ejection fraction is below 30%, cardiac output is below 1.5 L/m^2, and the mean pulmonary pressure is above 25 mm Hg, a cardiac transplant is often proposed as the only solution. Therefore, as long as myocardial biopsy eliminates the presence of associated degenerative cardiopathy coexistent with the ischemic cardiopathy, conservative surgery in this category of patients, who have a risk below 20%, brings definite hope for improvement that could be an alternative to cardiac transplantation, mainly in patients over 60 years old, diabetics, or those with respiratory insufficiency.

CONCLUSION

Endoventricular circular patch–plasty with septal exclusion is a safe and easily reproduced technique that improves ventricular function when combined with as complete coronary revascularization as possible. When associated with subtotal endocardiectomy, this technique affords excellent control of ventricular arrhythmias and should therefore be considered in the surgical treatment of left ventricular aneurysms.

REFERENCES

1. Cooley DA, Collins HA, Morris GC Jr, et al: Ventricular aneurysm after myocardial infarction: Surgical excision with use of temporary cardiopulmonary bypass. *JAMA* 167:557–560, 1958.
2. Froehlich RT, Falsetti HL, Doty DB, et al: Prospective study of surgery post left ventricular aneurysm. *Am J Cardiol* 45:923–931, 1980.
3. Cooley DA: Ventricular aneurysms and akinesia. *Cleve Clin Q* 45:130–132, 1978.
4. Jatene AD: Left ventricular aneurysmectomy: Resection or reconstruction. *J Thorac Cardiovasc Surg* 89:321–331, 1985.
5. Dor V, Kreitmann P, Jourdan J, et al: Interest of "physiological closure" (circumferential plasty on contractile areas) of left ventricle after re-

section and endocardiectomy for aneurysm or akinetic zone: Comparison with classical technique about a series of 209 left ventricular resections. *J Cardiovasc Surg* 26:73A, 1985.

6. Dor V, Saab M, Coste P, et al: Left ventricular aneurysm: A new surgical approach. *Thorac Cardiovasc Surg* 37:11–19, 1989.
7. Buckberg GD: Strategies and logic of cardioplegic delivery to prevent, avoid and reverse ischemic and reperfusion damage. *J Thorac Cardiovasc Surg* 93:127–139, 1978.
8. Fontan F: Transplantation of knowledge. *J Thorac Cardiovasc Surg* 99:113–118, 1990.
9. Dor V, Sabatier M, Di Donato M, et al: Late hemodynamic results after left ventricular patch repair associated with coronary grafting in patients with postinfarction akinetic or dyskinetic aneurysm of the left ventricle. *J Thorac Cardiovasc Surg* 110:1291–1301, 1995.
10. Di Donato M, Barletta G, Maioli M, et al: Early hemodynamic results of left ventricular reconstructive surgery for anterior wall left ventricular aneurysm. *Am J Cardiol* 69:886–890, 1992.
11. Louagie Y, Taoufik A, Lesperence J, et al: Left ventricular aneurysm completed by congestive heart failure: Analysis of long term results and risk factors of surgical treatment. *J Cardiovasc Surg* 30:648–655, 1989.
12. Fantini F, Barletta G, Baroni M, et al: Quantitative evaluation of left ventricular shape in anterior aneurysm. *Cathet Cardiovasc Diagn* 28:295–300, 1993.
13. Cox JL: Patient selection criteria and results of surgery for refractory ischemic ventricular tachycardia. *Circulation* 79:163S–177S, 1989.
14. Ostermeyer J, Kirklin JK, Borggref M, et al: Ten years of electrophysiologically guided direct operations for malignant ischemic ventricular tachycardia results. *Thorac Cardiovasc Surg* 37:20–27, 1988.
15. Dor V, Sabatier M, Montiglio F, et al: Results of nonguided subtotal endocardectomy associated with left ventricular reconstruction in patients with ischemic ventricular arrhythmias. *J Thorac Cardiovasc Surg* 107:1301–1308, 1994.

CHAPTER 3

Repair of Truncus Arteriosus

Miguel L. Barbero-Marcial, M.D.
Associate Professor, Chief of Pediatric Cardiac Surgery, Heart Institute, University of São Paulo Medical School, São Paulo, Brazil

Carla Tanamati, M.D.
Fellow, Cardiac Surgery, Heart Institute, University of São Paulo Medical School, São Paulo, Brazil

Truncus arteriosus, a relatively uncommon condition representing less than 3% of all congenital heart anomalies,[1] is characterized by the presence of a single arterial trunk that arises from the base of both ventricles by way of a semilunar (truncal) valve and gives origin to the coronary, systemic, and pulmonary circulations. Beneath the truncal valve is a ventricular septal defect (VSD).

Untreated patients have a poor prognosis, with 6-month and 1-year mortality rates of 65% and 75%, respectively.[2] The high mortality rate is related to the development of severe congestive heart failure caused by a large left-to-right shunt or progressive cyanosis as a result of accelerated pulmonary vascular obstructive disease.

The first surgical treatment proposed was banding of one or both pulmonary arteries.[3–5] The first successful intracardiac repair was performed in 1962 at the University of Michigan[6] and used a nonvalved Teflon conduit.

Notwithstanding progress in the correction of truncus arteriosus by the routine use of extracardiac conduits, results obtained in infants in the 1970s were not satisfactory. On the other hand, there was an immediate need to repair truncus arteriosus in the first days or months of life because of the high mortality rate.

The major progress in the repair of truncus arteriosus in children under 6 months of age was attributable to Ebert et al.,[7] who in 1984 published the results of repair in 100 infants, most of whom were younger than 6 months of age. The mortality rate was 11%. This motivated others to perform truncus repair in an elective manner during the neonatal period. Although not uniform, the results obtained demonstrated the feasibility of early repair.

Repair was done with the aid of extracardiac right ventricular to pulmonary artery conduits, which when used in children under 1 year of age necessitated repeat surgery because of internal obstruction or because the patient had outgrown the conduit. Eventually, the possibility for correction of truncus arteriosus without an extracardiac conduit became a reality, and this has been done in our institution since 1987.

HISTORICAL NOTE

The first case of truncus arteriosus was reported by Wilson[8] in 1798 and confirmed by clinical and autopsy examination in a 6-month-old infant by Buchanan[9] in 1864. Lev and Saphir[10] defined the basic morphological criteria for truncus arteriosus in 1942, and Collet and Edwards[11] reviewed previously reported cases and proposed a classification that is widely used.

As noted, the first successful intracardiac repair was performed in 1962 at the University of Michigan[6] and involved the use of a nonvalved Teflon conduit. Experimental work using valved ascending aortic allografts was reported by Arai and colleagues[12] in 1965 and by Rastelli et al.[13] in 1967. McGoon et al.[14] were the first to repair truncus arteriosus successfully and reported using a valved ascending aortic allograft in 1968. Binet[15] used a xenograft valve incorporated into a Dacron cylinder in 1971, and Bowman and associates[16] reported the use of a glutaraldehyde-treated porcine aortic valve in a Dacron cylinder in 1973.

The first repair using fresh homografts was reported in 1966 by Ross and Sommerville.[17] Recent promising results with aortic homografts, fresh and preserved by freezing, have resulted in a revival of the use of these conduits.

We reported the use of a valved conduit of bovine pericardium for right ventricle–pulmonary artery connections in 1995.[18] Earlier, in 1990, we reported the successful correction of truncus arteriosus without the use of extracardiac conduits.[19]

ANATOMICAL CONSIDERATIONS

CLASSIFICATION

The two major classifications used were proposed by Collet and Edwards[11] in 1949 and by Van Praagh and Van Praagh[20] in 1965.

TABLE 1.
Van Praagh and Van Praagh Classification

Type A (VSD Present)	Type B (VSD Absent)
1. Partially formed aorticopulmonary septum (main pulmonary segment present)	1. Partially formed aorticopulmonary septum (main pulmonary segment present)
2. Absence of aorticopulmonary septum (without main pulmonary segment)	2. Absence of one pulmonary artery from the common trunk
3. Absence of one pulmonary artery from the common trunk	3. Repeat as type A3
4. Underdeveloped aortic arch with large ductus arteriosus	4. Underdeveloped aortic arch with large ductus arteriosus

Abbreviation: VSD, ventricular septal defect.

Collet and Edwards subdivided truncus arteriosus into type I, in which the common trunk gives origin to a main pulmonary artery, which then bifurcates into pulmonary branches; type II, in which the left and right pulmonary arteries originate directly and closely to each other from the posterior truncus; type III, in which the branch pulmonary arteries arise from widely separated orifices on the lateral wall of the common trunk; and type IV, in which the pulmonary component of the trunk is absent, with the pulmonary blood supply derived from the collaterals of the descending aorta. This type of anomaly has been designated as type C pulmonary atresia with VSD.[21, 22]

Van Praagh and Van Praagh, who analyzed 57 autopsy cases of this anomaly, defined two basic types: type A, or truncus with VSD, and type B, or truncus without VSD. Groups A and B are subdivided into four subgroups (Table 1).

In our opinion, this classification stresses the presence of anomalies originating from the pulmonary arteries, which although not frequent, sometimes presents a surgical challenge.

THE VENTRICULAR SEPTAL DEFECT

The common trunk generally strides the defect, remaining about halfway in each ventricle.[23] Sometimes the common trunk arises almost exclusively from the left side or, less frequently, totally from the right ventricle.

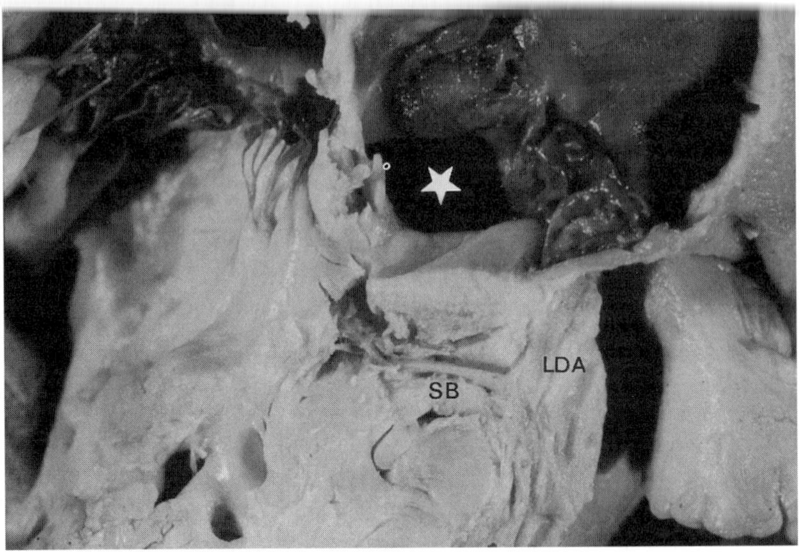

FIGURE 1.
Autopsy specimen from a 4-month-old patient with truncus arteriosus. The first septal branch of the left anterior descending coronary artery runs along the anterosuperior margin of the ventricular septal defect *(star). Abbreviations: LAD,* left anterior descending artery; *SB,* septal branch.

At the Heart Institute of the University of São Paulo we treated two patients with the aorta arising from the right ventricle, in addition to restrictive VSD. Such an association, although rare, leads to a delicate surgical problem. The VSD needs to be enlarged, and to achieve this, the anterosuperior band of the defect must be resected. Often, the first septal branch of the left anterior descending artery follows, at a few millimeters of depth, the anterosuperior margin of the defect (Fig 1). Therefore, enlargement of the VSD may damage the first septal branch and could provoke septal infarction and necrosis of its bundle and branches. The essence of the arterial supply to the atrioventricular conduction system is its duality.[24, 25] From its origin at the crux, the nodal artery reaches the atrioventricular node and can frequently supply its penetrating bundle. The other source of blood supply to the conduction system is the first or the second septal perforating artery of the anterior interventricular branch. In some variations of arterial anatomy, these perforating vessels could be the only blood supply of the conduction system.

The cause of death in two of our patients who underwent enlargement of a restrictive VSD and surgical correction without an extracardiac conduit was probably related to septal infarction and ischemia of his bundle.

The VSD in these cases is similar to that encountered in the tetralogy of Fallot except for the anatomy of its superior margin. The two limbs of the trabecula septomarginalis form the anterior and inferior margins of the defect. The posterior margin is formed by the ventriculo-infundibular fold that divides the truncal valve from the tricuspid valve. The ventriculo-infundibular fold merges with the posterior limb of the trabecula septomarginalis. In about two thirds of cases of truncus, this muscle is so well developed that the inferoposterior and posterior margins of the VSD exclusively consist of muscle and the defect is remote from the tricuspid annulus and the conduction system (Fig 2). In the remaining third these muscular portions are deficient and the septal defect is related to the tricuspid annulus, close to the conduction system (Fig 3). The superior margin is formed by the truncal annulus. The posterosuperior margin sometimes deviates more posteriorly and creates a sort of recess in this direction. When this recess is detected, a patch must be adequately tailored to fill this sometimes unsuspected ovoid-shaped VSD.

CORONARY ARTERIES

The pattern of coronary arteries encountered in a recent study of 22 specimens of truncus arteriosus at the Heart Institute of the University of São Paulo shows a number of coronary anomalies. In 17 specimens, anomalies of the coronary artery were found, the most frequent being (1) ostial stenosis (pinpoint) in 22.7%, (2) tangential origin in 22.7%, (3) intramural course in 13.6%, (4) a single ostium in 9.1%, and (5) a high ostial takeoff in 9.1%. The incidence and distribution of these anomalies in the two coronary systems are shown in Table 2. The relationship between the origin, course, and number of cusps of the truncal valve is illustrated in Figure 4.

In 85% of the specimens the origin of the sinus node artery came from the right coronary artery, and in 14% it came from the left coronary artery. In all cases in which the sinus node artery originated from the circumflex artery, the valves were quadricuspids.

Some of these anomalies may interfere with treatment and worsen the prognosis of such surgical patients.[26, 27] The high origin and ostial stenosis may be related to a deficiency in myocardial blood flow and, when associated with valvar truncal insufficiency, may cause problems with the administration of cardioplegic solution and therefore with myocardial protection.

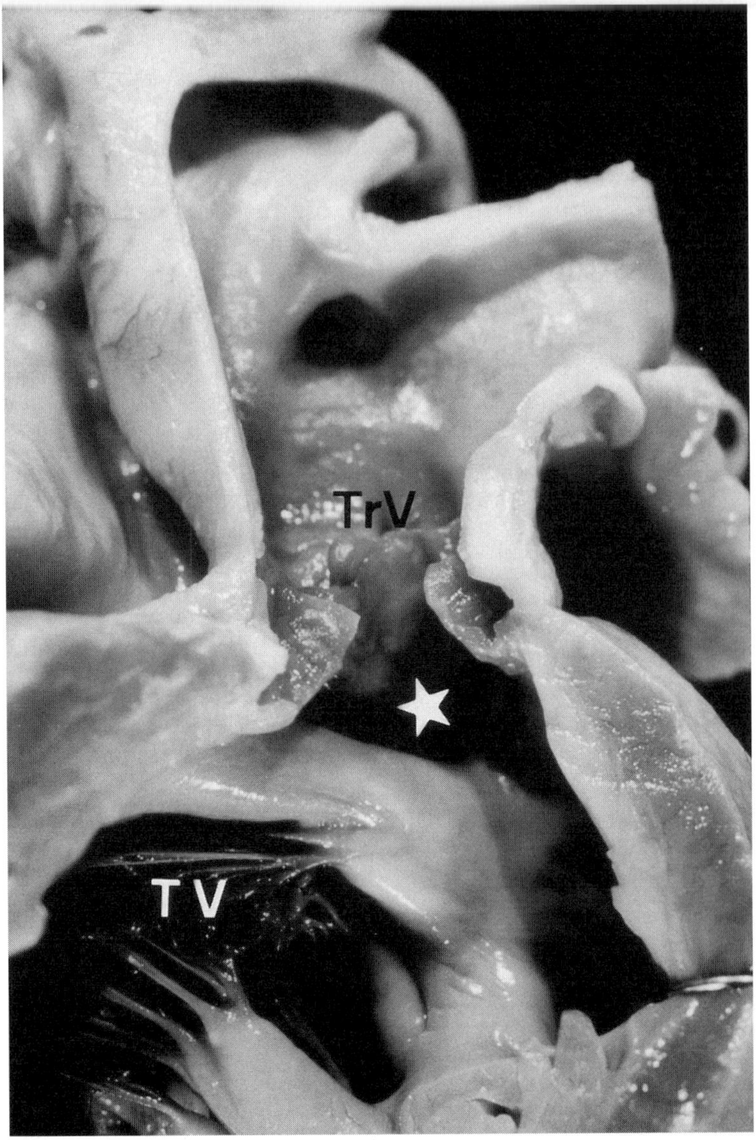

FIGURE 2.

Autopsy specimen from a 5-month-old patient with truncus arteriosus. The posterior margin of the ventricular septal defect *(star)* is made of muscle and the defect is remote from the tricuspid annulus and from the conduction system. *Abbreviations: TrV,* truncal valve; *TV,* tricuspid valve.

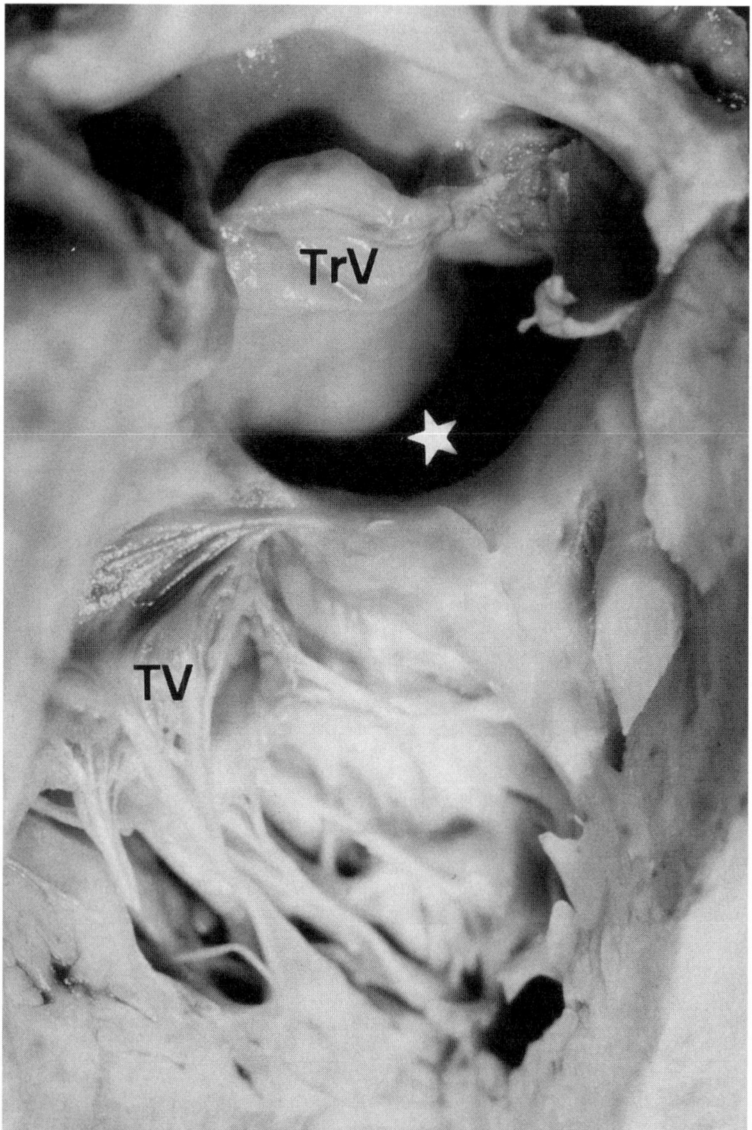

FIGURE 3.

Autopsy specimen from a 3-month-old patient with truncus arteriosus. The ventricular infundibular fold is poorly developed and therefore the ventricular septal defect *(star)* extends to the tricuspid annulus, close to the conduction system. *Abbreviations: TV,* tricuspid valve; *TrV,* truncal valve.

TABLE 2.
Distribution and Incidence of Anomalies of the Coronary System

Coronary Anomaly	Left Coronary	Right Coronary	Total
Ostial stenosis (pinpoint)	2	3	5 (22.7%)
Tangential origin	4	1	5 (22.7%)
Intramural course	3	0	3 (13.6%)
High ostial takeoff	1	1	2 (9.1%)
Single ostium	0	2	2 (9.1%)
Total	10	7	17 (77.2%)

Note: Study involving 22 specimens of truncus arteriosus types I and II from the Heart Institute in São Paulo, Brazil.

The right coronary artery can give rise to the anterior descending coronary artery, which often passes across the right ventricle (Fig 5). This can preclude non-conduit correction because it impedes right ventricular pulmonary artery anastomosis, as was seen in two patients in our series. An anomalous origin of the left coronary artery from the pulmonary component of the truncus can lead to an unperceived injury of the coronary artery during repair or lead to myocardial ischemia by compression.[28–30]

Whenever possible, preoperative angiography should be performed because it can be invaluable in detecting and thereby preventing some of these complications. When such a study cannot be performed, however, careful intraoperative assessment can facilitate the detection of coronary anomalies that may jeopardize the repair.

SEMILUNAR VALVE

In the 22 specimens under study, the truncal valve was bicuspid in 4 (18.2%), tricuspid in 10 (45.4%), and quadricuspid in 8 (36.4%). The degree of myxomatous thickening was severe in quadricuspid valves. Coincidentally, normal valves were encountered only in specimens with two or three cusps (Table 3). In only one of the specimens was severe valve stenosis present.

Other authors[31] report a correlation between the age of the patients and the incidence of abnormal valve cusps in the autopsy series. The incidence of severe myxomatous thickening was higher in neonates. These morphological alterations cause severe truncal valve regurgitation, early congestive heart failure, and death. Trun-

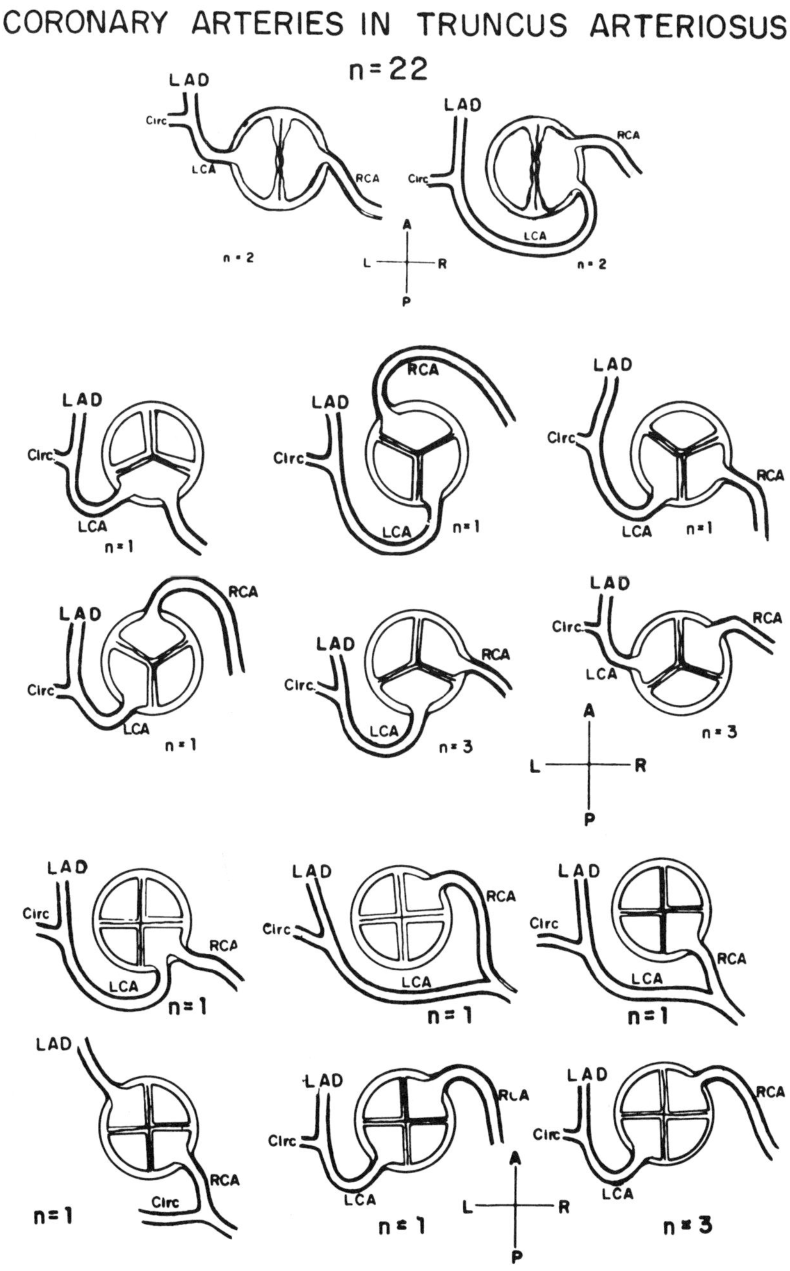

FIGURE 4.

Pattern of coronary arteries in relation to the number of cusps of the truncal valve in our study of 22 patients with truncus arteriosus. *Abbreviations: LCA,* left coronary artery; *RCA, right coronary artery; Circ,* circumflex coronary artery; *LAD,* left anterior descending coronary artery.

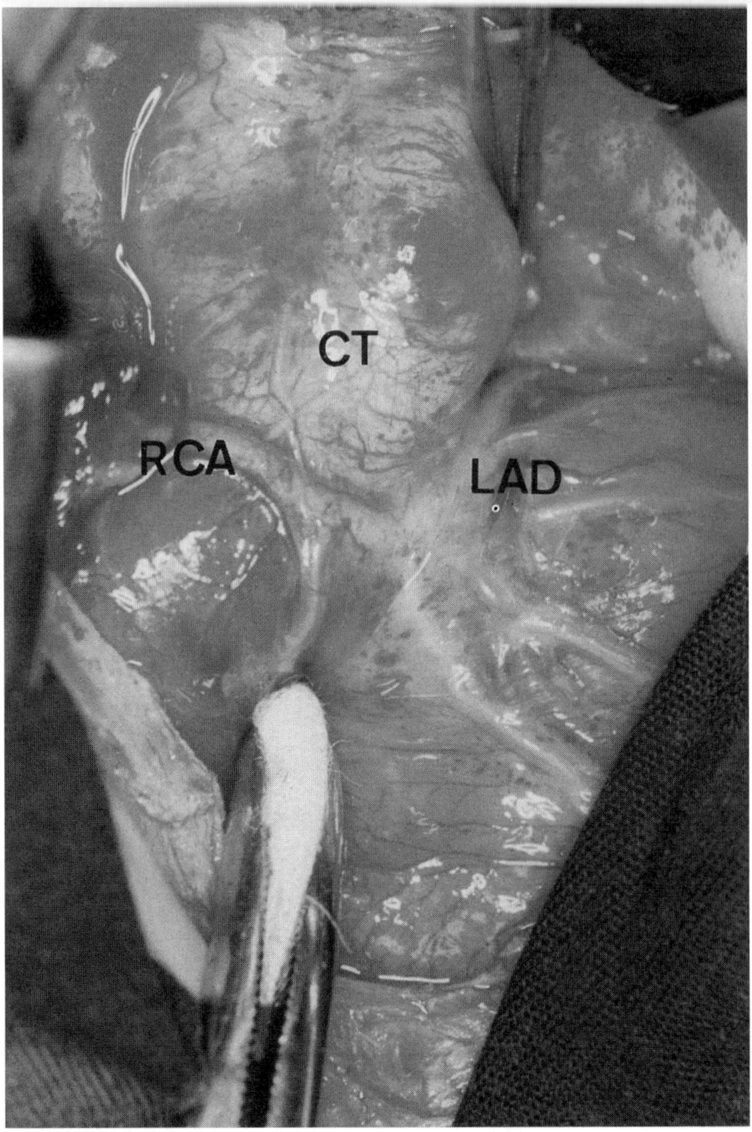

FIGURE 5.
Operative view of the heart of a 5-month-old infant with truncus arteriosus. The right coronary artery *(RCA)* gives origin to the anterior descending coronary artery, which courses anteriorly between the common trunk *(CT)* and the right ventricle. This anatomical variation precludes correction without extracardiac conduits. *Abbreviation: LAD,* left anterior descending coronary artery.

TABLE 3.
Incidence and Degree of Dysplasia Related to the Number of Truncal Valve Cusps

	Number of Cusps			
Degree of Dysplasia	**Bicuspid**	**Tricuspid**	**Quadricuspid**	**Total**
Without	2	3	0	5
Mild	0	4	0	4
Moderate	2	3	2	7
Severe	0	0	6	6
Total	4	10	8	22

Note: This anatomical study was done at the Heart Institute, University of São Paulo Medical School.

cal valve regurgitation was present in 20% of other series,[32] a fact that emphasizes the importance of this problem in the surgical treatment of these patients.

The specific etiology of the abundant mucoid connective tissue in the cusps is unknown. Furthermore, there is no explanation for the nonspecific fibrous proliferation in the malformed nodular margins of the valves.[33] Whether this malformation represents a developmental abnormality of the valve[34, 35] or an acquired alteration secondary to flow turbulence caused by the VSD in cusps that already have increased mucoid connective tissue is a controversial subject.

PULMONARY ARTERIES

The anatomy of the pulmonary arteries has a direct influence on the choice of surgical technique. The dividing line between types I and II is not distinct inasmuch as the wide range of variation in each type leads to a merger of one into the other. The total incidence of these two types ranges from 80% to 90%.[23] In our study, all specimens were of type I (22.7%) or type II (77.3%).

In approximately 10% of the autopsy cases, only one pulmonary artery arose from the common trunk.[32] There is nearly a consensus that the pulmonary artery is more frequently missing on the side opposite the aortic arch. However, others[36] report that the artery on the same side as the aortic arch is absent more frequently. The other pulmonary artery, when present, arises from the ductus arteriosus and is sometimes fibrotic, and the lumen of the pulmonary artery is found a few centimeters away from the pulmonary hilum.

In one of our patients, the left pulmonary artery arising from the ductus arteriosus supplied only the upper left lobe; the lower lobe was supplied by a pulmonary-systemic collateral. The right pulmonary artery originated from the left posterolateral wall of the truncal artery.

Bharati et al.[23] reported an atypical origin of the pulmonary arteries in 10 of 180 cases of truncus arteriosus. In 1 case there was a total absence of the right and left pulmonary arteries and the lungs. In 2 patients the right pulmonary artery was missing and the right lung was supplied by bronchial arteries. One patient had no left pulmonary artery, and the left lung was supplied by bronchial arteries. In the remaining 6 patients, the left and right pulmonary arteries originated from the ductus arteriosus.

ASSOCIATED ANOMALIES

Approximately 10% to 20% of patients with truncus arteriosus have associated cardiac and extracardiac anomalies.[32] The most frequent anomalies are right aortic arch (21% to 36%), interrupted aortic arch (11% to 19%), aberrant subclavian artery (4% to 10%), persistent left superior vena cava draining into the coronary sinus (4% to 9%), and the previously described absence of one pulmonary artery (10%).

NATURAL HISTORY

The incidence of truncus arteriosus ranges from 0.4% to 3.9% in autopsy studies of congenital heart defects.[1, 11] The natural evolution of truncus arteriosus is unfavorable because of the severe hemodynamic derangement early in life. Congestive heart failure frequently occurs in the first weeks of life and depends on the magnitude of the decrease in pulmonary resistance, which increases pulmonary blood flow. Truncal valve regurgitation and the presence of other associated anomalies are also factors that contribute to early death.

Without surgical treatment, mortality is about 80% during the first year of life,[37] only 50% survive beyond the neonatal period, and approximately 20% of these patients survive the first year; these "long-term" survivors die as a consequence of pulmonary vascular disease, which once established, appears to progress rapidly.[38] Other patients can succumb from cerebral abscess or bacterial endocarditis.[11]

Reports from the Mayo Clinic suggest that surgical repair in children 2 years and older is contraindicated when pulmonary vascular resistance is greater than 8 Wood units. Younger patients at this level of pulmonary resistance are accepted for surgical correction only if the resistance falls after ventilation with oxygen or vasodilator medication.[36, 39]

Approximately 5% of the patients with this anomaly can survive past the first 2 or 3 years of life with large left-to-right shunts without severe pulmonary arteriolar disease developing.

INDICATIONS FOR SURGERY

The policy at our institution is early primary repair, ideally within the first 3 months of age and, whenever possible, before 30 days of age. In view of the 50% mortality before 1 month, all effort must be made to correct the anomaly as early as possible. Unfortunately, a number of infants are referred to our service only after some months of age; usually they have extreme malnutrition secondary to severe congestive heart failure.

Failure of infants with truncus arteriosus to thrive can be attributed to the imbalance between caloric intake and energy expenditure; insufficient energy is left for normal growth. They have the classic sequelae of protein-calorie malnutrition, including subnormal growth, impaired immunocompetence, hypoalbuminemia, and atrophy of the respiratory muscles. These patients require nutritional support before and after surgery. Because many of these infants are unable to tolerate large volumes of milk, they need to be fed high-energy formulas gradually so that intake can be improved without overfeeding or fluid overload.

To increase caloric intake, several strategies are available, including a decrease in water intake and an increase in protein, carbohydrate, and fat intake. Requirements for an infant with congenital heart disease in the first year of life are as much as 140–170 kcal/kg/day. Approximately 30% of the total calories should come from fat and 70% from carbohydrates and protein. Many children with growth failure may have a limited tolerance to increases in feeding volume and concentration, so urine osmolarity should be monitored and not exceed 400 mOsm/L. Nutrition support may have to be increased progressively to reach an optimal level. To meet nutritional recommendations and the restrictions imposed by cardiac disease, tube feeding should be encouraged because it permits these patients to be fed during the night. Diuretics may help control the volume overload.

Pulmonary vascular disease in truncus arteriosus occurs early in life, but the pathogenesis is only partially known. Functional and structural changes in the walls of arterioles and precapillary arteries take place as a result of the release of substances by endothelial cells. The purpose of cardiac catheterization is to evaluate whether such changes are functional or structural, advanced or irreversible. At the Heart Institute of the University of São Paulo Medical School[40] we have adopted a protocol that measures mean pulmonary artery pressure, right and left atrial pressure, and right and left ventricular pressure. The pulmonary-systemic blood flow ratio and the pulmonary arteriolar resistance index are calculated by the Fick method. Changes in pressure and flow, under test conditions such as mask inhalation of oxygen and nitric oxide, are sometimes vital for determining the proper indication for surgery in patients with truncus arteriosus.

These tests involve the measurement of hemodynamic variables at baseline and during oxygen and nitric oxide intake. Children are considered operable when pulmonary vascular resistance falls below 8 Wood units in the 10 minutes subsequent to the administration of 100% oxygen or in the 20 minutes immediately after the administration 20 ppm nitric oxide. Pulmonary angiography is also performed. The transit time of contrast media and the type of small-artery tapering in the wedge angiogram are studied.

These parameters give additional information that could aid in determining the best approach to correct this defect and also how to manage the pulmonary artery postoperative hypertension crisis. In cases of severe pulmonary hypertension, lung biopsy may be required to assess both the severity and the potential reversibility of the obstructive arterial disease.

In patients with persistent truncus arteriosus, minimal proliferative lesions usually appear early in the natural history, even during the first year of life, and affect primarily the pre-acinar arteries. A morphometric approach to the arteries is important because it permits an assessment of the degree of dilatation of the intra-acinar vessels, as well as the number of arteries in relation to alveoli.[41] An increase in the number of vessels as a function of the age of the patient can be demonstrated by biopsy data.

Regression of arterial hypertrophy (Heath and Edwards[42] grade I and morphometric grade B) is always to be expected after repair of the cardiac anomaly.[43] The intimal proliferative lesions, on the other hand, can revert only partially, and patients with severe obstruction or dilatation injuries may exhibit progressive pulmonary hypertension, even after repair.

Early primary repair has acquired fundamental importance in our institution inasmuch as in all cases of truncus arteriosus with type I or II anatomy and no associated anomaly, we advocate the previously described repair, without extracardiac conduit. To achieve success with this technique, we believe that it is important to operate on patients with low pulmonary resistance, which is found only in the first months of life.

In children over 6 months of age or with signs of increased pulmonary resistance, we prefer to use the valved conduit procedure described by Rastelli because the use of a monocuspid valve in the pulmonary position is frequently followed by important residual pulmonary insufficiency.

SURGICAL TECHNIQUE

MYOCARDIAL PROTECTION

The preoperative heart failure condition in infants with truncus arteriosus is detrimental to mitochondria.[44] If such patients require preoperative catecholamine support, there could be a detrimental effect of decreased ventricular performance associated with the cardiac arrest, even under cardioplegic myocardial protection.

Biopsy of the myocardium at postischemic reperfusion shows injury to the mitochondria, intracellular edema, and a significant decrease in glycogen granules. We reported a correlation between the related myocardial alterations and the presence of low-output syndrome postoperatively.

Measures that may minimize postoperative myocardial deterioration are (1) early primary repair during the neonatal period; (2) induction with warm blood cardioplegia (20 mL/kg) followed by cold blood cardioplegia (20 mL/kg) at 4°C with maintenance cardioplegia every 20 minutes; (3) direct infusion of a cardioplegic solution at the coronary ostia in presence of truncal valve regurgitation; (4) if diameter and implantation ostial anomalies render the infusion of cardioplegia more difficult and unsafe, retrograde cardioplegia (pediatric RCSP cannula 94006/94106, DLP Meditronic, Grand Rapids, Mich) with an infusion pressure not above 40 mm Hg is appropriate; and (5) maintenance of myocardial temperature by myocardial cooling with cold saline solution. However, the possibility of paralysis of the phrenic nerve must be taken into account.

MYOCARDIAL ISCHEMIA AFTER INDUCTION OF ANESTHESIA

Truncus arteriosus is associated with a nonrestricted shunt between the pulmonary and systemic circulations.[45] This results in an interdependence of each of the vascular resistances. Therefore, an important decrease in systemic diastolic pressure may occur secondary to pulmonary vascular dilation provoked by anesthetic drugs.

On the other hand, there is increased ventricular myocardial wall tension secondary to dilation of the ventricular cavity (Laplace's law). This tension increases myocardial oxygen requirements. Because diastolic systemic pressure is often very low, coronary perfusion is affected, resulting in ischemia, which could have implications in postoperative cardiac function.

In our series of 80 cases of truncus arteriosus accumulated since 1987, we had at least 5 patients with significant ST-segment depression soon after induction of anesthesia. Two of them had cardiac arrest, which was reversed only after the initiation of cardiopulmonary bypass, although both died postoperatively. Apparently, the only efficient maneuver is temporary occlusion of the pulmonary artery to decrease pulmonary blood flow steal and thus increase systemic and coronary perfusion. Other efforts to increase systemic diastolic blood pressure such as volume loading or catecholamine administration were ineffective. Furthermore, maneuvers to decrease $F\text{IO}_2$ and increase $P\text{ACO}_2$ were almost ineffective in improving the ST-segment alterations in our patients.

OPERATIVE TECHNIQUES

Essentially there are two different techniques for the correction of truncus arteriosus:

With an extracardiac conduit—valved or nonvalved

Without an extracardiac conduit—reconstruction with a direct anastomosis between the right ventricle and the pulmonary arteries

Since 1962,[6] various types of conduit have been used: Dacron conduits without valves, Dacron conduits with porcine or other types of valves, and homografts. More recently, we reported the results of the use of valved conduits of crimped bovine pericardium.[18]

When conduits are used in infants, they must have a small diameter and are eventually outgrown by the patient. Other late complications frequently observed are valve calcification with stenosis in the Dacron conduits, stenosis in the proximal anastomosis, and stenosis in the tube itself. Even fresh aortic homografts may undergo late postoperative calcification. Currently, more surgeons are using homografts for the correction of truncus arteriosus, mainly

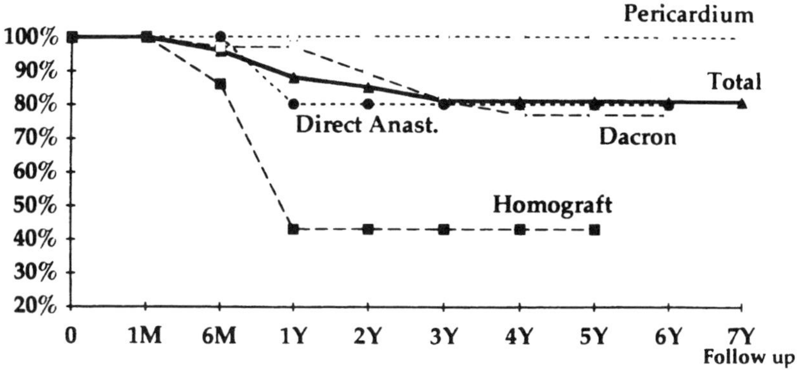

FIGURE 6.
Results of techniques of right ventricular outflow tract reconstruction. (Courtesy of Lacour-Gayet F, Serraf A, Komiya T, et al: Truncus arteriosus repair: Influence of techniques of right ventricular outflow tract reconstruction. *J Thorac Cardiovasc Surg* 111:849–856, 1996.)

to avoid a rigid prosthesis and because of easy suturing, improved hemostasis, and small bulk. The most important issue is whether the long-term results with this type of conduit will be better than the results with prosthetic conduits.

Kirklin et al.[46] reported good midterm results with the use of homografts. Cleveland et al.[47] reported that 45% of their patients with homografts needed a reoperation 5 years after homograft implantation between the right ventricle and the pulmonary artery. Lacour-Gayet et al.[48] reported an actuarial freedom from reoperation of 43% at 7 years of follow-up (Fig 6). These authors concluded that the use of homografts in neonates or infants correlates with an incremental risk for earlier reoperation. Razzouk et al.[49] reported a significantly higher rate of reoperation after the implantation of homografts than after the use of Dacron conduits. Heierman et al.[50] reported a significant difference between aortic and pulmonary homografts, the latter being relatively free of obstruction. In Brazil there is no adequate legislation for the commercialization of homografts, so the search for other types of material is ongoing.

Because of the aforementioned factors as well as the poor late results obtained with Dacron and homograft conduits, we decided to fashion conduits from crimped bovine pericardiac valves. Our good late results in the last 20 years with the use of bovine pericardium as patch material certainly influenced its selection for repairs. This type of conduit has a slim and flexible texture that facilitates suturing to the thin and fragile walls of the pulmonary arteries, thus improving homeostasis at the anastomosis.

We developed a special type of pericardium conduit by crimping the tube. This technique maintains the necessary, almost circular shape of the implant and allows the implant to be positioned in soft turns without kinking. Because the prosthesis is made of nonporous tissue and has no longitudinal and diametral restriction, it can be chosen at any time during surgery.[18]

Repair With Extracardiac Conduit

Repair with a conduit is conducted in the following sequence: after sternotomy the thymus gland is resected to facilitate exposure. The pericardium is opened longitudinally. If on ECG an ST-segment depression appears as a consequence of poor myocardial perfusion (see Myocardial Protection), the pulmonary arteries are dissected, snared, and partially occluded to increase diastolic systemic pressure.

Bicaval cannulation is performed with a purse-string suture at the junction between the inferior vena cava and the right atrium and at the right appendage of the superior vena cava. Cannulation of the aorta is done close to the origin of the brachiocephalic trunk in an attempt to leave sufficient space between the cannula and the pulmonary arteries of the common trunk.

After the onset of cardiopulmonary bypass, the pulmonary arteries are snared and occluded at their origin to avoid the outflow of systemic blood to the pulmonary circuit. The patient is cooled down to 20°C measured at the nasopharynx and at the rectum. Flow during cardiopulmonary bypass is set at 120 mL/kg/min.

Soon after the onset of cardiopulmonary bypass, the aorta is clamped and cardioplegic solution is infused (20 mL/kg, Saint Thomas solution). Infusion is done through the aorta. An aspirator is introduced into the right ventricle through the right atrium to decompress the left cavities.

In the presence of severe truncal valve insufficiency, palpation discloses that the pressure of the ascending aorta is low and the ventricles are distended. In such cases the common trunk is opened in the region where the pulmonary arteries will be removed and the cardioplegia is directly infused through cannulation of the ostia. Because of the position and orientation anomalies of the ostia, sometimes this maneuver is difficult and prolonged.

Next, the pulmonary arteries are removed from the common trunk (Fig 7, A) in an attempt to visualize the left coronary ostium so as not to cause injury. In general, the left coronary ostium is lo-

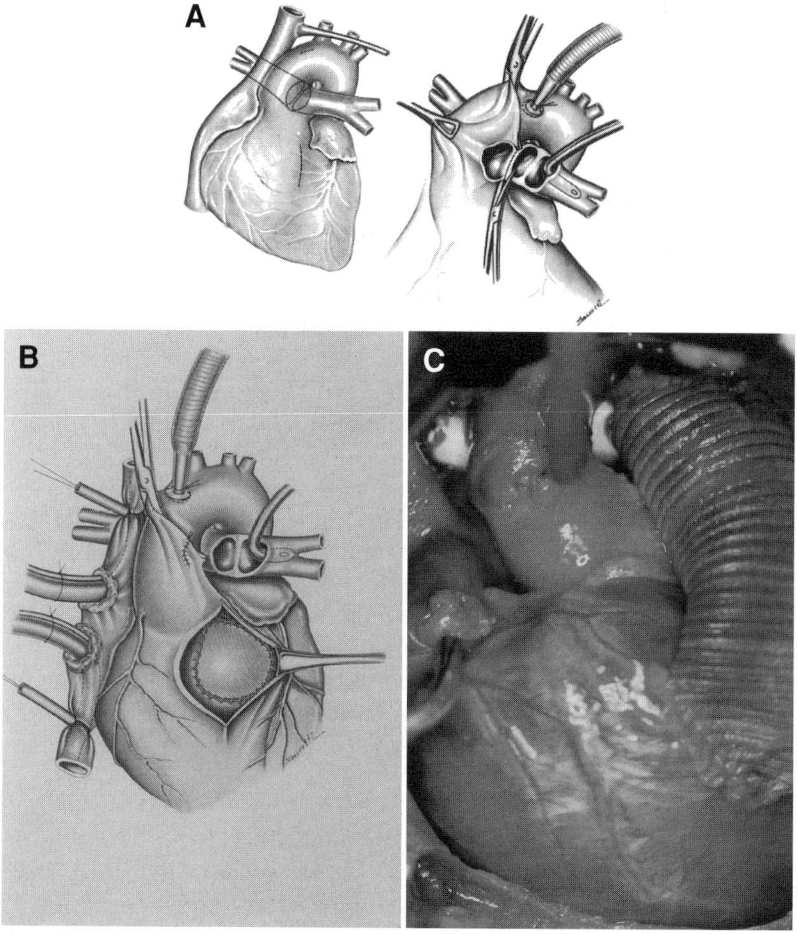

FIGURE 7.

Repair with an extracardiac conduit. **A,** the pulmonary arteries are withdrawn from the common trunk. **B,** closure of the ventricular septal defect is performed with a bovine pericardial patch. **C,** final aspect of the correction with a crimped bovine pericardial valve conduit.

cated between the root of the pulmonary arteries and the truncal annular level, often in a high position (over 1 cm above the valvar annulus).

In two cases the left coronary ostium was found in the pulmonary component. In these patients the ostium with a large flap of pulmonary tissue was moved into the proper position in the aortic component. After the aortic defect was closed with bovine pericardium, the right ventricle was opened by making a longitudinal incision of approximately 2 cm, commencing just below the truncal annulus level. The interventricular communication was closed with a patch of bovine pericardium and continuous suture with 6-0 Prolene reinforced with five equidistant stitches of 6-0 Prolene with a pledget (Fig 7, B). As described in the section on VSDs, sometimes there is a posterior recess in the interventricular communication that turns out to be larger than initially suspected. Usually we place a bovine pericardium patch larger than the diameter of the VSD and, if necessary, reduce it later.

A valve conduit of crimped bovine pericardium is selected. In children weighing less than 3 kg we prefer a conduit 10 mm in diameter; from 3 to 5 kg, one of 12 mm; and in those over 5 kg, a conduit 14 mm in diameter. Such conduit does not need precoagulation. The conduit is prepared so that the valve remains near the divided pulmonary end, and a continuous suture of 6-0 Prolene is used. The proximal end of the conduit is beveled so that a short rim of pericardium is left posteriorly to maintain the shape and diameter of the conduit. Continuous sutures of 5-0 and 6-0 Prolene are attached to a 4-mm–wide strip of bovine pericardium (Fig 7, C).

After aortic declamping, the ventricles are gently compressed to avoid distension, which is dependent on the degree of truncal valve regurgitation. Generally, after these maneuvers there is adequate myocardial recovery.

Repair Without an Extracardiac Conduit

The preliminary steps of the operation are identical to those previously described for repair with extracardiac conduits. The difference begins at the incision of the common trunk. A longitudinal incision is made in the left pulmonary artery, near its anterosuperior aspect, and is extended vertically toward the left sinus of Valsalva of the common trunk (Fig 8, A). After identification of the right pulmonary artery orifice and the left coronary ostium, a pericardial patch is sutured so that it divides the truncus arteriosus into two portions: aorta and pulmonary trunk (Fig 8, B). This is achieved by beginning the suture near the truncal valve ring, with the left sinus of Valsalva left in the pulmonary component. The posterior suture of the patch is placed between the left coronary ostium and the origin of the right pulmonary artery. Care is taken to ensure that the patch is not too large or the higher aortic pressure could obstruct the right pulmonary artery.

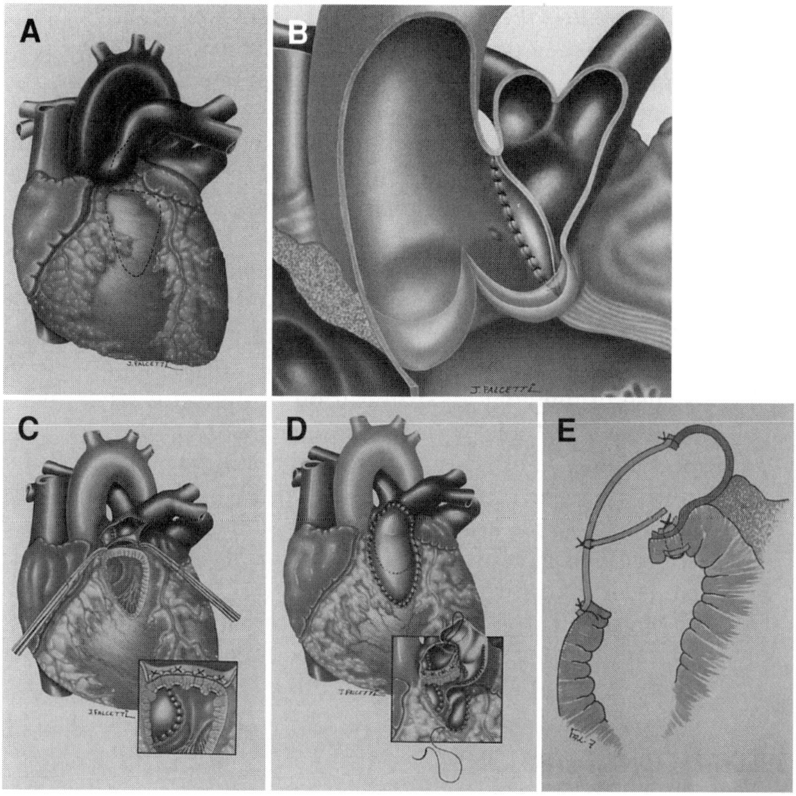

FIGURE 8.

Operative technique of correction without an extracardiac conduit. **A,** the proposed incision is indicated by the *dotted lines.* **B,** division of the truncus into the aorta and pulmonary arteries by insertion of the bovine pericardial patch. **C,** closure of the ventricular septal defect and the posterior anastomosis between the left superior pulmonary artery and the left superior oblique margin of the ventriculotomy with interrupted sutures. **D,** the *inset* shows the pericardial patch with the monocusp valve. The anterior wall is constructed with a bovine pericardial patch with a monocuspid valve. **E,** corrected position of the monocuspid valve during diastole.

The right ventricle is then incised immediately under the left sinus of Valsalva in an oblique direction with an inferior and leftward course. The muscular trabecula, which is usually present in the margins of the incision, is sectioned. The VSD is closed with a bovine pericardial patch (Fig 8, C). In two patients the restrictive VSD was enlarged in its anterosuperior portion.

Thereafter, the lower edge of the incision in the left pulmonary artery is pushed down and anastomosed to the left superior oblique margin of the ventriculotomy with separated U stitches to form an almost horizontal suture line.

Next, a bovine pericardial patch with a pericardial monocusp valve is sutured to the pulmonary artery and the ventricular edges to construct the anterior wall of the new right ventricular outflow tract (Fig 8, D).

In some patients with truncus arteriosus type II, a few technical modifications can be adopted. The pulmonary arteries, which arise from the posterior aspect of the common trunk, are divided with a bovine pericardial patch. In one of our patients, because of the great dextroposition of the trunk, the left ventricular–neoaortic tract was constructed with a double patch, one inferior and another superior, the resulting angle following the suture line and bulging into the right ventricle. The left atrial appendage was used to construct the posterior wall of the neopulmonary trunk, with the anterior wall being constructed just as in the previous patients.

More recently, in a large series of patients Norwood (personal communication, 1991) used this technique successfully for reconstruction of the right ventricle outflow tract.

SPECIAL CONSIDERATIONS

TRUNCAL VALVE REGURGITATION

Truncal valve regurgitation occurs in up to 50% of patients with truncus arteriosus.[51] In mild truncal valve regurgitation, operation is performed as usual. In cases with moderate or severe valve regurgitation, valvoplasty is mandatory. The insufficiency is usually secondary to cusp retraction or prolapse, annulus dilation, or abnormalities of the valve tissue.

At the time of surgery the valve is carefully inspected. The techniques of repair consist of suture of the minor cusp to another with better support, central triangular resection of the prolapsed cusp, lateral plication of the prolapsed cusp, and intercomissural plication; in some cases we have also used “transventricular annular plication” of the prolapsed cusp. This last maneuver was developed during closure of the VSD, looking at the ventricular side of the truncal annulus (Fig 9). The annulus is partially plicated with a continuous suture of 5-0 Prolene from one side of the edge of the VSD to the other. We used this technique in two patients with good results.

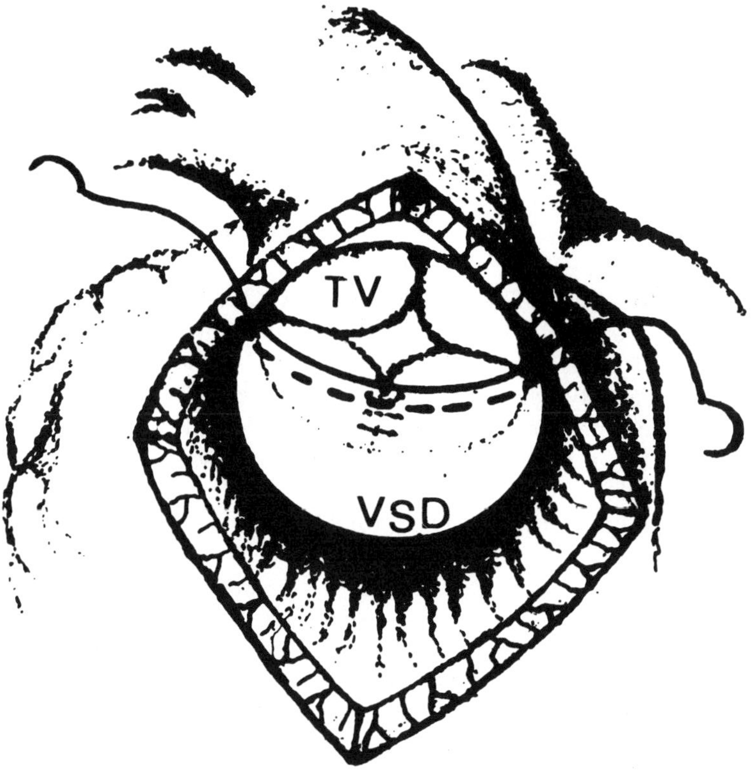

FIGURE 9.
Surgical illustration of "transventricular annular plication." The annulus is partially plicated with a continuous side-to-side suture of the edge of the ventricular septal defect *(VSD). Abbreviation: TrV,* truncal valve.

HEMITRUNCUS

In cases of hemitruncus, the pulmonary vascular disease progresses more rapidly in the lung connected to the common trunk;[52] thus the repair should be done as early as possible. Pulmonary angiography is important for locating the other pulmonary artery and facilitates correction. The operation consists of reconstruction of the pulmonary circulation by direct reimplantation of the pulmonary artery or by interposition of a tubular graft.

In four of the five cases of hemitruncus seen in our institution we performed direct reimplantation, and in the other, a polytetrafluoroethylene graft was necessary to reconstruct the pulmonary arteries. Probably the presence of residual ductus tissue led to stenosis of the reimplanted pulmonary artery in two patients and necessitated reintervention. In view of these cases, interposition of the graft might be more appropriate.

If one pulmonary artery is missing,[23] the repair must be done by connecting the existent pulmonary artery to the right ventricular outflow tract, which in the long term could increase the risk of pulmonary vascular disease.

RESULTS

REPAIR WITHOUT AN EXTRACARDIAC CONDUIT

From 1987 to 1996 at our institution, 45 nonconsecutive patients with truncus arteriosus type I or II underwent correction by direct reconstruction of the right ventricle–pulmonary arteries continuity. The hospital mortality rate was 24.4%. In a follow-up of up to 10 years, two noncardiac late deaths occurred (4.4%).

Early and midterm results of correction of truncus arteriosus without an extracardiac conduit have been reported in the last several years. Norwood (personal communication, 1996) reported his experience with type I and II truncus arteriosus at the Children's Hospital of Philadelphia; an overall mortality rate of 10% was observed.

At the Birmingham Children's Hospital, a technical modification was introduced by Brown (personal communication, 1996). A large button of truncal wall is excised. The opening into the truncus is closed by a patch. The posterior wall of the pulmonary arteries, surrounded by tissue, is anastomosed at the upper edge of the right ventriculotomy on the right side of the aorta. Then the anterior wall of the new right ventricle outflow tract is constructed by using a pericardial patch without a monocusp valve.

Nakae et al.[53] reported good early and late results in neonates and small infants when using an autologous arterial flap for primary correction instead of conduit repair. These authors emphasize the importance of developing surgical methods that allow growth of the pulmonary tract. When the distance between the pulmonary arteries and the ventricular edge of the ventriculotomy is too large, as in truncus type III, interposition of the left atrial appendage was also done to construct the posterior wall of the right ventricle–pulmonary artery pathway.

Lacour-Gayet et al.[48] in 1996 published a study about the effect of different techniques on reconstruction of the right outflow tract. Direct anastomosis between the right ventricle and the pulmonary arteries was associated with higher hospital mortality when compared with other techniques. The higher mortality rate observed in the direct anastomosis group correlated with more complex associated anomalies, low weight, and nonavailability of cryopreserved homograft conduit. The homograft conduit in turn correlated with an increased risk of early reoperation, 40% at 5 years, when compared with patients treated by direct anastomosis, 20% at 6 years.

REPAIR WITH EXTRACARDIAC CONDUITS

In our institution from 1987 to 1997, 35 nonconsecutive patients with truncus arteriosus type I, II, or III underwent repair with an extracardiac conduit. Until 1990 we constructed the valve out of bovine pericardium in the operating room within a Dacron tube.

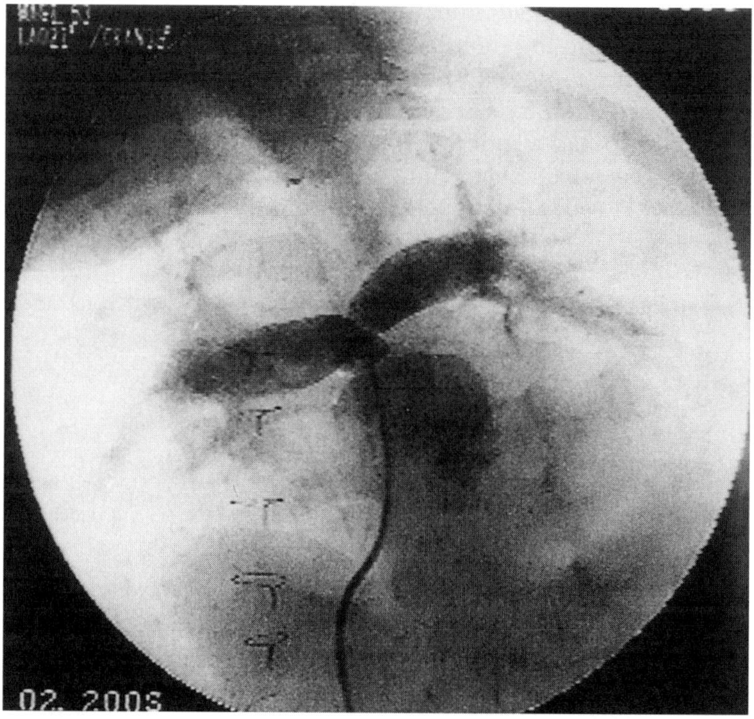

FIGURE 10.

Postoperative angiography of a patient with right ventricular outflow tract obstruction 2 years after correction without an extracardiac conduit. Right ventricle injection shows stenosis at the level of the right ventricle–pulmonary artery anastomosis and at the origin of the left pulmonary artery. This was the third and last patient who underwent a reoperation to relieve pulmonary stenosis.

To construct the valve, the Dacron tube was totally inverted and one Hegar dilator of adequate size was introduced inside to keep the tube completely expanded. Afterward, one of the sides of the strip of bovine pericardium was sutured around the entire circumference of the inverted tube. Three other equidistant sutures were placed from the sutured border to the free margin, as described by Oliveira et al.[54] The tube was reinverted to the original position with the valve left inside. Easy to construct in the operating room, this valved tube is stentless and costs very little.

Since 1991, motivated by the significant incidence of Dacron tube obstruction at midterm follow-up (Fig 10), we began using crimped bovine pericardial conduits with bovine pericardial valves, which were inserted in 25 patients in our series (Fig 11). Their ages ranged from 2 months to 7 years (median age, 12.5 months), and the internal diameter of the conduits ranged from 10 to 18 mm. Follow-up ranged from 2 months to 72 months. Serial echocardiography showed stenosis in 3 cases. One 12-year-old patient who had a pulmonary gradient pressure of 52 mm Hg 1 year after the repair successfully underwent pulmonary artery angioplasty. A second patient, a 1-year-old girl who had an obstruction

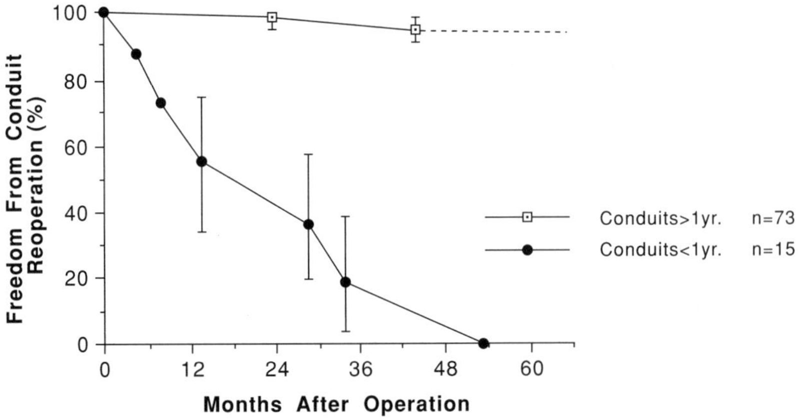

FIGURE 11.

Actuarial freedom from reoperation for allograft valved conduit dysfunction as a function of months after surgery. *Vertical bars* represent 70% confidence intervals. *Dashed lines* represent patients monitored beyond the last event. (Courtesy of Hawkins JA, Bailey WW, Dillon T, et al: Midterm results with cryopreserved allograft valved conduits from the right ventricle to the pulmonary arteries. *J Thorac Cardiovasc Surg* 104:910–916, 1992.)

and a pulmonary gradient pressure of 36 mm Hg, underwent dilatation of the obstruction and attained a final gradient of 21 mm Hg. A third patient, who has a gradient pressure of 80 mm Hg inside the conduit, is awaiting reintervention or angioplasty.

Two patients who had fungal endocarditis *(Candida albicans)* 6 and 9 months after correction underwent conduit replacement and had a satisfactory postoperative course.

In conclusion, the results of the present study on the use of valved crimped bovine pericardial conduits seem promising. The merits of this conduit will be evaluated as the length of follow-up increases.

PREOPERATIVE RISK FACTORS FOR DEATH AFTER REPAIR

In the last several years consensus has been reached on early primary repair before 3 months of age. Factors that favor the performance of early primary repair are (1) the higher incidence of pulmonary hypertensive crises in the postoperative period in older children, (2) the improved operative and postoperative management of complex cardiac anomalies, (3) the feasibility of using small homografts, and (4) the even more promising possibility of repair by direct anastomosis between the right ventricle and the pulmonary arteries without the use of an extracardiac conduit.

In our experience, preoperative risk factors in patients with truncus arteriosus are older age at surgery, truncal valve regurgitation, interrupted aortic arch, coronary artery anomalies, and hemitruncus.

OLD AGE AT SURGERY

There is a significant correlation between age and mortality rate when repair is conducted without using extracardiac conduits. Hospital mortality in the neonatal period was 12.5% without the exclusion of patients with complex cardiac anomalies, 15.7% in patients 1–3 months of age, and 35.5% in patients 3–6 months of age.

Reconstruction of the right ventricular outflow tract with autologous tissue can cause some degree of pulmonary regurgitation. In older patients (over 3 months of age), pulmonary vascular resistance is higher and pulmonary hypertensive crises are more frequent and severe. Thus in our institution we prefer repair in the neonatal period, before 3 months of age, a time when it is more difficult to find and place an extracardiac conduit. After 5 months of age we prefer correction with extracardiac conduits.

The type, size, position, and manufacture of monocuspid valves are important factors. In the presence of "ideal" factors, pulmonary regurgitation is almost nonexistent. Recently we have been using a commercially available bovine pericardial monocusp with a large internal diameter ranging from 8 to 12 mm. This monocusp valve must be positioned as high as possible in the right ventricular outflow tract so that during closure its free margin is placed against the posterior spur corresponding to the ventricle–pulmonary artery anastomosis.

Other risk factors—*truncal valve regurgitation, interrupted aortic arch, coronary artery anomalies,* and *hemitruncus*—were previously discussed.

ACKNOWLEDGMENT

We thank the Heart Institute Scientific Department, Dr. Jane Oba, Dr. Estela Azeka, Dr. Vera D. Aiello, and Miss Daniela for their contribution to this chapter.

REFERENCES

1. Keith JD, Rowe RD, Vlad P: *Heart Disease in Infancy and Childhood,* ed 3. New York, Macmillan, 1978.
2. Butto F, Lucas RV, Edwards JE: Persistent truncus arteriosus: Pathologic anatomy in 54 cases. *Pediatr Cardiol* 7:95–101, 1986.
3. Armer RM, De Oliveira PF, Lurie PR: True truncus arteriosus: Review of 17 cases and report of surgery in 7 patients. *Circulation* 24:878A, 1961.
4. Heilbrunn A, Kittle CF, Diehl AM: Pulmonary arterial banding in the treatment of truncus arteriosus. *Circulation* 29:102, 1964.
5. Smith GW, Thompson WM, Damman JF, et al: Use of the pulmonary artery banding procedure in treating type II truncus arteriosus. *Circulation* 29:108S, 1964.
6. Behrendt DM, Kirsch MM, Stern A, et al: The surgical therapy for pulmonary artery–right ventricular discontinuity. *Ann Thorac Surg* 18:122, 1974.
7. Ebert PA, Turley K, Stanger P, et al: Surgical treatment of truncus arteriosus in the first six months of life. *Ann Surg* 200:451–456, 1984.
8. Wilson J: A description of a very unusual malformation of the human heart. *Philos Trans R Soc Lond Biol* 18:346, 1798.
9. Buchanan A: Malformation of the heart: Undivided truncus arteriosus. Heart otherwise double. *Trans Pathol Soc Lond* 15:89, 1864.
10. Lev M, Saphir O: Truncus arteriosus communis persistens. *J Pediatr* 20:74, 1943.
11. Collet RW, Edwards JE: Persistent truncus arteriosus: A classification according to anatomic types. *Surg Clin North Am* 29:1245–1270, 1949.

12. Arai T, Tsuzuki Y, Nazi M, et al: Experimental study on bypass between the right and left ventricle and aorta by means of homograft with valve. *Bull Heart Inst Jpn* 9:49, 1965.
13. Rastelli GC, Titus JL, McGoon DC: Homograft of ascending aorta and aortic valve as a right ventricular outflow. *Arch Surg* 95:698–708, 1967.
14. McGoon DC, Rastelli GC, Ongley PA: An operation for the correction of truncus arteriosus. *JAMA* 205:59–73, 1968.
15. Moore CH, Martelli V, Ross DN: Reconstruction of right ventricular outflow tract with a valved conduit in 75 cases of congenital heart disease. *J Thorac Cardiovasc Surg* 71:11, 1976.
16. Bowman FOG, Hancock WD, Malm JR: A valve-containing Dacron prosthesis: Its use in restoring pulmonary artery–right ventricular continuity. *Arch Surg* 107:724–728, 1973.
17. Ross DN, Sommerville J: Correction of pulmonary atresia with a homograft aortic valve. *Lancet* 2:1446–1447, 1966.
18. Barbero-Marcial M, Baucia JA, Jatene A: Valved conduits of bovine pericardium for right ventricle to pulmonary artery connections. *Semin Thorac Cardiovasc Surg* 7:148–153, 1995.
19. Barbero-Marcial M, Riso A, Atik E, et al: A technique for correction of truncus arteriosus types I and II without extracardiac conduits. *J Thorac Cardiovasc Surg* 99:364–369, 1990.
20. Van Praagh R, Van Praagh S: The anatomy of common aorticopulmonary trunk (truncus arteriosus communis) and its embryonic implications: A study of 57 necropsy cases. *Am J Cardiol* 16:406–425, 1965.
21. Thiene G, Bortolotti U, Galluci V, et al: Anatomical study of truncus arteriosus communis with embryological and surgical considerations. *Br Heart J* 38:1109–1123, 1976.
22. Crupi G, Macartney FJ, Anderson RH: Persistent truncus arteriosus: A study of 66 autopsy cases with special reference to definition and morphogenesis. *Am J Cardiol* 40:569–578, 1977.
23. Bharati S, McAllister H , Rosenquist GC, et al: The surgical anatomy of truncus arteriosus communis. *J Thorac Cardiovasc Surg* 67:501–510, 1974.
24. Davies MJ, Anderson RH, Becker AE: *Blood Supply of the Conduction System of the Heart.* London, Butterworths, 1983, pp 74–80.
25. Suzuki A, Ho YS, Anderson RH, et al: Coronary arterial and sinusal anatomy in hearts with a common arterial trunk. *Ann Thorac Surg* 48:792–797, 1989.
26. De la Cruz M, Cayre R, Angelini P, et al: Coronary arteries in truncus arteriosus. *Am J Cardiol* 66:1482–1486, 1990.
27. Lenox CC, Debich DE, Zuberbuhler JR: The role of coronary artery abnormalities in the prognosis of truncus arteriosus. *J Thorac Cardiovasc Surg* 104:1728–1742, 1992.

28. Anderson KR, McGoon DC, Lie JT: Surgical significance of the coronary arterial anatomy in truncus arteriosus communis. *Am J Cardiol* 41:76–81, 1978.
29. Daskapoulous DA, Edwards WD, Driscoll DJ, et al: Coronary artery compression with fatal myocardial ischemia: A rare complication of valved extracardiac conduit in children with congenital heart disease. *J Thorac Cardiovasc Surg* 85:546–551, 1983.
30. Daskapoulous DA, Edwards WD, Driscoll DJ, et al: Fatal pulmonary artery banding in truncus arteriosus with anomalous origin of circumflex coronary artery from right pulmonary artery. *Am J Cardiol* 52:1363–1367, 1983.
31. Kirklin JW, Barratt-Boyes BG: *Cardiac Surgery. Morphology, Diagnostic Criteria, Natural History, Techniques, Results, and Indications,* ed 2. New York, Churchill Livingstone, 1993, pp 1131–1151.
32. Calder L, Van Praagh R, Van Praagh S, et al: Truncus arteriosus communis: Clinical, angiocardiographic, and pathologic findings in 100 patients. *Am Heart J* 92:23–38, 1976.
33. Gelband H, Van Meter S, Gersony WM: Truncal Valve abnormalities in infants with persistent truncus arteriosus: A clinicopathologic study. *Circulation* 40:397–403, 1972.
34. Motta C: Tronco arterioso comum permanente com endocardite chronica fetal. *Ann Fac Med São Paulo* 7:125, 1932.
35. Becker AE, Becker MJ, Edwards JE: Pathology of the semilunar valve in persistent truncus arteriosus. *J Thorac Cardiovasc Surg* 62:16–26, 1971.
36. Mair DD, Ritter DG, Davis GD, et al: Selection of patients with truncus arteriosus for surgical correction: Anatomic and hemodynamic considerations. *Circulation* 59:144–151, 1974.
37. Marcelletti C, McGoon DC, Mair DD: The natural history of truncus arteriosus. *Circulation* 54:108–111, 1976.
38. Juaneda E, Haworth SG: Pulmonary vascular disease in children with truncus arteriosus. *Am J Cardiol* 54:1314–1320, 1984.
39. Keck EW: Pulmonary hypertension and pulmonary vascular disease in congenital heart defects. *Z Kardiol* 78:65S–73S, 1989.
40. Azeka E, Auler JOC, Kajita L, et al: The use of nitric oxide and its complications on the evaluation of pulmonary arterial hypertension in children. *Intensive Care Med* 23:19S, 1997.
41. Rabinovitch M, Haworth SG, Castaneda AR, et al: Lung biopsy in congenital heart disease: A morphometric approach to pulmonary vascular disease. *Circulation* 58:1107–1122, 1978.
42. Heath D, Edwards JE: The pathology of hypertensive pulmonary vascular disease. *Circulation* 18:533–544, 1958.
43. Wagenvoort CA, Wagenwoort N, Draulans-Noe Y: Reversibility of plexogenic pulmonary arteriopathy following banding of the pulmonary artery. *J Thorac Cardiovasc Surg* 87:876–886, 1984.

44. Sawa Y, Matsuda H, Shimazaki Y, et al: Ultrastructural assessment of the infant myocardium receiving crystalloid cardioplegia. *Circulation* 76:141S–145S, 1987.
45. Wong RS, Baum VC, Sangwan S: Truncus arteriosus: Recognition and therapy of intraoperative cardiac ischemia. *Anesthesiology* 74:378–380, 1991.
46. Kirklin JW, Blackstone EH, Maehara T, et al: Intermediate-term fate of cryopreserved allograft and xenograft valve conduits. *Ann Thorac Surg* 44:598–606, 1987.
47. Cleveland DC, Williams WG, Razzouk A, et al: Failure of cryopreserved homograft valved conduits in the pulmonary circulation. *Circulation* 86:150S–153S, 1992.
48. Lacour-Gayet F, Serraf A, Komiya T, et al: Truncus arteriosus repair: Influence of techniques of right ventricular outflow tract reconstruction. *J Thorac Cardiovasc Surg* 111:849–856, 1996.
49. Razzouk AJ, Williams WG, Cleveland DC, et al: Surgical connections from ventricle to pulmonary artery: Comparison of four types of valved implants. *Circulation* 86:154S–158S, 1992.
50. Heinemann MK, Hanley FL, Fenton KN, et al: Fate of small homograft conduits after early repair of truncus arteriosus. *Ann Thorac Surg* 55:1409–1412, 1993.
51. DiDonato RM, Fyfe DA, Puga FJ, et al: Fifteen-year experience with surgical repair of truncus arteriosus. *J Thorac Cardiovasc Surg* 89:414–422, 1985.
52. Mair DD, Ritter DG, Danielson GK, et al: Truncus arteriosus with unilateral absence of a pulmonary artery: Criteria for operability and surgical results. *Circulation* 55:641–647, 1977.
53. Nakae S, Kasahara S, Kuroyama N, et al: Correction of truncus arteriosus with autologous arterial flap in neonates and small infants. *Ann Thorac Surg* 62:123–129, 1996.
54. Oliveira JB, Souza LCB, Arnoni AS, et al: Conduto valvulado: Nova técnica. *Arq Bras Cardiol* 46:401–406, 1986.

CHAPTER 4

Neurologic Injury During Coronary Revascularization: Etiology and Management*

John M. Murkin, M.D., F.R.C.P.C.
Professor of Anesthesia; Director, Cardiac Anesthesia, University Campus, London Health Sciences Center, University of Western Ontario, London, Ontario, Canada

In a recent prospective clinical trial evaluating 2,108 patients undergoing coronary artery bypass (CAB) surgery at 24 U.S. institutions, adverse cerebral outcomes consisting of focal injury, stupor, or coma; or seizures, memory deficit, or deterioration in intellectual function occurred overall in 6.1% of patients. Age, proximal aortic atherosclerosis, and history of neurologic disease were all strongly correlated with these adverse neurologic outcomes.[1] The relative importance of neurologic morbidity associated with CAB surgery and the risk of perioperative death have increased over the past two decades. Data from the Cleveland Clinic have shown that in the early 1970s, fewer than 10% of patient deaths after cardiac surgery were due to primary neurologic injury. However, in their series a decade later, over 20% of the deaths after coronary bypass were due to primary neurologic injury—stroke.[2] When one considers the type of patients now undergoing coronary revascularization, it is apparent that they have also changed fundamentally over the last decade.

Data from Emory University cardiac center comparing their experience with over 1,500 CAB patients in 1981 vs. 1987 demonstrated an increase in the number of patients over age 70—from less than 10% to over 20%.[3] Similarly, the number of patients with con-

*Adapted with permission from CD-ROM interactive, J.M. Murkin, *The Brain at Risk: Neurological Complications after Cardiopulmonary Bypass.* London, Ontario, E-Media Medical Educationals, 1997.

comitant diabetes increased from less than 1 in 6 to over 1 in 4. The incidence of poor ventricular function, defined as an ejection fraction less than 0.4, had also risen—from less than 25% to over 33% of patients. One result of these changes was that the perioperative stroke rate went from less than 1.5% to 2.8%. This is consistent with other data in the literature. In our own recently published series assessing postoperative neurobehavioral sequelae in over 300 CAB patients, the stroke rate was 2.5%, 33% of all CAB patients demonstrated cognitive dysfunction, and a further 18% demonstrated abnormal neurologic signs 2 months postoperatively.[4] In a preliminary 3-year follow-up report of 97 of these same patients, 22% had cognitive impairment and a further 18% again demonstrated abnormal neurologic signs.[5] It is apparent that we are now operating on older and sicker patients and that the resultant neurologic morbidity associated with cardiac surgery in this population, of which clinical stroke is only the most obvious form of neurologic injury, has increased dramatically over the last decade.

Tuman and colleagues in Chicago undertook a prospective survey of over 2,000 patients undergoing coronary bypass surgery and found that there was a direct correlation between patient age and associated neurologic morbidity.[6] They demonstrated that in patients less than 65 years of age the risk of stroke after CAB surgery is less than 1%. However, in patients over 65 years of age, the stroke rate rises to approximately 5%, and for patients over 75 years of age, 1 patient in 11 will have a perioperative stroke.[6] This stroke rate may seem high and may be influenced by the relatively small number of patients in the over-75 age group, but it is strikingly consistent with the data reported by Gardner et al. over a decade ago.[7] In that retrospective study of 3,279 patients who underwent CAB surgery from 1974 through 1983, the overall stroke rate was 1.7%, and they showed a very significant age-associated risk of stroke that rose from an incidence of 1.3% in patients between 51 and 60 to 3% in patients in their 60s and to 6.2% in patients over age 70. For those patients older than 75 years, the stroke rate was 7.1%. Both of these studies thus demonstrate a consistent and very strong correlation between risk of stroke after CAB surgery and age of the patient.

One interesting aspect of the Tuman data is that the postoperative myocardial infarction rate and low–cardiac output state were not age associated, so these patients often do very well postoperatively from a cardiovascular standpoint. Despite their primary cardiac disease, patients will not necessarily have an increased age-associated risk of poor ventricular function or myocardial infarction postoperatively. As shown in Figure 1, however, the risk of

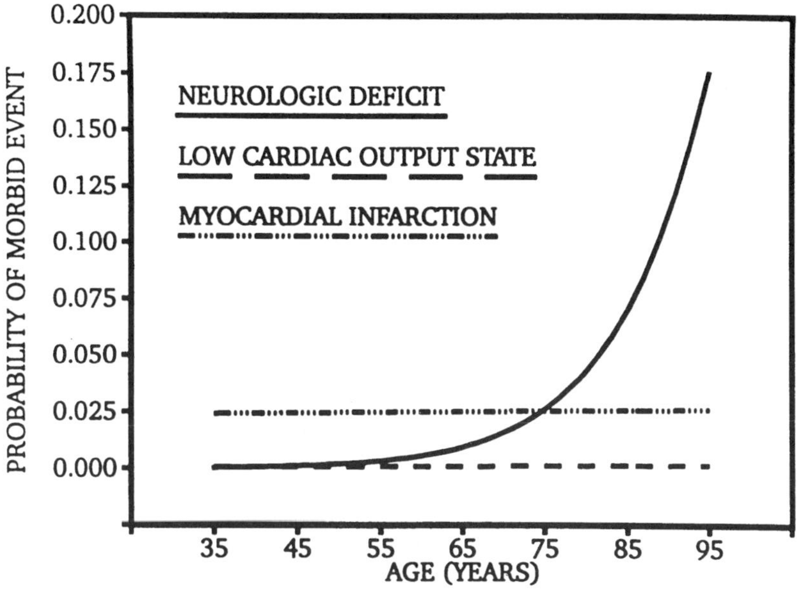

FIGURE 1.

For both myocardial infarction and low cardiac output, there is not an appreciable effect of age on probability of an adverse event. For neurologic deficit, however, there is an exponential increase in the risk of morbidity associated with increasing age. (Courtesy of Tuman KJ, McCarthy RJ, Najafi H, et al: Differential effects of advanced age on neurologic and cardiac risks of coronary artery operations. *J Thorac Cardiovasc Surg* 104:1510–1517, 1992.)

stroke is very directly related to age and rises exponentially in patients over age 65.[6] Data from our own center as of 1995 indicate that there has been a greater than 50% increase in the number of patients undergoing cardiac surgery who are over the age of 70 years. In the years from 1991 to 1995, analysis of the ages of patients undergoing CAB surgery indicate that the percentage of patients over 70 years increased from 20% to more than 30%, as shown in Figure 2. It is apparent that similar changes in patient demographics have been seen in all North American cardiac centers.

CEREBRAL ATHEROEMBOLI

In addition to age, other risk factors are associated with coronary bypass procedures. Data from Blauth and colleagues from a study of 200 patients who died after cardiac or vascular surgery indicate that there was a strong correlation between age of the patient, pres-

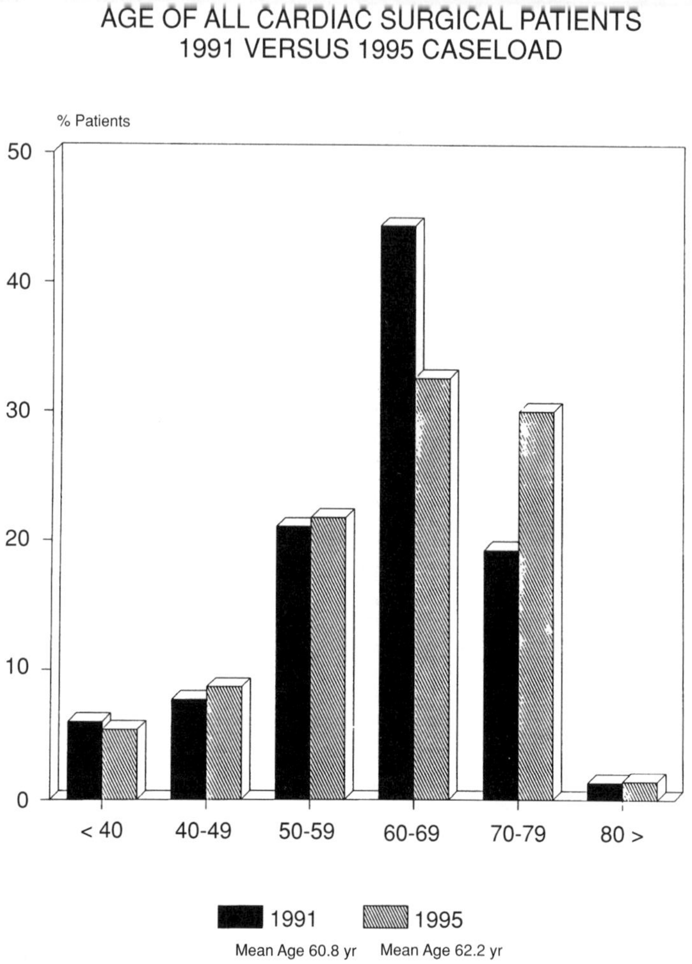

FIGURE 2.
Comparative percentages of patients having coronary bypass surgery by age in years at a single cardiac referral center in 1991 and 1995.

ence of peripheral vascular disease or concomitant diabetes, and atheroemboli.[8] Patients with these risk factors were significantly more likely to have evidence of atheroembolism in the brain and other organs on postmortem examination. They found that patients who had no evidence of peripheral vascular disease had a slight, but significant age-related increase in the incidence of atheroemboli in the brain, kidneys, heart, and other organs. However, as shown in Figure 3, in patients with peripheral vascular disease the association between age and atheroemboli was very strong.

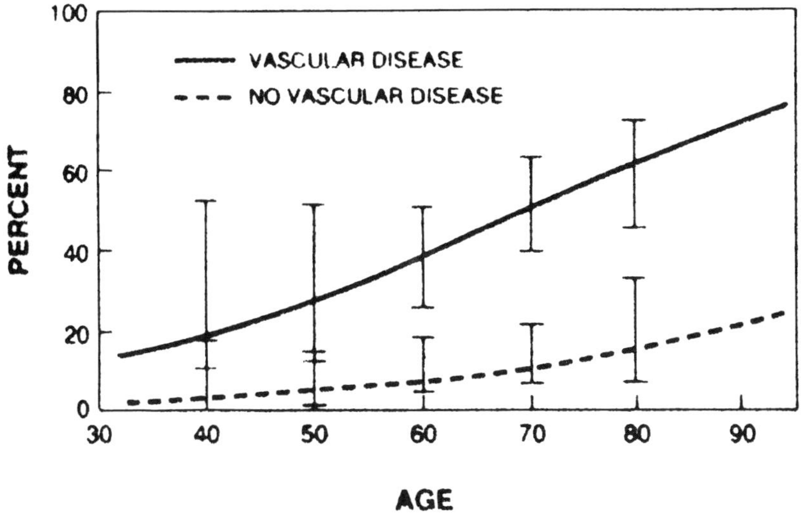

FIGURE 3.
Probability of atheroembolism relative to age with and without severe atherosclerosis of the ascending aorta. (Courtesy of Blauth CI, Cosgrove DM, Webb BW, et al: Atheroembolism from the ascending aorta. *J Thorac Cardiovasc Surg* 103:1104–1112, 1992.)

Patients with atheroemboli also had the highest incidence of ascending aortic atherosclerosis. Atheroemboli were detected in 46 of 123 patients with severe disease of the ascending aorta (37.4%), but in only 2 of 98 patients (2%) without significant ascending aortic disease. Forty-six of 48 patients (95.8%) who had evidence of atheroemboli had severe atherosclerosis of the ascending aorta. They also observed a direct correlation between age, severe atherosclerosis of the ascending aorta, and atheroemboli.[8] In a separate report of 120 consecutive necropsy studies in general hospital patients ranging in age from 29 to 94 years, arterial thromboemboli were observed in 33%.[9] Embolism was again significantly correlated with evidence of atherosclerotic disease of the ascending aorta and aortic arch.

Using intraoperative epiaortic B-mode ultrasound imaging of the ascending aorta, Davila-Roman and colleagues demonstrated an exponential increase in the incidence of ascending aortic atherosclerosis in CAB patients (Fig 4)—data that are virtually superimposable on the postoperative stroke data reported by Tuman and colleagues (see Fig 1).[10] It is therefore becoming apparent that in the context of cardiac surgery, stroke risk is most strongly correlated with ascending aortic atherosclerosis because of the risk of

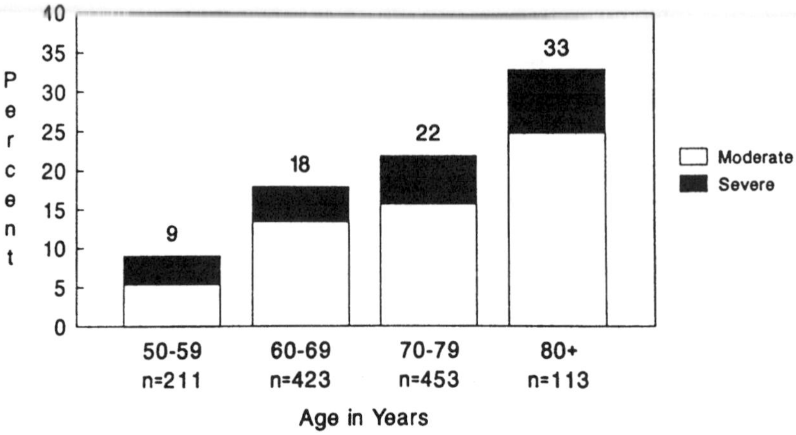

FIGURE 4.
Relationship between age and atherosclerosis of the ascending aorta detected by ultrasonic imaging. (Data modified from Davila-Roman VG, Barzilai B, Wareing TH, et al: Intraoperative ultrasonographic evaluation of the ascending aorta in 100 consecutive patients undergoing cardiac surgery. *Circulation* 84:47S–53S. Copyright 1991, American Heart Association.)

plaque disruption and cerebral embolization as a result of aortic instrumentation. Advancing age, peripheral vascular disease, and diabetes mellitus act as surrogate markers for the presence of significant aortic atherosclerotic disease and should alert the clinician to the increased stroke risk in such patients.

Not only does stroke occur in the context of aortic instrumentation for cardiac surgery, but stroke has also been reported to be associated with the presence of mobile atheroma during coronary angiography.[11] Additionally, it is also clear that cerebral microemboli occurring as a consequence of perfusion through a proximal aortic cannula with resultant scouring of the atherosclerotic lumen are also significantly increased in the presence of ascending aortic atheromatous disease.[12]

In an intraoperative study of 18 patients, blood velocity within the aortic arch was assessed by epiaortic scanning to determine peak forward flow velocity in the presence of either a short (1.5 cm) cannula or a long (7.0 cm) aortic perfusion cannula.[13] Use of the long cannula resulted in a significant decrease in forward flow velocity and turbulence in the aortic arch when compared with the short cannula. In a report comparing closed-tip and various-length end-hole cannulas, significantly lower exit force and a lower-velocity, more diffuse flow pattern was seen with the closed-tip cannulas.[14, 15] In a series of 19 patients with severe calcific ascending aortic and arch disease, use of a rounded cannula tip mounted on a retractable-blade introducer was associated with no operative mortality or postoperative neurologic deficits.[16] Currently, no prospective outcome studies have evaluated the clinical efficacy of changes in cannula design.

That ascending aortic atherosclerosis is a significant risk for stroke during CAB surgery is not surprising inasmuch as several clinical series have demonstrated a strong correlation between stroke risk and ascending aortic disease in contexts other than CAB surgery. In a series of 334 nonsurgical patients admitted with stroke, transesophageal echocardiography (TEE) was used to assess aortic atheromatous disease and stroke risk.[17] Over the course of a 2- to 4-year follow-up period, the risk of further vascular events was highest among patients with noncalcified plaque of 4 mm or more, a relative risk index of 10.3. This implies that absence of aortic calcification on chest radiographs or on direct intraoperative palpation does not lower the likelihood of significant risk of atheroemboli and stroke during cannulation and clamping of the aorta. Noncalcific "cheesy" atheroma is difficult to detect by palpation but more likely to embolize during manipulation—the usual clinical assessment by palpation will not detect noncalcific aortic plaque.

In a further study of 1,200 cardiac patients, epiaortic scanning was used to assess the correlation between the presence or absence of atherosclerotic aortic disease of the ascending aorta and arch and previous neurologic events.[18] Atherosclerotic aortic disease was significantly and independently associated with the occurrence of previous neurologic events and was second only to hypertension as a risk factor, showing an even greater correlation with stroke than with atrial fibrillation. It is clear, then, that the greatest single risk factor for stroke in cardiac surgical patients is atheromatous disease of the ascending aorta and aortic arch.

DIRECT AORTIC PALPATION AND ASSESSMENT OF ATHEROSCLEROTIC DISEASE

In most cardiac centers, intraoperative palpation of the aorta is still the standard of care for detection of aortic atheroma and selection of cannulation and aortic clamp sites. In a clinical study of 100 consecutive patients undergoing CAB surgery, Davila-Roman and colleagues compared intraoperative palpation of the aorta with direct epiaortic ultrasonic scanning for the detection of significant atherosclerotic disease.[19] Thirty-eight percent of the ultrasound studies were normal, mild atherosclerosis was shown in 33%, moderate atherosclerosis was present in 19%, and severe atherosclerosis was noted in 10% of the patients. Seventy percent of the patients with severe disease (7/10) were not detected by palpation. The operative procedure was altered to reduce the risk of embolization in 17% of these patients overall. Two strokes were reported in this series, both in patients with minimal atherosclerotic disease and apparently occurring in the postoperative period after episodes of protracted hypotension.

Ribakove and associates compared TEE in 97 patients greater than 65 years of age with intraoperative aortic palpation for assessment and grading of atherosclerotic change within the ascending aorta.[20] Seventy-six patients were thought to have normal aortas by palpation, yet 16 of these demonstrated severe disease on TEE. Overall, severe atheromatous disease was detected by TEE in 35 patients, whereas another 33 demonstrated extensive intimal thickening. Of 20 patients showing severe disease on TEE, 80% (16/20) were judged to have normal aortas by palpation. The stroke rate was 4.1%, all in patients judged to have normal aortas by palpation and who underwent surgery with standard operative approaches, yet 3 of these 4 patients had unappreciated mobile atheroma within the aortic lumen.

In a further study of 130 patients undergoing cardiac surgery, the same group reported that 23 of 130 patients undergoing cardiac surgery had protruding ascending aortic atheromas, 12 of which had a mobile component.[21] As outlined schematically in Figure 5, of the 12 patients with mobile atheroma, modification of intraoperative technique was undertaken in 5 patients, all of whom recovered uneventfully and had no neurologic sequelae. The remaining 7 patients were treated with standard intraoperative techniques and 3 (43%) awoke from anesthesia with a stroke. Wareing and colleagues similarly reported that in a series of 500 patients in whom intraoperative epiaortic scanning was used, significant disease was detected ultrasonographically in 68, but in only 38% (26 patients) did palpation identify atheromatous disease, and even then manual palpation still underestimated the severity of disease in those patients.[22]

In a recent series of ten patients undergoing CAB surgery, St Amand and colleagues reported that epiaortic scanning resulted in a change in cannulation site in two patients, one after detection of unrecognized atheroma and the other after ultrasonic identification

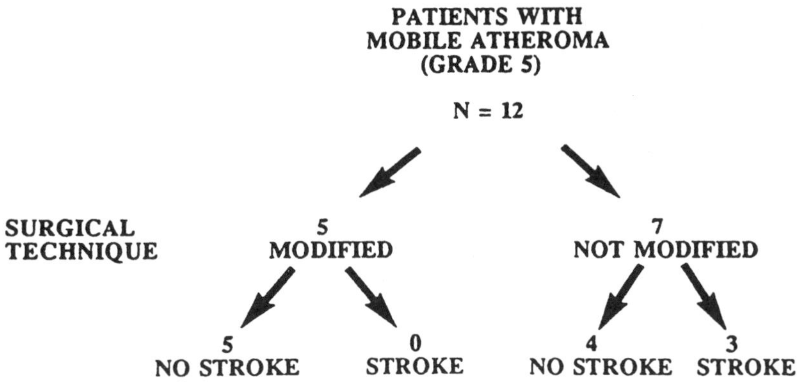

FIGURE 5.

Influence on neurologic outcome of altering operative technique on the basis of the finding of mobile atheromas on transesophageal echocardiography. (Reprinted with permission from the American College of Cardiology, from Katz ES, Tunick PA, Rusinek H, et al: Protruding aortic atheromas predict stroke in elderly patients undergoing cardiopulmonary bypass: Experience with intraoperative transesophageal echocardiography. *J Am Coll Cardiol* 20:70–77, 1992.)

of a section of disease-free aorta in a patient in whom diffuse aortic atherosclerosis had been determined by palpation.[23] None of these patients experienced a postoperative stroke. Similarly, Nicolosi and colleagues compared the sensitivity of intraoperative epiaortic scanning and manual palpation of the aorta for detection of atherosclerotic disease in 89 cardiac surgical patients.[24] Operative techniques were modified to avoid plaque detected on scanning in 11.2% of the patients. The sensitivity of palpation in comparison to scanning was 0.46. There were two strokes in this group, one in a patient with minimal aortic atherosclerotic disease and the other in a patient with extensive aortic calcification.

INTRAOPERATIVE ASSESSMENT OF AORTIC ATHEROSCLEROSIS: TRANSESOPHAGEAL ECHOCARDIOGRAPHY VS. EPIAORTIC SCANNING

Because of repeated demonstration of the failure of aortic palpation to detect the presence of significant atheromatous changes within the ascending aorta, ultrasonic assessment of the ascending aorta before cannulation and cross-clamping is increasingly being used to noninvasively determine the degree of atherosclerosis and thus the risk of cerebral atheroemboli from within the ascending aorta.[25] As shown in Figure 6, a typical epiaortic scan of a high-

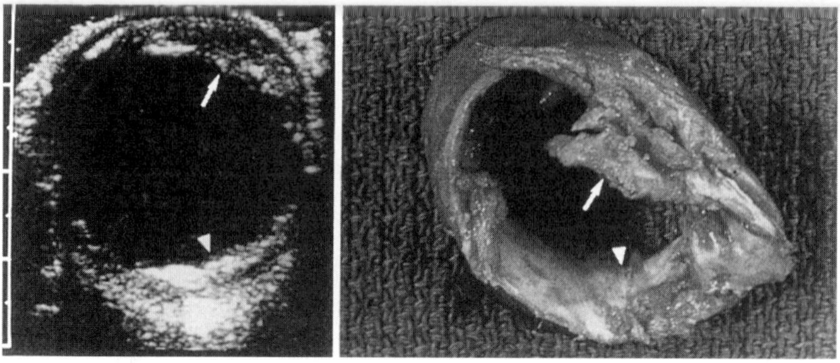

FIGURE 6.
Transverse ultrasonic image of the ascending aorta and the corresponding segment of aorta in a patient with severe atherosclerosis. Note the calcification *(triangle)* and the projection of atheroma *(arrow)* into the lumen. (Courtesy of Wareing TH, Davila-Roman VG, Barzilai B, et al: Management of the severely atherosclerotic ascending aorta during cardiac operations. *J Thorac Cardiovasc Surg* 103:453–462, 1992.)

risk patient demonstrates large ulcerated plaque protruding into the aortic lumen within the ascending aorta. This segment of ascending aorta was replaced electively, and the pathology specimen shows the anatomical correlates of what was seen with an intraoperative epiaortic ultrasonic scan.[22]

In most centers, aortic cannulation is preceded by manual palpation of the aorta, during which the aorta is assessed manually to determine suitable sites for cannulation and placement of aortic clamps. This is currently the standard of care in many cardiac centers in North America and Europe. It is well documented that between 30% and 70% of significant atherosclerotic plaque is not identified with this approach, however.[19–24] As indicated earlier, there is now increasing interest in the use of intraoperative B-mode ultrasonic imaging to assess the aorta for optimal sites for cannulation and clamping. Figure 7 shows a patient with protruding anterior atherosclerotic plaque that was present at the proposed cannulation site. Having identified this abnormality intraoperatively before aortic instrumentation, the cannulation site was changed and the patient recovered uneventfully without overt neurologic sequelae.

B-mode Doppler ultrasound imaging is being evaluated in several centers to assess the extent of aortic atherosclerotic plaque as a guide to selection of the optimal cannulation site. Marschall and colleagues used TEE to evaluate and grade the extent of aortic ath-

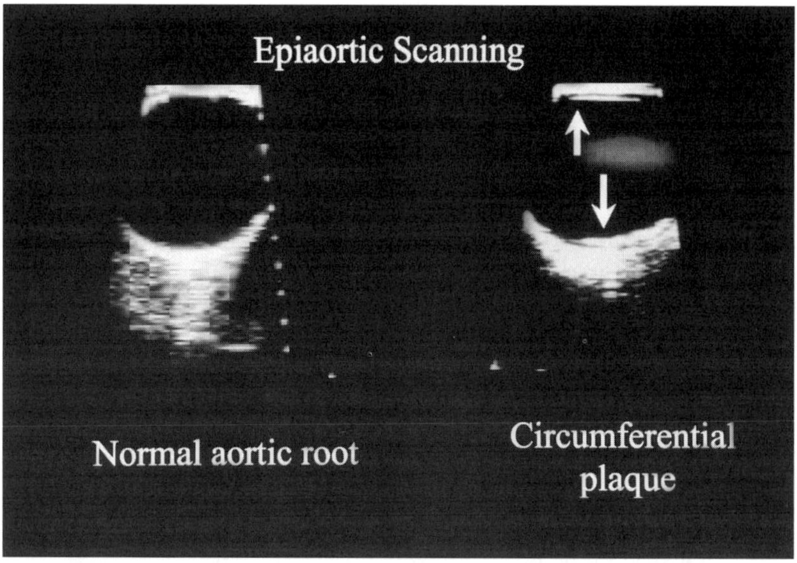

FIGURE 7.

Two scanning images of the midsegment of the ascending aorta in different patients. The patient on the *left* has a normal aortic root with no atherosclerosis, whereas the patient on the *right* has evidence of circumferential atherosclerotic plaque in both the anterior and posterior aspects of the aorta as indicated by the two *arrows*. The area in the middle of the lumen on the right is a reflected light artifact.

erosclerosis.[25] They demonstrated a strong correlation between increasing age and severity of aortic disease—a 20% incidence of severe disease in patients over age 70—and a corresponding association between perioperative stroke and severe aortic arch disease.

Concern has been raised about the ability of TEE to adequately assess the ascending aorta in the region of greatest interest for cannulation and clamping, however. In the mid and upper thirds of the ascending aorta the relationship between the distal ascending aorta and the esophagus is altered by interposition of the right main-stem bronchus and trachea and overlying lung tissue, which renders the aorta impervious to TEE examination via the esophagus in this critical region.

In a recent comparison of TEE vs. epiaortic scanning conducted in 100 patients undergoing cardiac surgery, Sylviris et al. demonstrated that manual palpation and TEE were equally unreliable for detection of severe atheroma of the mid and distal ascending aorta in comparison to epiaortic scanning.[26] Overall, 90% of the patients had atheroma detected by ultrasound techniques whereas only 16% were detected by manual palpation. In the proximal third of the aorta, there was no significant difference between TEE and epiaortic scanning, whereas palpation significantly underestimated atheroma grade in this region in 69 of 100 cases. In the mid and distal segments of the ascending aorta, however, both manual palpation and TEE significantly underestimated atheroma grade in 53 and 51 of 100 cases, respectively. These investigators concluded that TEE is an insensitive technique for such evaluations and is of little value in guiding surgical manipulations such as aortic cannulation and cross-clamping.[26] Very similar results showing a very low sensitivity of TEE (29% detection rate) vs. epiaortic scanning were reported by Konstadt et al.[27] In a study of 27 patients in whom TEE was used for assessment of aortic disease, concomitant epiaortic scanning was undertaken in 14 patients. Of the patients who underwent both TEE and epiaortic scanning, severe atherosclerotic plaque (more than 3 mm thick) was not seen on TEE in 5 patients but was detected in all 5 by epiaortic scanning.

Davila-Roman and colleagues also compared intraoperative epiaortic scanning, TEE, and manual palpation for assessment of aortic disease in 44 cardiac surgical patients.[28] They similarly showed that epiaortic scanning was far more accurate than TEE for identification of atherosclerosis of the ascending aorta, particularly in the distal ascending segment, and that when compared with both epiaortic scanning and biplane TEE, palpation significantly underestimated the presence and severity of aortic atherosclerosis.

TECHNICAL MODIFICATIONS IN THE PRESENCE OF AORTIC ATHEROSCLEROSIS

With the possibility of enhancing the detection of significant aortic atheromatous disease by using epiaortic ultrasound scanning, a variety of alternative surgical approaches have been developed to avoid the risks of instrumentation of a severely diseased aorta. In a series of 13 patients with extensive calcification of the ascending aorta operated on before the ready availability of intraoperative ultrasonic scanning, Culliford and colleagues used selective cannulation of either the femoral artery or the ascending aorta or transverse aortic arch with a long cannula that had its tip distal to the left subclavian artery, profound core cooling and circulatory arrest, and atherectomy of the ascending aorta.[29] With the exception of 1 patient in whom occipital lobe infarcts occurred and in whom aortic calcification was discovered after application of the clamp, all other 12 patients recovered without neurologic complications. A similar approach using femoral or distal aortic arch cannulation, circulatory arrest, and aortic arch débridement was advocated by Ribakove and associates.[20]

In a series of 1,200 patients in whom intraoperative epiaortic scanning was used, moderate (3–5 mm thick) or severe (more than 5 mm thick or ulcerations, circumferential aortic involvement, or mobile atheroma) ascending aortic atherosclerotic disease was found in 231 (19.3%) patients.[30] In 27 patients with severe atherosclerotic disease, the ascending aorta was replaced, with no strokes occurring in this group. In 168 patients with less extensive disease, technical modifications included the use of femoral or distal aortic arch cannulation sites, no aortic clamping or more proximal placement of aortic clamps, delivery of cardioplegia retrogradely through the coronary sinus or hypothermic fibrillatory arrest, and more proximal placement of proximal anastomoses or the use of skip grafts without proximal aortic anastomoses. This same group published an algorithm for management of aortic atherosclerosis, as shown in Table 1, that is based on their initial experience with intraoperative epiaortic ultrasound scanning in a series of 500 patients.[22]

A further series of ten cardiac surgical patients with severely calcified aortas in whom radical aortic endarterectomy was successfully undertaken via hypothermic circulatory arrest without postoperative stroke has also been recently reported from Scandinavia.[31]

In a series of 792 patients undergoing CAB surgery, intraoperative TEE detected 114 patients in whom significant ascending aortic atherosclerotic disease was present.[32] Modification of surgical technique, including femoral artery cannulation and fibrillatory arrest, cannulation distal to the atheroma, or aortic débridement and atherectomy with retrograde cerebral perfusion, resulted in no perioperative strokes in this group. The overall stroke rate was 0.76%.

Whether or not extensive débridement or replacement of the ascending aorta is required in severe cases of aortic atheromatous disease, epiaortic ultrasonic scanning for selection of a disease-free cannulation site—in the distal aortic arch or the femoral or axillary arteries—and directing the aortic cannula tip distal to the origin of the great vessels of the head appear to be relatively easily attainable modifications of surgical technique that show promise

TABLE 1.
Algorithm for Management of Atherosclerotic Ascending Aorta Based on Ultrasonography

Normal Aorta or Mild Aortic Disease*	Moderate Aortic Disease†	Severe Aortic Disease‡
Standard operative procedure	Distal Third of Aorta Femoral artery cannulation Placement of aortic clamp more proximally or hypothermic fibrillation without aortic clamping Middle Third of Aorta Vein graft anastomosis to another site (usually more proximal aorta) Relocation of cardioplegic needle or retrograde cardioplegia	Femoral artery cannulation Hypothermic circulatory arrest Graft replacement of ascending aorta

*Intimal thickening, ≤3 mm.
†Focal areas of moderate or severe atherosclerosis, >3-mm intimal thickening.
‡Multiple areas of severe artherosclerosis or circumferential involvement.
(Adapted from Wareing TH, Davilla-Roman VG, Barzilai B, et al: Management of the severely atherosclerotic ascending aorta during cardiac operations. *J Thorac Cardiovasc Surg* 103:453–462, 1992.)

of decreasing strokes associated with aortic instrumentation. Conservatively, it can be estimated that such modifications could decrease the perioperative stroke rate by 50%. Whether the use of technical improvements such as three-dimensional imaging will further enhance intraoperative diagnostic efficacy and improve patient outcomes remains to be seen.[33]

As a study of therapeutic efficacy, 195 consecutive CAB surgery patients underwent intraoperative epiaortic scanning; the results obtained were compared with those of 164 consecutive patients operated on in the preceding 12-month period.[34] Significant aortic disease was detected in 2% (3) of the control group patients in whom fibrillatory arrest without clamping was used; there was a 3.6% mortality rate and 3.0% ($n = 5$) stroke rate in this group overall. In 195 patients in the epiaortic scanning group, normal or minimal disease was detected in 168 patients, moderate disease was detected in 20, and severe disease was found in 7. Modification of surgical technique involving hypothermic fibrillatory arrest with no cross-clamping and left ventricular venting was employed in 14 patients, modification of the aortic cannulation site or single cross-clamping in 3 patients, and modification in placement of the proximal anastomoses or the use of all arterial grafts in 2 patients resulted in an overall operative mortality rate of 2.6%, with no perioperative strokes occurring in the scanned group.[34]

MICROGASEOUS EMBOLI FROM CARDIOPULMONARY BYPASS EQUIPMENT

Not only are emboli from the ascending aorta a major risk factor, but it is also apparent that cerebral embolization is occurring diffusely throughout the duration of cardiopulmonary bypass (CPB). Blauth and colleagues used fluorescein retinal angiography during CPB and were able to demonstrate retinal microemboli occurring at various times during CPB in those patients in whom a bubble oxygenator was used; on the other hand, use of a membrane oxygenator was able to significantly decrease the number of retinal embolizations.[35]

The introduction of transcranial Doppler devices to measure flow velocity within the middle cerebral arteries, as shown in Figure 8, has not only allowed an assessment of the indices of cerebral blood flow (CBF) but can also be used to detect the presence of emboli within the middle cerebral artery. By insonation of the middle cerebral artery, audible changes in the characteristics of the reflected Doppler signal can indicate changes in the composition of the blood column being insonated. Excluding artifact, this is most commonly due to either microparticulate or microgaseous emboli occurring during bypass. Certain features of the change in Doppler signal allow one to reliably discriminate between an embolus and noise artifact. Characteristically, cerebral emboli result in a chirpy, high-pitched, relatively short-duration sound that is biphasic when the flow velocity profile is examined. Figure 9 shows representative examples of tracings from patients who had aortic valve replacement and demonstrates whited-out areas that represent saturation of the ultrasonic filter. Air has a high reflec-

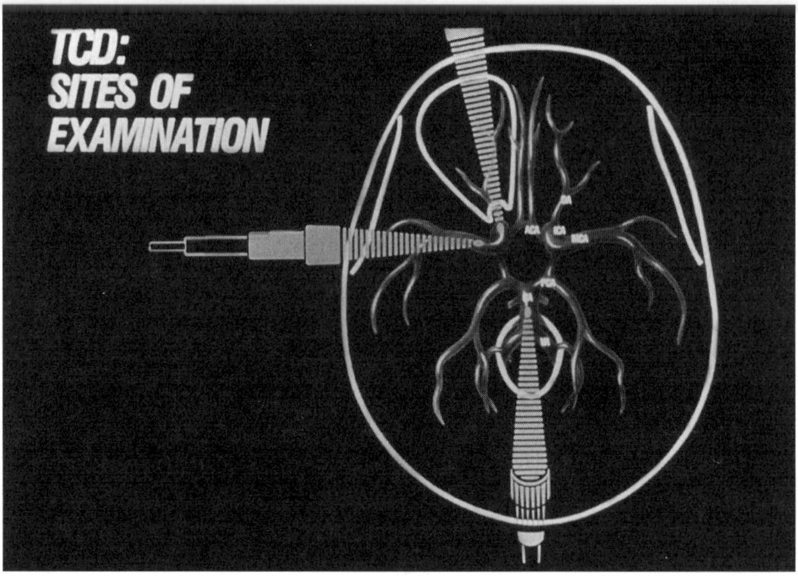

FIGURE 8.
Transcranial Doppler *(TCD)* insonation of the left middle cerebral artery via a left transcranial window.

tance coefficient such that the returning signals overdrive the system amplifier and Doppler signals are shut out at these times. The upper panel illustrates massive embolization, most likely air, occurring in this patient with release of the aortic cross-clamp after aortic valve replacement. The lower panel shows a similar patient after separation from CPB. Here, there is a very high-intensity signal buried within the velocity profile, indicative of an embolus that is probably particulate because of its high-intensity and lower-frequency signal.

Equipment can also have an impact on the generation and delivery of emboli into the cerebral circulation. Padayachee and colleagues were able to demonstrate with the use of an unfiltered bubble oxygenator that emboli were detected in the middle cerebral artery diffusely throughout CPB, as seen in Figure 10.[36] With the use of a membrane oxygenator, however, there are effectively no emboli detected within the middle cerebral artery, consistent with the retinal microembolization data from Blauth et al.[35] Selection of a membrane oxygenator over a bubble oxygenator and use of an arterial line filter can thus substantially reduce the delivery of microemboli into the cerebral circulation.

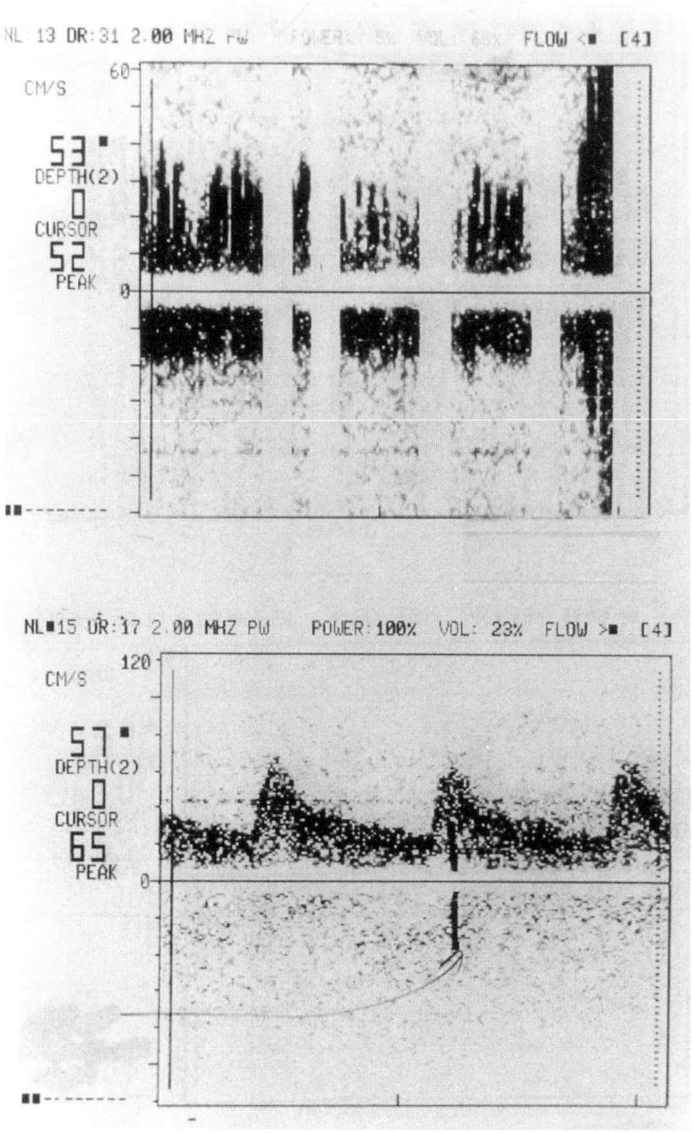

FIGURE 9.

Transcranial Doppler images of two patients. The *upper* display indicates massive air embolism occurring with release of the aortic cross-clamp as indicated by the *whited-out areas* on the graph. The *lower* image represents another patient after separation from cardiopulmonary bypass with an embolus detected within the flow envelope during systole. Increased density of this embolic signal suggests that it may be particulate in nature.

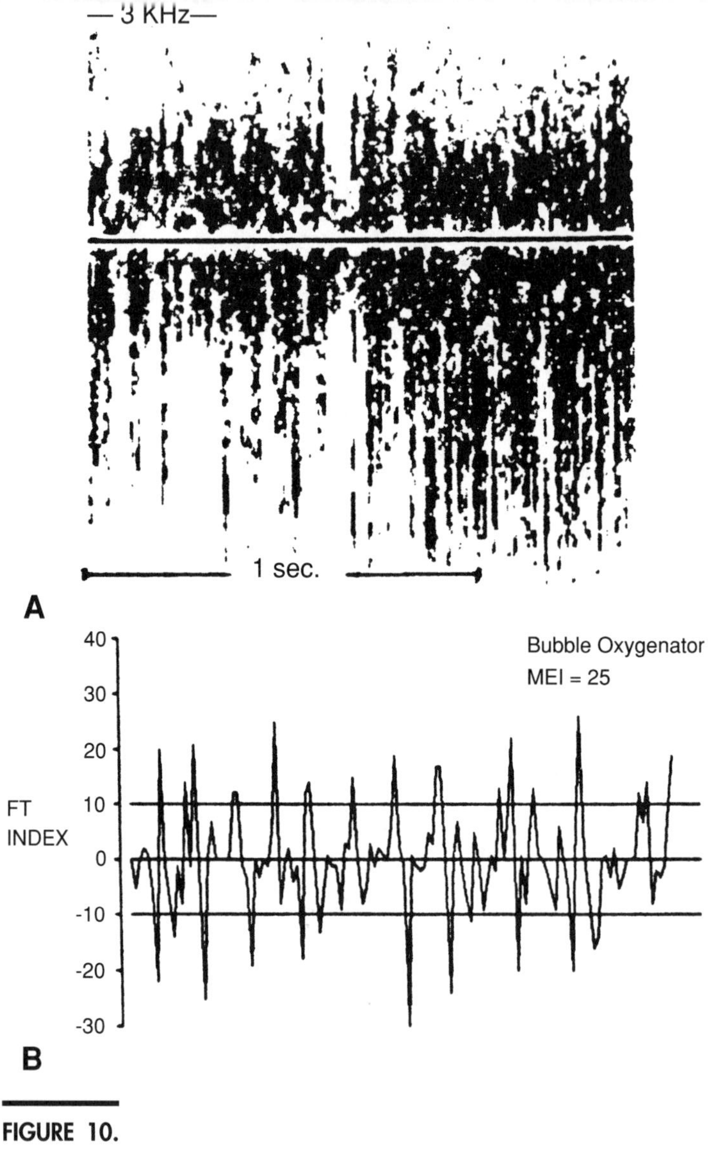

FIGURE 10.
Sonograms **(A)** and computed ultrasound microemboli index *(MEI)* **(B)** from a patient on cardiopulmonary bypass with a bubble oxygenator. The FT index spikes represent embolic events detected within the middle cerebral artery. (Reprinted with permission from the Society of Thoracic Surgeons, courtesy of Padayachee TS, Parsons S, Theobold R, et al: The detection of microemboli in the middle cerebral artery during cardiopulmonary bypass: A transcranial Doppler ultrasound investigation using membrane and bubble oxygenators. *Ann Thorac Surg* 44:298–302, 1987.)

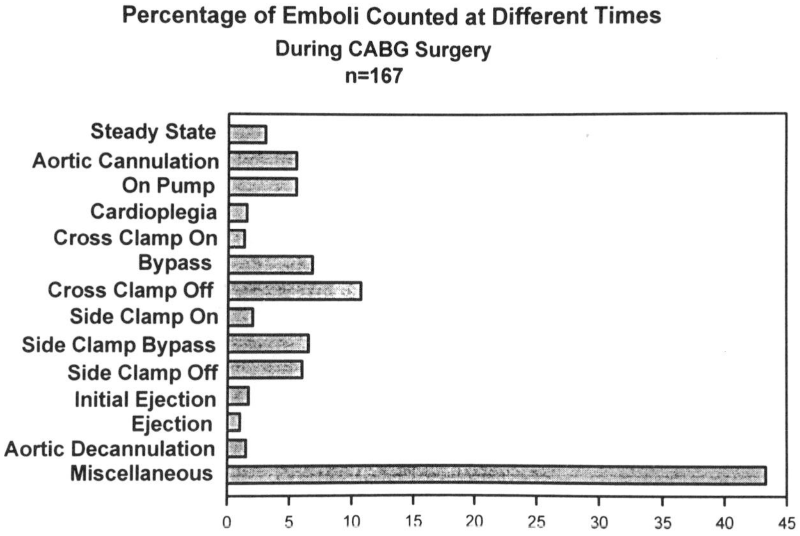

FIGURE 11.

Fifty-eight percent of the embolic signals detected during cardiopulmonary bypass grafting *(CABG)* surgery were associated with specific surgical manipulations or time intervals. Forty-two percent of the embolic signals were not associated with any of the 13 categories listed in the figure. The *miscellaneous* events were often spontaneous and few in number. Embolic signals associated with surgical maneuvers were often detected in greater numbers (n = 196). (Courtesy of Stump DA, Newman SP: Emboli detection during cardiopulmonary bypass, in Tegler CH, Babikian VL, Gomez CR [eds]: *Neurosonology.* St Louis, Mosby, 1996, pp 252–255.)

Data from Stump and Newman at Bowman-Gray University have graphically demonstrated the various stages during cardiac surgery during which emboli are occurring and showed that approximately 50% are associated with instrumentation of the aorta.[37] For example, Figure 11 shows that with application of the aortic cross-clamp, removal of the cross-clamp, side clamping, etc., emboli are detected within the middle cerebral artery. Of interest, however, they also showed that approximately 40% to 50% of these embolic events occur diffusely throughout CPB, so they are not all directly associated with aortic instrumentation. From the data of St Amand et al., it is likely that a significant number of these emboli are microparticulate atheromatous debris occurring as a result of the jet of blood from the aortic perfusion cannula scouring the aortic lumen and dislodging associated atherosclerotic plaque.[12]

HISTOLOGIC DEMONSTRATION OF CEREBRAL MICROEMBOLI

Not only is there evidence of cerebral emboli from transcranial Doppler signals and retinal fluorescein imaging, but there are some interesting data from histologic studies by Moody and colleagues.[38] They used a thick-section histologic preparation to look at animals exposed to either CPB or sham surgery, as well as to examine the cerebral microvasculature of patients who died after cardiac surgery or after noncardiac surgery. What is important regarding the histologic preparation they used is that it consisted of thick-section slices. Rather than a standard 8- to 20-μm histologic section, they used 100- to 150-μm sections so that they could focus up and down along the length of these cerebral arterioles. As shown in Figure 12, in sections of the cerebral arterioles after perfusion during CPB there are a series of dilatations termed *SCADs,*

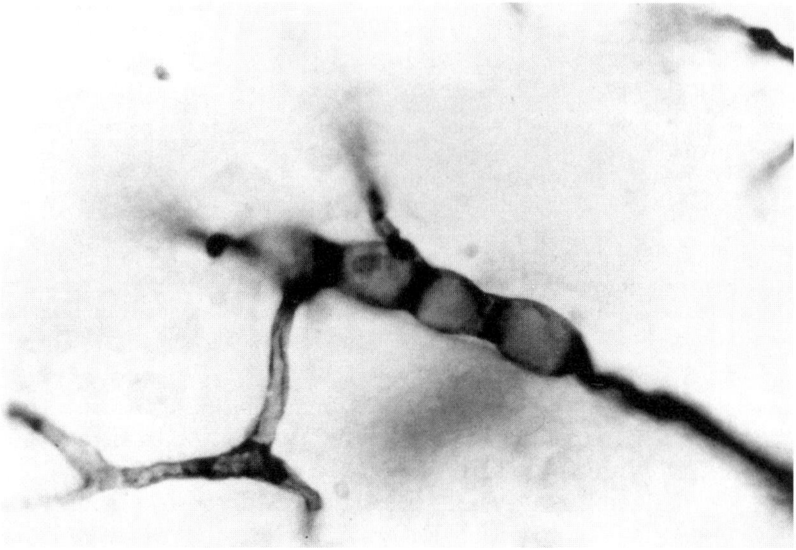

FIGURE 12.

Sausage-like dilations in a medium-sized arteriole from the white matter of a patient who had recently undergone cardiopulmonary bypass. These putative emboli are 40 μm in diameter and are probably more dangerous than the smaller ones. Notice that blood elements are displaced out of the lumen at the site of the clear swellings. Another of these emboli is seen in a smaller arteriole (100-μm-thick colloidin section stained for alkaline phosphatase). (Reprinted from *Annals of Neurology,* courtesy of Moody DM, Bell MA, Challa VR, et al: Brain microemboli during cardiac surgery or aortography. *Ann Neurol* 28:477–486, 1990, by permission of Little, Brown and Company, Inc.)

or small capillary and arteriolar dilatations. Because of the staining techniques used, these are vacuolated and thus it is not possible to determine the former content of these dilatations, but it is thought that they may be the footprint of emboli similar to those detected by retinal fluorescein angiography or with transcranial Doppler. In a further series of elegant studies, these investigators have proceeded to characterize when such emboli are occurring.[39] Using black or white microspheres injected either immediately before or after CPB, they were able to time-lock the development of the SCADs. They found that in all the animals studied, there was a similar anatomical relationship between the microspheres and SCADs. With the microspheres distributed in a proximal-to-distal

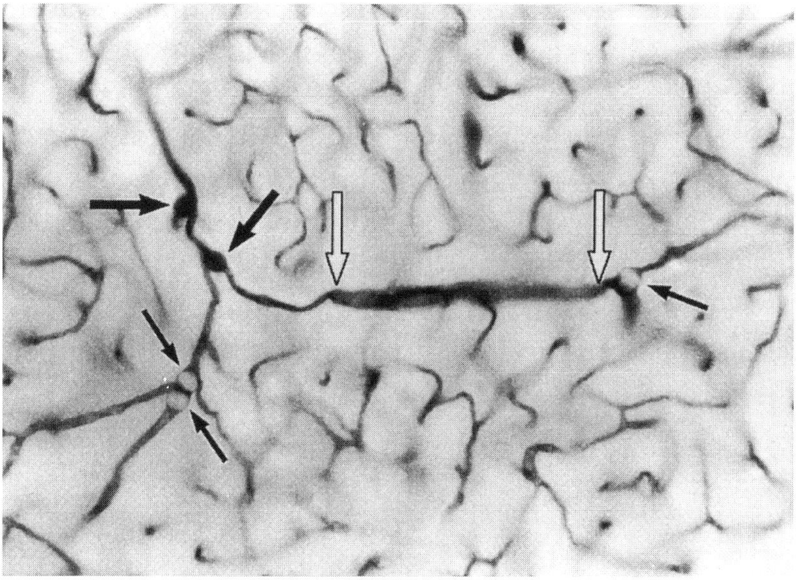

FIGURE 13.

Microemboli *(white arrows)* bracketed in time by sequentially injected microspheres of different colors. Clear microspheres *(small black arrows)* and black microspheres *(large black arrows)* can be seen in a distal-to-proximal order in a single arteriolar complex. In this experiment, clear spheres were injected into the carotid artery of a dog, followed in succession by an injection of corn oil and then black spheres. The direction of blood flow in the arteriole is from top to bottom (alkaline phosphatase–stained 100-μm-thick colloidin section; microspheres = 15 μm). (Reprinted with permission from the Society of Thoracic Surgeons, courtesy of Brown WR, Moody DM, Stump DA, et al: Dog model for cerebrovascular studies of the proximal-to-distal distribution of sequentially injected emboli. *Ann Thorac Surg* 59:1304–1307, 1995.)

progression along a cerebral arteriole, one would always find those colored microspheres injected before bypass, followed by the SCADs, followed by the microspheres injected after bypass, as shown in Figure 13. Although that complete sequence did not occur in all the cerebral microcirculatory beds examined, of those that were scanned, there was always a similar temporal relationship indicating that the development and generation of SCADs are definitely associated with CPB.

EMBOLIC LOAD AND NEUROBEHAVIORAL OUTCOMES

Whether from data obtained by using fluorescein retinal angiography, histologic brain sections, or transcranial Doppler, it is apparent that there is evidence from multiple diverse sources for cerebral emboli associated with CPB. Until recently, however, there was very little indication that in the absence of clinical stroke these had any measurable negative impact on postoperative neurobehavioral outcomes. However, in a paper by Pugsley et al., the relationship between the magnitude of the embolic load and postoperative cognitive performance was assessed by preoperative and postoperative neuropsychological testing.[40] These investigators were able to show that patients with the lowest number of emboli as detected by transcranial Doppler had a relatively low (below 10%) incidence of neurobehavioral dysfunction on postoperative psychometric testing. However, as the embolic load increased, over 40% of the patients who had greater than 1,000 emboli detected intraoperatively demonstrated postoperative cognitive impairment. Accordingly, they showed a direct relationship between embolic load and postoperative outcome, and because they were using arterial line filters to reduce the embolic counts, they found that use of an arterial line filter decreased the embolic load and therefore resulted in an improved outcome postoperatively. These data help further confirm the association between intraoperative cerebral embolization and postoperative neurobehavioral outcome and demonstrate the positive role that judicious equipment modifications can have on postoperative outcome.

Similar data were also reported by Stump et al. from Bowman-Gray.[41] They found a relationship between intraoperative embolic counts and neuropsychological outcome. Using carotid Doppler, they demonstrated that patients who had 79 or fewer emboli had a much lower risk of neuropsychological impairment postoperatively—less than 27%. On the other hand, if the number of emboli increased to an average of 156, i.e., double the number of emboli, 73% of the patients in whom this occurred would have postoperative neurobehavioral impairment.[41] This helps further establish the relationship between the magnitude of embolic load and the risk of postoperative cognitive impairment.

CEREBRAL EMBOLI AND RETROGRADE VS. ANTEROGRADE CORONARY PERFUSION

Of interest in these data on cerebral emboli is the recent demonstration that not only can the perfusion equipment itself influence the generation and delivery of emboli into the cerebral circulation, but even the cardioplegic technique can have a profound impact on cerebral embolization rates. This may appear surprising, for although cardioplegic technique might obviously be expected to influence myocardial performance, one would not expect an association between it and emboli occurring within the cerebral circulation.

A study by Baker and colleagues in Toronto evaluated patients in whom either anterograde or retrograde cardioplegia was used along with transcranial Doppler to detect the occurrence of cerebral emboli.[42] Within all cardioplegia groups, aortic cross-clamping was associated with the greatest number of embolic events. In itself, this is neither surprising nor new.[37, 43] What is of interest, however, is that when they looked at both the cold anterograde and warm anterograde cardioplegic groups, they found that the incidence of emboli associated with release of the aortic cross-clamp was significantly lower in those groups in which anterograde cardioplegia was used than in the group administered retrograde cardioplegia. Retrograde cardioplegia was associated with significantly more emboli after release of the aortic cross-clamp. This implies that with retrograde cardioplegia there may be flushing of intracoronary air and atherosclerotic debris within the coronary circulation into the aortic root such that with release of the aortic cross-clamp, these embolic particles are delivered into the cerebral circulation. As yet there have been no outcome data assessing the impact of cardioplegia techniques on cognitive functioning, but once again, it is suggested that in the context of CPB there is an intimate link between manipulation of the heart and subsequent delivery of emboli into the cerebral circulation.

pH MANAGEMENT AND CEREBRAL OUTCOME IN CORONARY ARTERY BYPASS SURGERY

We have previously used xenon radioisotopic studies in cardiac surgical patients to examine the influence of pH management and carbon dioxide management on CBF and cerebral physiology during CPB.[44] Patients were randomized to either alpha-stat management, i.e., non-temperature–corrected blood gas management, or pH-stat management, in which the temperature-corrected Pa_{CO_2} is maintained at approximately 40 mm Hg by the addition of exogenous CO_2. The difference in Pa_{CO_2} between these two management strategies at 28°C is approximately 15 mm Hg. As shown in Figure 14, the pH-stat group shows no relationship between CBF and cerebral oxygen consumption. Normally, there is very tight linkage between CBF and cerebral oxygen consumption. This loss of flow/metabolism coupling is a consequence of the addition of exogenous CO_2, i.e., pH-stat. However, in patients during alpha-stat management there was a direct relationship between CBF and cerebral oxygen consumption such that as cerebral oxygen consumption increased, CBF also increased, thus demonstrating preservation of flow/metabolism coupling. Similarly, in the pH-stat group, the relationship between CBF and perfusion pressure can best be described as pressure passive. As cerebral perfusion pressure increases, so does CBF. This suggests that with pH-stat, cerebral autoregulation is lost. With alpha-stat pH management there was no relationship between cerebral perfusion pressure and CBF over the range of pressure from about 20 to 100 mm Hg. This is consistent with other studies by Govier et al.[45] and Prough et al.[46] and demonstrates that cerebral autoregulation is preserved with alpha-stat management. There was no neurologic outcome study associated with this investigation, but given the evidence of emboli occurring diffusely throughout CPB, we were concerned that any unnecessary elevation in CBF such as may attend pH-stat management may further increase the delivery of microemboli to the cerebral circulation and result in adverse neurologic outcomes.[44]

Subsequently, we published the results of an outcome study assessing postoperative neurobehavioral performance as related to intraoperative pH management. Three hundred sixteen patients undergoing CAB surgery with CPB were randomized to either alpha-stat or pH-stat management intraoperatively.[4] Patients were stratified by surgeon so that each of the four surgeons and their various surgical techniques were represented in all study groups. These patients were also randomized to pulsatile or nonpulsatile perfusion during bypass. Preoperative neurologic and neuropsychological assessments were performed as a baseline and again at 24 hours postoperatively, 7 days postoperatively, and 2 months after discharge from the hospital. The neurologic examination was performed in a standardized manner to allow quantitation and scoring of the neurologic examination and to enable detection of any subtle abnormalities such as development of primitive reflexes, areas of hypoes-

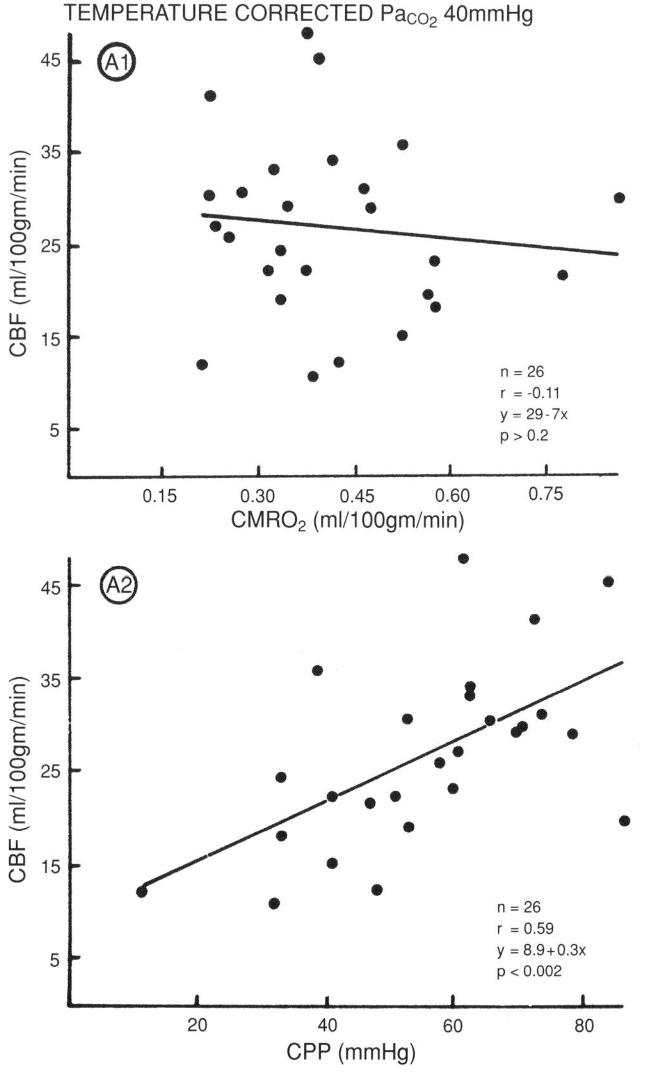

FIGURE 14.

Simple linear regression of cerebral blood flow *(CBF)* vs. cerebral perfusion pressure *(CPP)* or cerebral oxygen consumption *(CMRO$_2$)* for temperature-corrected and non–temperature-corrected groups. In the *upper panel* there is no significant correlation between CBF and CMRO$_2$ in the temperature-corrected group *(A1),* whereas CBF significantly correlates with CMRO$_2$ in the non–temperature-corrected group *(B1).* In the *lower panel,* CBF is significantly correlated with CPP in the temperature-corrected group *(A2),* whereas CBF is independent of CPP in the non–temperature-corrected group *(B2).* (Courtesy of Murkin JM, Farrar JK, Tweed WA, et al: Cerebral autoregulation and flow/metabolism coupling during cardiopulmonary bypass: The influence of PaCO_2. *Anesth Analg* 66:825–832, 1987.)

(continued)

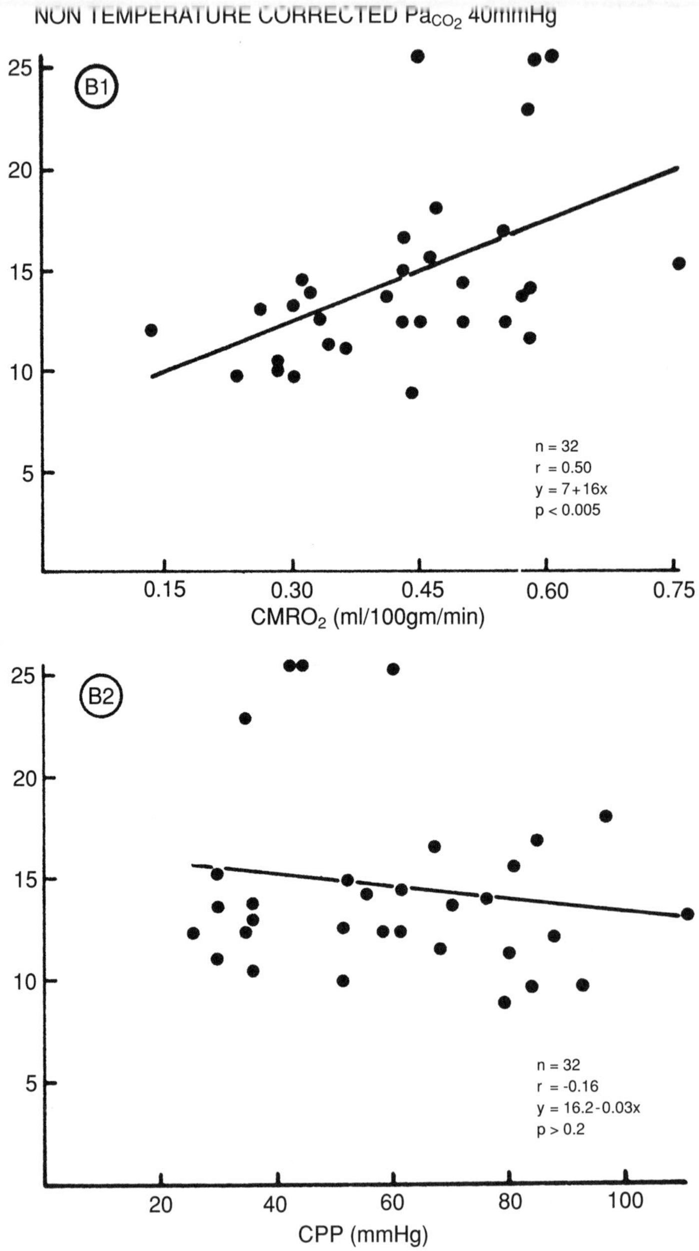

FIGURE 14. (continued)

thesia, and abnormal motor or sensory function. All patients acted as their own controls to allow measurement of subtle changes in the neurologic examination from the preoperative to the postoperative period. At the same time, we also administered a series of cognitive tests to assess short-term memory, hand–eye coordination, and various other subtle skills of cognitive performance. At 7 days postoperatively, over 85% of the patients had evidence of some deterioration in their performance relative to their preoperative status. Of these patients, approximately 79% had a decrement in neuropsychological performance on this battery of cognitive tests—an incidence similar to that detected by Shaw et al. in their series of 312 CAB patients in 1985.[47] More than 30% of these patients also had subtle changes on neurologic examination. Also of interest is that there was no complete overlap between cognitive and neurologic abnormalities, so we now feel quite strongly that in order to do a complete assessment of postoperative central nervous system (CNS) functioning, both cognitive testing and a standardized neurologic examination should be used.

More important was the incidence of dysfunction that was detected 2 months postoperatively. This was a postconvalescence assessment; patients were now at home after having ostensibly recovered from their major surgery, yet at this time over 45% of these patients still had not regained their level of preoperative baseline performance on cognitive testing or they demonstrated abnormal neurologic signs. Approximately a third of these patients demonstrated cognitive abnormalities, and 18% demonstrated subtle neurologic abnormalities.[4] In looking at the influence of intraoperative changes in pH management, at 2 months postoperatively there was a trend toward a reduction in the incidence of cognitive dysfunction overall in the group that received alpha-stat management. These results did not achieve statistical significance, however. When this group was further categorized into patients who were on bypass for longer than 90 minutes—in this case approximately half of the overall study group—there was a significant reduction in the incidence of cognitive impairment, from 44% in the pH-stat group to 27% in the alpha-stat group as shown in Figure 15.[4]

In retrospect, this is not surprising inasmuch as we used a filtered arterial line and membrane oxygenator to maximally decrease the generation of emboli during CPB. Because all of these patients are exposed to the same risks of emboli during aortic instrumentation, cross-clamping, cannulation, etc., and because it has been shown that these events are associated with approximately 50% of the emboli that are generated during bypass, changes in pH man-

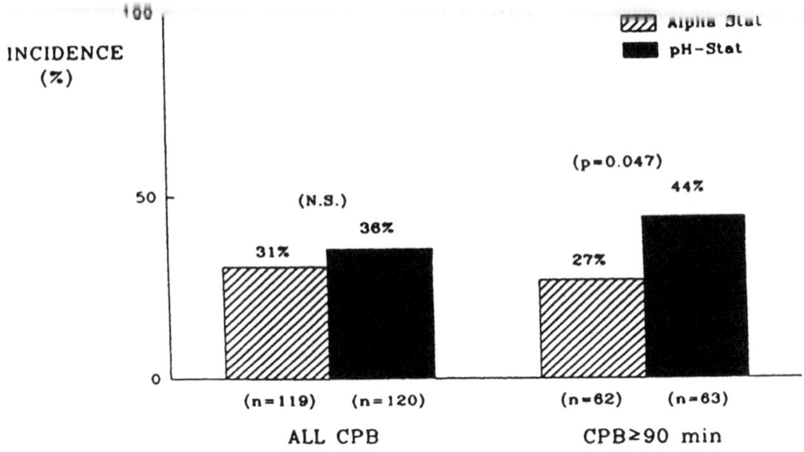

FIGURE 15.
Incidence of cognitive dysfunction 2 months after surgery for all patients in the cardiopulmonary bypass *(CPB)* and for those in whom the duration of CPB was 90 minutes or greater, excluding those in whom 7-day assessment was not available. Dysfunction was significantly greater in the pH-stat group in comparison to the alpha-stat group for those patients undergoing CPB for 90 minutes or longer. (Courtesy of Murkin JM, Martzke JS, Buchan AM, et al: A randomized study of the influence of perfusion technique and pH management strategy in 316 patients undergoing coronary artery bypass surgery. II Neurologic and cognitive outcomes. *J Thorac Cardiovasc Surg* 110:349–362, 1995.)

agement could only possibly influence the delivery of roughly 50% of emboli that occur randomly throughout bypass. Thus, only with prolonged exposure to CPB, in this case 90 minutes or greater, can the impact of changes in CBF (i.e., prevention of cerebral hyperemia as occurs with pH-stat management) become effective in reducing the delivery of emboli into the cerebral circulation, which was manifested in this study as a favorable neurobehavioral outcome 2 months postoperatively.[4] In several smaller studies, similar results also favoring alpha-stat over pH-stat management have now been reported.[48, 49] An important aspect of this demonstration is that this is a very cost-effective intervention. Merely turning down CO_2 levels to the pump oxygenator during moderate hypothermic (28°C—nasopharyngeal temperature) bypass has this dramatic effect of reducing cognitive impairment 2 months postoperatively.

In addition to studying these patients at 2 months postoperatively, a representative subset of 100 patients have now been ex-

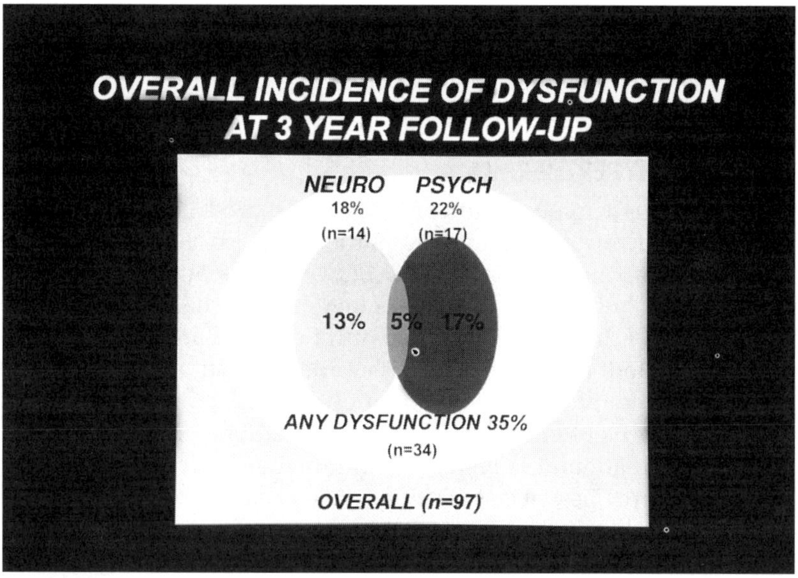

FIGURE 16.
Overall incidence of neurobehavioral dysfunction at the 3-year follow-up in 97 patients after coronary bypass surgery. The overall incidence of any form of neurologic or cognitive dysfunction was 35%, with 22% of the patients manifesting cognitive impairment and 18% manifesting neurologic abnormalities. Note that the majority of patients manifest either neurologic or cognitive impairment, with relatively few patients manifesting both forms of dysfunction.

amined an average of 3 years postoperatively. A similar battery of neurologic and cognitive testing was used, and we found that at the 3-year follow-up, nearly 35% of these patients again showed measurable dysfunction manifested as either cognitive impairment or change in neurologic examination.[5] Interestingly, once again there was not much overlap between patients with neurologic abnormalities and those with cognitive abnormalities. As shown in Figure 16, approximately 22% of the patients demonstrated cognitive abnormalities whereas 18% demonstrated neurologic abnormalities, but only about 5% of the patients had both. The implication is that the incidence of neurobehavioral impairment seen at 2 months postoperatively is effectively the same as the incidence 3 years postoperatively. Not only are cerebral emboli being showered into the brain during CPB, but reducing the magnitude of cerebral emboli can also have an important effect on decreasing the incidence of neurobehavioral impairment postoperatively. If patients remain impaired 3 months postoperatively, however, it is likely that this is a permanent injury.

CEREBRAL HYPERTHERMIA

Although many clinicians have observed cerebral hyperthermia during rewarming after hypothermic CPB and some have speculated about a potential link between this and postbypass impairment,[50, 51] until now this phenomenon has been poorly documented. In attempting to quantify clinical practice with respect to the extent of cerebral hyperthermia, a recent survey by Nathan and Lavallee provided some important indicators regarding current standards of practice.[52] In 24 of 28 centers responding to their survey, an attempt is made to monitor some surrogate of cerebral temperature, i.e., either nasopharyngeal or esophageal temperatures; this is less reassuring when it is recognized that in the context of cardiac surgery and CPB, esophageal temperature—representing as it does a heterogeneous measure that is variably influenced by core body temperature as well as blood temperature from the aortic inflow cannula and iced slush or fluid within the pericardium—is not reliably representative of temperatures of any specific organ system.[53] When viewed from this perspective, only about half of these cardiac centers routinely monitor a site, i.e., nasopharynx, that provides even a moderately reliable index of brain temperature. Furthermore, Nathan and Lavallee reported that even in those centers monitoring nasopharyngeal temperature, brain temperatures routinely exceed 38°C, as shown in Figure 17. Transient cerebral hyperthermia is thus the rule rather than the exception for most patients currently undergoing moderate hypothermic CPB.

It could be argued de facto that this transient hyperthermia is innocuous, given that it apparently occurs in a majority of CAB patients who do not obviously manifest clinically overt neurologic syndromes. Recently, however, several centers have observed postoperative seizures in "fast-track" CAB patients extubated shortly after hypothermic CPB. Although the etiology of these seizures has not been conclusively documented, those clinicians involved indicated that careful avoidance of cerebral hyperthermia during rewarming subsequently eliminated the problem. It appears entirely likely that avoidance of high dosages of benzodiazepines and narcotics, combined with elimination of postoperative paralysis and ventilation in order to facilitate early extubation, unmasked these "febrile" seizures that were occurring as a result of intraoperative

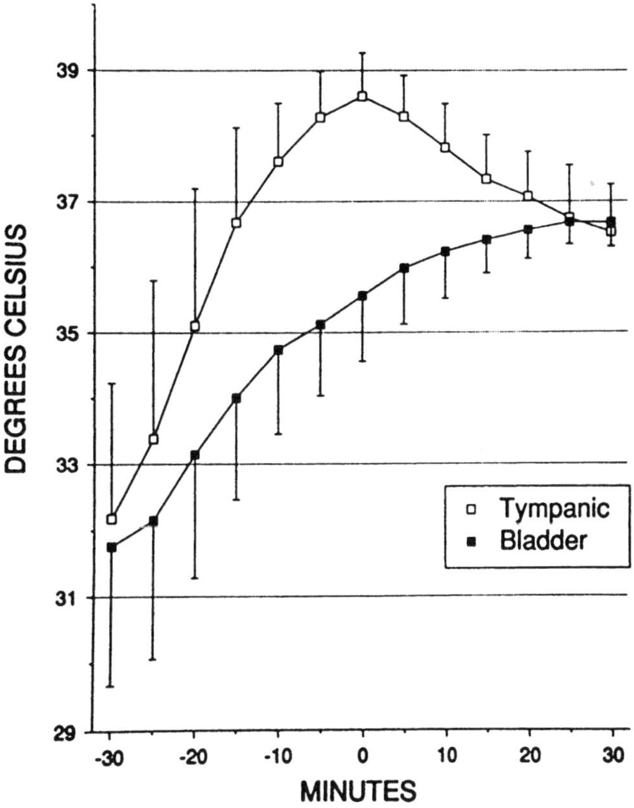

FIGURE 17.

Tympanic and bladder temperatures during rewarming. Time 0 is the maximum tympanic temperature achieved. Mean temperatures with standard deviation are shown. (Courtesy of Nathan HJ, Lavallee G: The management of temperature during hypothermic cardiopulmonary bypass: I. Canadian survey. *Can J Anaesth* 42:669–671, 1995.)

cerebral hyperthermia. In addition, there is now a growing body of evidence indicating wide-ranging subtle cerebral dysfunction occurring after bypass. Shaw et al.,[47] Smith and colleagues,[54] and Venn et al.,[49] as well as ourselves,[4] in studies that have cumulatively assessed over 700 CAB patients, have documented incidences of new subtle cognitive and neurologic impairment ranging from 50% to 80% in patients within 1 week after CAB surgery. Even months after surgery, upward of 30% of patients are still performing at cognitive levels significantly below their preoperative baselines.[4, 49]

The question is therefore how much of this CNS dysfunction is due to cerebral hyperthermia superimposed on a brain suffused with focal ischemic lesions?[55] It is known that the vulnerability of the normothermic brain to focal ischemic insult is surprisingly variable in the presence of small gradations in temperature. Busto et al.[56] demonstrated that at 33°C, expression of cerebral ischemia was virtually eliminated when compared with controls maintained at 36°C. In fact, a large measure of the apparent cerebroprotective efficacy of the glutamate receptor antagonist MK-801 in global ischemia was demonstrated by Buchan and Pulsinelli to be mediated by just such a small secondary decrease in brain temperature.[57] Conversely, small increases in brain temperature, e.g., 39°C—increments such as are occurring daily during CAB surgery—have been shown to profoundly enhance the susceptibility of the brain to focal ischemic insult and result in ischemic lesions of much greater extent in comparison to controls at 37°C.[58]

NORMOTHERMIA VS. HYPOTHERMIA FOR CORONARY SURGERY

The demonstration of apparently improved myocardial performance after normothermic CPB has prompted several outcome studies to assess the efficacy of this therapy, with particular focus now centered on CNS outcomes. In a prospective study of 1,732 patients undergoing CAB surgery and randomized to normothermic or hypothermic CPB, a decreased incidence of low-output syndrome and lower levels of cardiac isoenzyme fractions in the warm group were not associated with any difference in stroke rates in comparison to the hypothermic CPB group, 1.6% vs. 1.5%, respectively.[59]

In contrast, a study by Martin et al. of 1,001 patients similarly randomized to warm or cold CPB again demonstrated marginally better myocardial protection with warm CPB but found a significantly higher rate of stroke in the warm group than in the hypothermic CPB group, 3.1% vs. 1.0%, respectively.[60] Although reasons for this striking difference in stroke rate with two ostensibly similar techniques at different centers are not apparent, it does appear as though the group reported by Martin et al. were at higher risk because there were more diabetics (25% vs. 5.5%, respectively) and more of their patients had undergone prior CAB surgery (14.5% vs. 8% prior vascular surgery, respectively) than in the other trial. One further note is that retrograde cardioplegia was used in the majority of patients in the normothermic group but not the hypothermic group in the study reported by Martin et al.[60] In contrast, few patients in either the normothermic or hypothermic groups in the study reported by The Warm Heart Investigators[59] underwent retrograde cardioplegia.

It is unclear whether these differences in modes of administration of cardioplegia between these two studies account for the significant difference in stroke rates in the normothermic groups, as may be inferred from the cerebral embolization data of Baker et al.,[42] but the striking disparity in outcomes between two such ostensibly similar studies is noteworthy.

HYPOPERFUSION

The extent to which hypoperfusion is contributing to postoperative cerebral morbidity is unclear, but it is apparent that a greater understanding of the specific factors influencing cerebral physiology during CPB is essential. In a recent study using a hypothermic CPB model, Schwartz et al.[61] demonstrated that changes in mean arterial pressure (MAP) below the apparent cerebral autoregulatory range were shown to influence CBF directly. Conversely, profound reductions in pump flow rate produced no significant effects on CBF, provided that MAP was preserved. Other studies, both clinical and experimental, have suggested such effects, but generally either the variables in these studies were altered over a fairly limited range or flow rate and perfusion pressure interacted and were not kept as totally independent variables. The data of Schwartz et al. effectively confirmed the primacy of perfusion pressure over flow rates; the clinical implications of this information and the implications for further investigations should be considered. We and others have shown that CBF in patients is not affected by changes in pump flow rates over the range from 2.2 to 1.0 $L/m^2/min$.[62, 63]

Clinically, these data suggest that when flow reductions are required during CPB, efforts must be made to maintain cerebral perfusion pressure to preserve CBF. Similarly, even when hypotension is accompanied by high pump flow rates—such as sometimes occurs during normothermic CPB—the adequacy of cerebral perfusion cannot be assumed.

Specifically what perfusion pressure should be used has not yet been adequately addressed. A recent clinical outcome trial in 248 coronary bypass patients was able to show a significant decrease in cumulative adverse outcomes involving mortality (1.6% vs. 4.0%), stroke rate (2.4% vs. 7.2%), and cardiovascular complications (2.4% vs. 4.8%) in a group in whom MAP was maintained at 80–100 mm Hg vs. one in which systemic pressure averaged 50–60 mm Hg.[64]

The larger, physiologic question of whether the limits of cerebral autoregulation are extended during moderate hypothermic CPB, as several clinical studies have suggested,[44, 45] remains unclear. Cerebral autoregulation does appear to be lost at extremes of hypotension.[61] There is evidence from the meticulous work of Newman, Croughwell, and colleagues that during nonpulsatile CPB, cerebral autoregulation exhibits a small pressure dependence such that a 20–mm Hg increase in MAP results in approximately a 10% increase in CBF.[65] Further studies from this group have shown that hypotension (MAP less than 50 mm Hg) and rapid rewarming during CPB contributed significantly to postoperative cognitive dysfunction in elderly CAB patients.[66]

As such, it would appear that the clinician cannot blithely accept hypotension, even during hypothermia with high flow rates, with any confidence of maintaining adequate CBF. By default, maintaining pressures at the normal lower limit of cerebral autoregulation—50 mm Hg—or higher appears judicious. Cerebral perfusion pressure, like coronary perfusion pressure, must be maintained.

CONCLUSION

Overall, in various controlled clinical trials the factors that have been found to be associated with CNS dysfunction after CBP include the use of normothermic rather than hypothermic bypass, lack of arterial line filtration, advanced age, duration of CPB, severity of aortic atherosclerosis, and the use of pH-stat rather than alpha-stat management. The tremendous efficacy and therapeutic potential of intraoperative ultrasonic scanning for the assessment of aortic cannulation and clamp sites would now seem to be clearly established, and intraoperative ultrasonic scanning offers significant promise of decreasing intraoperative stroke rates in this ever-older and ever-sicker surgical population.

REFERENCES

1. Roach GW, Kanchuger M, Mora Mangano C, et al: Adverse cerebral outcomes after coronary bypass surgery. *N Engl J Med* 335:1857–1863, 1996.
2. Cosgrove DM, Loop FD, Lyttle BW, et al: Primary myocardial revascularization: Trends in surgical mortality. *J Thorac Cardiovasc Surg* 88:673–684, 1984.
3. Jones EL, Weintraub WS, Craver JM, et al: Coronary bypass surgery: Is the operation different today? *J Thorac Cardiovasc Surg* 101:108–115, 1991.

4. Murkin JM, Martzke JS, Buchan AM, et al: A randomized study of the influence of perfusion technique and pH management strategy in 316 patients undergoing coronary artery bypass surgery: II. Neurologic and cognitive outcomes. *J Thorac Cardiovasc Surg* 110:349–362, 1995.
5. Murkin JM, Baird DL, Martzke JS, et al: Long-term neurological and neuropsychological outcome 3 years after coronary artery bypass surgery. *Anesth Analg* 82:328S, 1996.
6. Tuman KJ, McCarthy RJ, Najafi H, et al: Differential effects of advanced age on neurologic and cardiac risks of coronary artery operations. *J Thorac Cardiovasc Surg* 104:1510–1517, 1992.
7. Gardner TJ, Horneffer PJ, Manolio TA, et al: Stroke following coronary artery bypass grafting: A ten-year study. *Ann Thorac Surg* 40:574–581, 1985.
8. Blauth CI, Cosgrove DM, Webb BW, et al: Atheroembolism from the ascending aorta. *J Thorac Cardiovasc Surg* 103:1104–1112, 1992.
9. Khatibzadeh M, Mitusch R, Stierle U, et al: Aortic atherosclerotic plaques as a source of systemic embolism. *J Am Coll Cardiol* 27:664–669, 1996.
10. Davila-Roman VG, Barzilai B, Wareing TH, et al: Intraoperative ultrasonic evaluation of the ascending aorta in 100 consecutive patients undergoing cardiac surgery. *Circulation* 84:47S–53S, 1991.
11. Shmuely H, Zoldan J, Sagie A, et al: Acute stroke after coronary angiography associated with protruding mobile thoracic aortic atheromas. *Neurology* 49:1689–1691, 1997.
12. St Amand MA, Murkin JM, Menkis AH, et al: Aortic atherosclerotic plaque identified by epiaortic scanning predicts cerebral embolic load in cardiac surgery. *Can J Anaesth* 44:A7, 1997.
13. Grossi EA, Kanchuger MS, Schwartz DS, et al: Effect of cannula length on aortic arch flow: Protection of the atheromatous arch. *Ann Thorac Surg* 59:710–712, 1995.
14. Groom RC, Hill AG, Akl BF, et al: Cannula length and arch flow erosion (letter). *Ann Thorac Surg* 61:773–774, 1996.
15. Muehrcke DD, Cornhill JF, Thomas JD, et al: Flow characteristics of aortic cannulae. *J Card Surg* 10:514–519, 1995.
16. Razi DM: The challenge of calcific aortitis. *J Card Surg* 8:102–107, 1993.
17. Cohen A, Tzourio C, Bertrand B, et al: Aortic plaque morphology and vascular events: A follow-up study in patients with ischemic stroke. FAPS Investigators. French Study of Aortic Plaques in Stroke. *Circulation* 96:3838–3841, 1997.
18. Davila-Roman VG, Barzilai B, Wareing TH, et al: Atherosclerosis of the ascending aorta: Prevalence and role as an independent predictor of cerebrovascular events in cardiac patients. *Stroke* 25:2010–2016, 1994.
19. Davila-Roman VG, Barzilai B, Wareing TH, et al: Intraoperative ultrasonographic evaluation of the ascending aorta in 100 consecu-

tive patients undergoing cardiac surgery. *Circulation* 84:178–538, 1991.
20. Ribakove GH, Katz ES, Galloway AC, et al: Surgical implications of transesophageal echocardiography to grade the atheromatous aortic arch. *Ann Thorac Surg* 53:758–763, 1992.
21. Katz ES, Tunick PA, Rusinek H, et al: Protruding aortic atheromas predict stroke in elderly patients undergoing cardiopulmonary bypass: Experience with intraoperative transesophageal echocardiography. *J Am Coll Cardiol* 20:70–77, 1992.
22. Wareing TH, Davila-Roman VG, Barzilai B, et al: Management of the severely atherosclerotic ascending aorta during cardiac operations. *J Thorac Cardiovasc Surg* 103:453–462, 1992.
23. St Amand MA, Murkin JM, Baird D, et al: The influence of epiaortic scanning on aortic cannulation for cardiac surgery. *Can J Anaesth* 43:A6, 1996.
24. Nicolosi AC, Aggarwai A, Almassi GH, et al: Intraoperative epiaortic ultrasound during cardiac surgery. *J Card Surg* 11:49–55, 1996.
25. Marschall K, Kanchuger M, Kessler K, et al: Superiority of transesophageal echocardiography in detecting aortic arch disease: Identification of patients at increased risk of stroke during cardiac surgery. *J Cardiothorac Vasc Surg* 8:5–13, 1994.
26. Sylviris S, Calafiore P, Matalanis G, et al: The intraoperative assessment of ascending aortic atheroma: Epiaortic imaging is superior to both transesophageal echocardiography and direct palpation. *J Cardiothorac Vasc Anesth* 11:704–707, 1997.
27. Konstadt S, Reich D, Kahn R, et al: Transesophageal echocardiography can be used to screen for ascending aortic atherosclerosis. *Anesth Analg* 81:225–228, 1995.
28. Davila-Roman VG, Phillips KJ, Daily BB, et al: Intraoperative transesophageal echocardiography and epiaortic ultrasound for assessment of atherosclerosis of the thoracic aorta. *J Am Coll Cardiol* 28:942–947, 1996.
29. Culliford AT, Stephen BC, Rohrer K, et al: The atherosclerotic ascending aorta and transverse arch: A new technique to prevent cerebral injury during bypass. Experience with 13 patients. *Ann Thorac Surg* 41:27–35, 1986.
30. Wareing TH, Davila-Roman VG, Daily BB, et al: Strategy for the reduction of stroke incidence in cardiac surgical patients. *Ann Thorac Surg* 55:1400–1407, 1993.
31. Koul B, Wierup P, Englund E, et al: Radical endarterectomy of severely calcified ascending aorta prevents stroke during open-heart surgery. *Scand Cardiovasc J* 31:33–37, 1997.
32. Trehan N, Mishra M, Dhole S, et al: Significantly reduced incidence of stroke during coronary artery bypass grafting using transesophageal echocardiography. *Eur J Cardiothorac Surg* 11:234–242, 1997.

33. Kasprzak JD, Salustri A, Yosir Y, et al: Three-dimensional echocardiography of the thoracic aorta. *Eur Heart J* 17:1584–1592, 1996.
34. Duda AM, Letwin LB, Sutter FP, et al: Does routine use of aortic ultrasonography decrease the stroke rate in coronary artery bypass surgery? *J Vasc Surg* 21:98–109, 1995.
35. Blauth CI, Smith PL, Arnold JV, et al: Influence of oxygenator type on the prevalence and extent of microembolic retinal ischemia during cardiopulmonary bypass. *J Thorac Cardiovasc Surg* 99:61–69, 1990.
36. Padayachee TS, Parsons S, Theobold R, et al: The detection of microemboli in the middle cerebral artery during cardiopulmonary bypass: A transcranial Doppler ultrasound investigation using membrane and bubble oxygenators. *Ann Thorac Surg* 44:298–302, 1987.
37. Stump DA, Newman SP: Emboli detection during cardiopulmonary bypass, in Tegler CH, Babikian VL, Gomez CR (eds): *Neurosonology.* St Louis, Mosby, 1996, pp 252–255.
38. Moody DM, Bell MA, Challa VR, et al: Brain microemboli during cardiac surgery or aortography. *Ann Neurol* 28:477–486, 1990.
39. Brown WR, Moody DM, Stump DA, et al: Dog model for cerebrovascular studies of the proximal-to-distal distribution of sequentially injected emboli. *Ann Thorac Surg* 59:1304–1307, 1995.
40. Pugsley W, Klinger L, Paschalis C, et al: The impact of microemboli during cardiopulmonary bypass on neuropsychological functioning. *Stroke* 25:1393–1399, 1994.
41. Stump DA, Rogers AT, Hammon JW, et al: Cerebral emboli and cognitive outcomes after cardiac surgery. *J Cardiothorac Vasc Anesth* 10: 113–119, 1995.
42. Baker AJ, Naser B, Benaroia M, et al: Cerebral microembolism during coronary artery bypass using different cardioplegia techniques. *Ann Thorac Surg* 59:1187–1191, 1995.
43. Barbut D, Hinton RB, Szatrowski TP, et al: Cerebral emboli detected during bypass surgery are associated with clamp removal. *Stroke* 25:2398–2402, 1994.
44. Murkin JM, Farrar JK, Tweed WA, et al: Cerebral autoregulation and flow/metabolism coupling during cardiopulmonary bypass: The influence of $Paco_2$. *Anesth Analg* 66:825–832, 1987.
45. Govier ASAV, Reves JG, McKay RD, et al: Factors and their influence on regional cerebral blood flow during nonpulsatile cardiopulmonary bypass. *Ann Thorac Surg* 38:592–600, 1984.
46. Prough DS, Stump DA, Roy RC, et al: Response of cerebral blood flow to changes in carbon dioxide tension during hypothermic cardiopulmonary bypass. *Anesthesiology* 64:576–581, 1986.
47. Shaw PJ, Bates D, Cartlidge NEF, et al: Early neurological complications of coronary artery bypass surgery. *BMJ* 291:1384–1387, 1985.
48. Stephan H, Weyland A, Kazmaier S, et al: Acid-base management during hypothermic cardiopulmonary bypass does not affect cerebral me-

tabolism but does affect blood flow and neurological outcome. *Br J Anaesth* 69:51–57, 1992.
49. Venn GE, Patel RL, Chambers DJ: Cardiopulmonary bypass: Perioperative cerebral blood flow and postoperative cognitive deficit. *Ann Thorac Surg* 59:1331–1339, 1995.
50. Murkin JM: Hypothermic cardiopulmonary bypass—time for a more temperate approach? *Can J Anaesth* 42:663–668, 1995.
51. Drummond JC: Brain protection during anesthesia: A reader's guide. *Anesthesiology* 79:877–880, 1993.
52. Nathan HJ, Lavallee G: The management of temperature during hypothermic cardiopulmonary bypass: I. Canadian survey. *Can J Anaesth* 42:669–671, 1995.
53. Muravchick S: Deep body thermometry during general anesthesia. *Anesthesiology* 58:271–275, 1983.
54. Smith PLC, Newman SP, Ell PJ, et al: Cerebral consequences of cardiopulmonary bypass. *Lancet* 1:823–825, 1986.
55. Moody DM, Brown WR, Challa VR, et al: Brain microemboli associated with cardiopulmonary bypass: A histologic and magnetic resonance imaging study. *Ann Thorac Surg* 59:1304–1307, 1995.
56. Busto R, Dietrich WD, Globus MY-T, et al: The importance of brain temperature in cerebral injury. *Stroke* 20:1113–1114, 1989.
57. Buchan A, Pulsinelli WA: Hypothermia but not the *N*-methyl-D-aspartate antagonist, MK-801, attenuates neuronal damage in gerbils subjected to transient global ischemia. *J Neurosci* 10:311–316, 1990.
58. Chopp M, Knight R, Tidwell CD, et al: The metabolic effects of mild hypothermia on global cerebral ischemia and recirculation in the cat: Comparison of normothermia to hyperthermia. *J Cereb Blood Flow Metab* 9:141–148, 1989.
59. The Warm Heart Investigators: Randomised Trial of Normothermic Versus Hypothermic Coronary Bypass Surgery. *Lancet* 343:559–563, 1994.
60. Martin TD, Craver JM, Gott JP, et al: Prospective, randomized trial of retrograde warm blood cardioplegia: Myocardial benefit and neurologic threat. *Ann Thorac Surg* 57:298–304, 1994.
61. Schwartz AE, Sandhu AA, Kaplon RJ, et al: Cerebral blood flow is determined by arterial pressure and not cardiopulmonary bypass flow rate. *Ann Thorac Surg* 60:165–170, 1995.
62. Murkin JM, Farrar JK, Cleland CP, et al: The influence of perfusion flow rates on cerebral blood flow and oxygen consumption during hypothermic cardiopulmonary bypass. *Anesthesiology* 67:A9, 1987.
63. Rogers AT, Prough DS, Roy RC, et al: Cerebrovascular and cerebral metabolic effects of alterations in perfusion flow rate during hypothermic cardiopulmonary bypass in man. *J Thorac Cardiovasc Surg* 103:363–368, 1992.
64. Gold JP, Charlson ME, Williams-Russo P, et al: Improvement of outcomes after coronary artery bypass: A randomized trial comparing in-

traoperative high versus low mean arterial pressure. *J Thorac Cardiovasc Surg* 110:1302–1314, 1995.
65. Newman MF, Croughwell ND, Blumenthal JA, et al: Predictors of cognitive decline after cardiac surgery. *Ann Thorac Surg* 59:1326–1330, 1995.
66. Newman MF, Kramer D, Croughwell ND, et al: Differential effects of mean arterial pressure and rewarming on cognitive dysfunction after cardiac surgery. *Anesth Analg* 81:236–242, 1995.

CHAPTER 5

Retrograde Cardioplegia

Richard N. Gates, M.D.
Assistant Clinical Professor of Surgery, Division of Cardiothoracic Surgery, UCLA School of Medicine, UCLA Medical Center, Los Angeles, California; Children's Hospital of Orange County, Orange, California

Hillel Laks, M.D.
Professor and Chief, Division of Cardiothoracic Surgery; Director, Heart and Heart–Lung Transplant Program, UCLA Medical Center, Los Angeles, California

Widespread clinical use of the retrograde approach to cardioplegia delivery began in the late 1980s and early 1990s with development of the transatrial coronary sinus cannula. Buckberg at UCLA and Gundry at Loma Linda were instrumental in the design of these cannula. Interestingly, many surgeons were enticed to begin using retrograde cardioplegia by early reports of improved myocardial protection achieved by warm continuous blood cardioplegia techniques.[1] It was quickly appreciated that the retrograde approach allowed for continuous delivery of cardioplegia regardless of the position of the heart. Such was not the case with antegrade delivery, where aortic insufficiency frequently developed with positioning of the heart for lateral and inferior coronary anastomosis. Although use of the warm continuous technique for myocardial protection appears to be waning, clinical use of the retrograde approach to cardioplegia delivery continues to grow.

As such, a good deal of research has been focused on retrograde cardioplegia distribution, techniques, and clinical results. In this manuscript, we will attempt to review this information. Additionally, we present our clinical techniques for both adult and pediatric retrograde cardioplegia within the framework of "an integrated approach to myocardial protection." Initially, we begin with a short review of the basic concepts of myocardial protection to place retrograde cardioplegia within proper perspective.

Advances in Cardiac Surgery®, vol. 10

CONCEPTS IN MYOCARDIAL PROTECTION

PRIMARY GOALS

Every cardiac surgeon appreciates the value of good myocardial protection. However, it should always be remembered that myocardial protection is an adjunct to the operative procedure. Performance of a technically precise and expedient operation is the prime determinant of both short- and long-term results. Thus, the approach to myocardial protection should be individualized and planned so that it facilitates conduct of the operation, not the reverse.

PHASES OF MYOCARDIAL PROTECTION

For the purpose of devising strategies for myocardial protection, it is useful to divide the process into five phases: (1) pre-arrest period, (2) induction of arrest, (3) maintenance of arrest, (4) reperfusion, and (5) postreperfusion period (Table 1). During the pre-arrest period every attempt should be made to optimize cardiopulmonary dynamics. Maneuvers to decrease pressure and volume loads on the heart, improve the metabolic status of myocytes, and reduce hypoxia should be aggressively sought. Myocytes that enter into a cardioplegic arrest in a glycogen- or high-energy phosphate–depleted state are far more susceptible to injury upon subsequent reperfusion.[2]

Buckberg has championed the importance of the initiation of cardiac arrest. An initial arrest with "resuscitation" or "induction" warm blood cardioplegia containing amino acid enhancement is directed at repleting high-energy phosphate–depleted myocytes. In metabolically depleted and injured myocardium, such an approach significantly improves subsequent postoperative myocardial function.[3, 4] For patients with metabolically intact myocardium, the initial arrest need not be "resuscitation" cardioplegia. In all initial arrests, one should focus on complete decompression of the heart along with maximum cardioplegic distribution.[5, 6]

The approach to maintenance cardioplegia should be planned so as to minimize or optimally avoid myocardial ischemia in the period between arrest and reperfusion. Because this is the period in which the intracardiac or extracardiac portion of the operation is being performed, approaches to maintenance cardioplegia should be tailored to the specific operation being performed. Intermittent or continuous, warm, tepid, or cold techniques may be used. The approach used should facilitate the operation and allow for a technically optimal result. In all cases, maintenance of arrest and complete decompression of the heart are essential. Taken to-

TABLE 1.
Phases of Myocardial Protection With Related Strategies to Improve Myocardial Function

Phase and Goals	Clinical Strategies
1. *Pre-arrest:* Maximize oxygen supply and reduce demand by optimizing cardiopulmonary status	Optimize cardiopulmonary dynamics Optimize anesthetic induction Early institution of partial CPB
2. *Arrest:* Replete myocardial substrate and energy stores if necessary; achieve complete electromechanical arrest of the decompressed heart	Warm substrate-enhanced "resuscitation" cardioplegia if necessary Hyperkalemic arrest with maximum cardioplegic distribution
3. *Maintenance:* Minimize development of ischemia; provide optimal operative field	Hypothermic intermittent oxygenated cardioplegia with maximum distribution
4. *Reperfusion:* Limit calcium and oxygen free radical–mediated reperfusion injury	Warm substrate-enhanced hypocalcemic cardioplegia Leukocyte depleting Free radical scavenging
5. *Postarrest:* Maximize oxygen supply and reduce demand by optimizing cardiopulmonary status; reduce free water gain	Optimize cardiopulmonary dynamics Unload damaged myocardium (i.e., IABP, LVAD, ECMO) Modified ultrafiltration

Abbreviations: CPB, cardiopulmonary bypass; *IABP,* intra-aortic balloon pumping; *LVAO,* left ventricular assist device; *ECMO,* extracorporeal membrane oxygenation.

gether, arrest and decompression reduce 90% of the myocardial oxygen demand. Cooling from 37°C to 10°C reduces demand from 10% to 3%.[7]

Reperfusion occurs when the cross-clamp is removed and the heart is subjected to corporeal blood. At the time of reperfusion, any myocytes that have become ischemic and energy depleted are subject to "reperfusion" injury. Factors involved in reperfusion injury are protean and include activated neutrophils and oxygen free radicals.[8] The end result of a reperfusion injury is "stunned" and dysfunctional myocardium.[9] The degree of dysfunction is related to both the amount of ischemia suffered and the exposure to injurious blood components upon reperfusion. To reduce reperfusion injury, Buckberg and others have purposed "controlled reperfusion."[10] Controlled reperfusion occurs by giving blood through a cardioplegia circuit modified to reduce reperfusion injury and enhance metabolic recovery. During controlled reperfusion, the heart should remain decompressed and the initial perfusion pressures kept in the range of 50–60 mm Hg.[11] Modification of the blood can include substrate enhancement, hypocalcemia, leukocyte depletion, free radical scavenging, and other techniques. In the postreperfusion period the myocardium must now maintain cardiac output while repairing any cellular injury that occurred during ischemia and reperfusion. If myocardial stunning and dysfunction are significant, placing excessive functional demands on the myocardium may further exacerbate injury or hinder expedient recovery. As such, early institution of intra-aortic balloon pumping or ventricular assist should be considered for the dysfunctional heart.

WARM AND COLD CARDIOPLEGIA

Warm cardioplegic conditions promote aerobic metabolism and should be used in scenarios where continuous cardioplegia administration is feasible and does not interfere with the technical performance of the operation. For procedures or parts of procedures in which intermittent cardioplegia delivery is desired, cold cardioplegia techniques should be used. For most procedures, a cardioplegic strategy that involves both warm continuous and cold intermittent cardioplegia can be developed.

DISTRIBUTION

The critical importance of complete and uniform distribution of the cardioplegic solution to the myocardium has only recently been appreciated. In models of acute complete coronary artery occlusion, it has been demonstrated that the retrograde delivery approach improves myocardial protection.[12, 13] Experimental data regarding the distribution of retrograde cardioplegia will be presented in detail later. Initially it was anticipated that retrograde cardioplegia would be useful in two predominant ways: first, to ensure cardioplegic distribution to regions where antegrade coronary artery flow is minimal or nil, and second, to allow for cardioplegia delivery in situations where antegrade delivery is cumbersome or impossible (i.e., an initial arrest with severe aortic insufficiency, during warm continuous cardioplegia for coronary surgery when positioning of the heart renders the aortic valve incompetent, for an anomalous coronary artery arising from the pulmonary artery, etc.). However, recent experimental work has suggested that the use of both antegrade and retrograde cardioplegia together results in superior cardioplegic distribution over antegrade cardioplegia alone. This appears to be true even in hearts without obstruction to antegrade coronary artery flow.[14, 15] The inability of antegrade cardioplegia to completely perfuse all capillary beds, even in normal hearts, may be due to arteriolar autoregulation with selective arterio-venous-venous shunting. Such autoregulation of the microvasculature is well known,[16] and retrograde cardioplegia offers another anatomical approach to such regulated capillary beds. Enhanced microvascular perfusion achieved by combining antegrade and retrograde cardioplegia may partly explain the excellent clinical results reported when using combined approaches.[17, 18]

RETROGRADE CARDIOPLEGIA DISTRIBUTION

BASIC ANATOMY

To plan effective strategies for myocardial protection via retrograde cardioplegia, one needs to anatomically understand where the retrogradely delivered cardioplegia flows and how this is affected by the delivery technique used. The coronary sinus drains 60% to 83% of the blood delivered to the heart.[19, 20] The remaining venous drainage occurs by the thebesian veins.[21] The thebesian veins are small venous passages that drain directly into the chambers of the heart. They occur predominantly in the right ventricle but also to a small degree in the papillary muscle of the left ventricle.[22] Thus, nearly all blood perfused through the left main coronary artery exits the coronary sinus. However, the vast majority of blood that perfuses the right coronary artery drains by thebesian veins, not the coronary sinus. Unlike coronary arteries, coronary veins are rich with venovenous anastomoses. Such venovenous anastomoses are numerous and connect the anterior intraventricular vein (LAD vein), the middle cardiac vein (Parsonnet), and the posterior intraventricular vein (PDA vein). Additionally, venovenous anastomoses occur between these epicardial veins and the thebesian vein system, and the greatest connections to the thebesian system are from the PDA vein.[23, 24] It is extremely important to note that the PDA vein generally enters the coronary sinus only 1–3 cm from the coronary sinus ostium.

These venovenous pathways allow for ligation of the coronary sinus and total cardiac venous drainage through thebesian veins.[25] They also explain why simultaneous antegrade and retrograde cardioplegia can be safely delivered. Cardioplegia drainage occurs through thebesian veins directly into the body of the ventricles.[26, 27] Unfortunately, these pathways (coronary sinus to coronary vein to thebesian vein to ventricular cavity) scuttled the brilliant and imaginative work of Beck et al. in their attempts to treat coronary artery disease by arterialization of the coronary sinus.[28] Indeed, only 14% to 25% of the normal oxygen requirements could be delivered by arterialization of the coronary sinus.[29]

EXPERIMENTAL WORK

With such complex venous drainage of the heart, it would be rather naive to assume that cardioplegia delivered by a transatrial coronary sinus cannula would be evenly distributed to all regions of the heart and that all delivered cardioplegia solution would provide capillary (or nutrient) flow. Indeed, very early in our experience with retrograde cardioplegia we noted two interesting findings during aortic valve replacement when the coronary ostia were easily observed: (1) only a fraction of the delivered cardioplegia solution exited the coronary ostia, and (2) the cardioplegia solution that did egress from the aortic root did so predominantly from the left coronary ostium. This suggested to us that most of the retrogradely delivered cardioplegia was not providing nutrient flow, and the left ventricle appeared to be receiving significantly more flow than the right ventricle.

The notion that coronary sinus–delivered solutions predominantly or exclusively perfused the left ventricle was well established in animal models.[30–33] However, in animals the thebesian system is more developed than in humans and the posterior descending vein does not always empty into the coronary sinus.[30] To study retrograde distribution in humans, we developed the model of the explanted human heart during 1992.[34] In this model, human hearts were arrested in situ with cold antegrade cardioplegic solution and excised with their coronary sinus collecting system intact. The hearts were immediately transferred to the laboratory and prepared for study within 20 minutes to mimic the clinical situation.

In our initial study, a retroperfusion cannula was placed into the coronary sinus and a purse-string suture was used to occlude the sinus opening. The left and right coronary ostia were cannulated to drain and measure the effluent. Warm blood cardioplegia was then infused at 30–40 mm Hg. Left coronary, right coronary, and thebesian effluents were measured (Table 2). We found that 67% ± 6% of the cardioplegia solution drained through thebesian veins, 29% ± 6% drained from the left coronary artery, and 4% ±

TABLE 2.

Gross Results (Effluents)

Heart	Rt CA (mL/min)	Lt CA (mL/min)	Thebs (mL/min)	% Rt CA	% Lt CA	% Thebs	Weight (g)	Rt CA (mL/min/g)	Lt CA (mL/min/g)	Thebs (mL/min/g)	Total CPG mL/min	Total CPG mL/min/g
1	4	80	162	1.6	32.5	65.9	570	0.0070	0.14	0.28	246	0.43
2	6	79	174	2.3	30.5	67.3	520	0.012	0.15	0.33	259	0.50
3	4	62	95	2.5	38.5	59.0	332	0.012	0.19	0.29	161	0.48
4	26	70	176	9.6	25.7	64.7	562	0.046	0.12	0.31	272	0.48
5	8	65	152	3.6	28.9	67.5	504	0.016	0.13	0.30	225	0.45
6	3	38	151	1.6	19.8	78.6	350	0.0086	0.11	0.43	192	0.54
Mean ± SD	8.5 ± 8.8	65.7 ± 15.4	151.7 ± 29.7	3.5 ± 3.1	29.3 ± 6.3	67.2 ± 6.4	473 ± 105.4	0.017 ± 0.015	0.14 ± 0.027	0.32 ± 0.055	225.8 ± 42.4	0.48 ± 0.041

Abbreviations: Rt, right; *CA,* coronary artery; *Lt,* left; *Thebs,* thebesian; *CPG,* cardioplegia.

(Reprinted with permission from the Society of Thoracic Surgeons, courtesy of Gates RN, Laks H, Drinkwater DC, et al: Gross and microvascular distribution of retrograde cardioplegia in explanted human hearts. *Ann Thorac Surg* 53:410–417, 1993.)

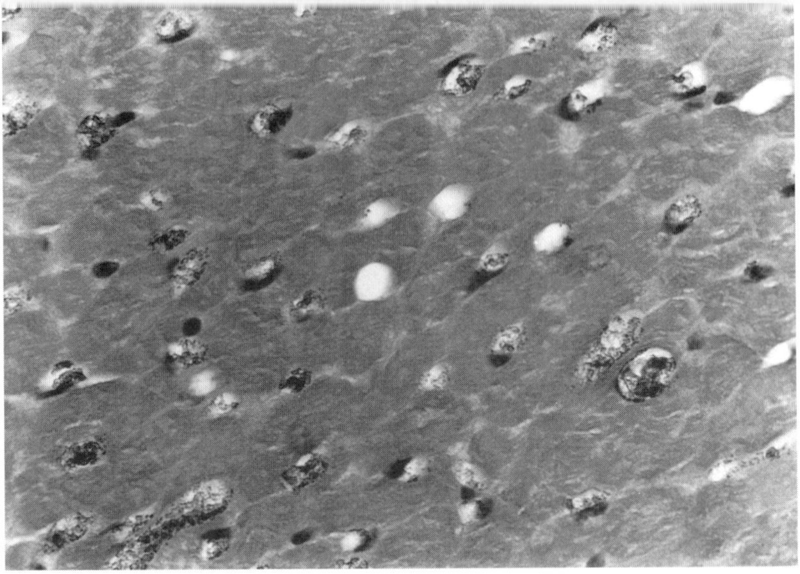

FIGURE 1.
Photomicrograph of a section of right ventricular myocardium after retrograde fixation and NTB-2 perfusion. NTB-2 is seen filling most capillaries (magnification, ×161.1).

3% drained from the right coronary artery.[30] Subsequently, an inert intracapillary marker (NTB-2) was infused retrogradely after retrograde glutaraldehyde fixation. Capillary perfusion was documented in all regions of both the left and right ventricles (Fig 1). From this study we concluded that (1) capillary perfusion occurs in all regions of the myocardium when retrograde cardioplegia is delivered with an occluded coronary sinus, (2) the majority (67%) of a retrograde cardioplegia dose bypassed the ventricular capillary beds and dumped into the ventricular cavities, and (3) a much greater amount, 29% vs. 4%, of capillary cardioplegia flow occurred in the left ventricle as opposed to the right ventricle.

These data suggested that with retrograde cardioplegia, relatively less capillary perfusion was occurring in the right ventricle. To more closely examine true microvascular flow we performed an addition study on explanted human hearts given retrograde cardioplegia in which the solution contained colored microspheres. This cardioplegia was delivered through a cardioplegia cannula placed well into the coronary sinus but without coronary ostial occlusion. The results of this study indicated that approximately four times greater capillary blood flow was occurring in the left ventricle than the right.[35] These results were quite similar to those of contrast echocardiography experiments published by Allen et al.[36] and Aronson and associates.[37]

During this time, we began to routinely use retrograde cardioplegia during congenital heart procedures. Because these operations were generally done with the right atrium open, the coronary sinus was cannulated under direct vision. We noted that a significant amount of the cardioplegic dose regurgitated back out the coronary sinus. To prevent this, we began placing a purse-string suture about the coronary sinus. This purse-string suture must be carefully placed within the base of the sinus to avoid the atrioventricular node. With placement of the purse-string suture we noted several changes: (1) lower volumes of cardioplegia solution could be given to effect the same coronary sinus pressure, (2) the PDA vein was more tensely distended and to a pressure equivalent to that of the LAD vein, and (3) more cardioplegia solution was noted to exit the aortic root, particularly the right coronary ostium.

We documented these findings by using the explanted human heart model and colored microspheres.[38] Cardioplegia efficacy was improved inasmuch as 1.06 ± 0.32 mL of cardioplegia solution per gram of heart tissue vs. 1.74 ± 0.40 mL of cardioplegia solution per gram of heart tissue was required to maintain coronary sinus pressure with the coronary sinus closed vs. open, respectively. Additionally, the percentage of nutrient flow (that cardioplegia solution that has traversed capillaries and exited the coronary arteries) to total cardioplegia flow increased from 32.3 ± 15.1 to 61.3 ± 7.9 with the sinus closed vs. open, respectively. Most significantly, the capillary flow per gram of heart tissue to the right ventricle equaled that to the left ventricle with the coronary sinus occluded (Table 3).

One common misconception is the notion that coronary sinus regurgitation can be eliminated and improved right ventricular distribution achieved by using a transatrial retroperfusion cannula that is manually inflated as opposed to auto-inflated. This is simply not true during routine transatrial retrograde cardioplegia administration. The reason for this is simple and anatomical (Fig 2). Because the entrance of the PDA vein to the coronary sinus is generally 1–3 cm from the coronary sinus ostium, either auto-inflating or manually inflating cannulas generally lie well past the PDA vein in the body of the coronary sinus. As such, cardioplegia solution that reaches the PDA vein does so through venovenous connections from more distal (with respect to the cannula tip in the body of

TABLE 3.
Microvascular Data (Coronary Sinus Open vs. Closed)

	Anterior	Lateral/Mid	Posterior	____
LV	0.34 ± 0.32 vs. 0.25 ± 0.30*	0.20 ± 0.26 vs. 0.10 ± 0.07*	0.11 ± 0.13 vs. 0.26 ± 0.28*	0.12 ± 0.18 vs. 0.30 ± 0.29*
RV	0.20 ± 0.21 vs. 0.21 ± 0.19*	0.05 ± 0.03 vs. 0.17 ± 0.13†	0.04 ± 0.03 vs. 0.18 ± 0.13†	0.11 ± 0.07 vs. 0.23 ± 0.12†
IVS	0.12 ± 0.31 vs. 0.26 ± 0.20*	0.11 ± 0.08 vs. 0.24 ± 0.17*	0.02 ± 0.01 vs. 0.19 ± 0.10†	0.14 ± 0.12 vs. 0.35 ± 0.23†

Note: All flows are expressed in milliliters per gram myocardium.
*$P > 0.05$.
†$P < 0.05$.
Abbreviations: LV, left ventricle: *RV,* right ventricle: *IVS,* intraventricular septum.

the coronary sinus) veins. Because there is direct communication from the low-pressure right atrium to the proximal coronary sinus to the PDA vein, a good deal of delivered cardioplegia flow is siphoned off in this manner back to the right atrium. This gives the appearance that leakage is occurring around the balloon tip of the retroperfusion cannula, but it is truly draining of the PDA vein. This is why with routine transatrial retroperfusion the PDA vein is generally less distended than the LAD vein. It is also likely to explain why right ventricular perfusion is one fourth left ventricular perfusion. The only reliable way to prevent coronary sinus ostial regurgitation and equalize right and left ventricular perfusion with retrograde cardioplegia administration is to do so through an open atrium with a purse-string suture about the coronary sinus.

SUMMARY

The distribution and efficacy of retrogradely delivered cardioplegia depends on whether the cardioplegia is delivered with a transatrial cannula or with the right atrium open and the coronary sinus ostium occluded with a purse-string suture. With transatrial cannulation, approximately a third of the delivered cardioplegia dose is nutrient flow and capillary flow is approximately four times greater per gram of heart muscle in the left vs. the right ventricle. With a purse-string suture about the coronary sinus, approximately

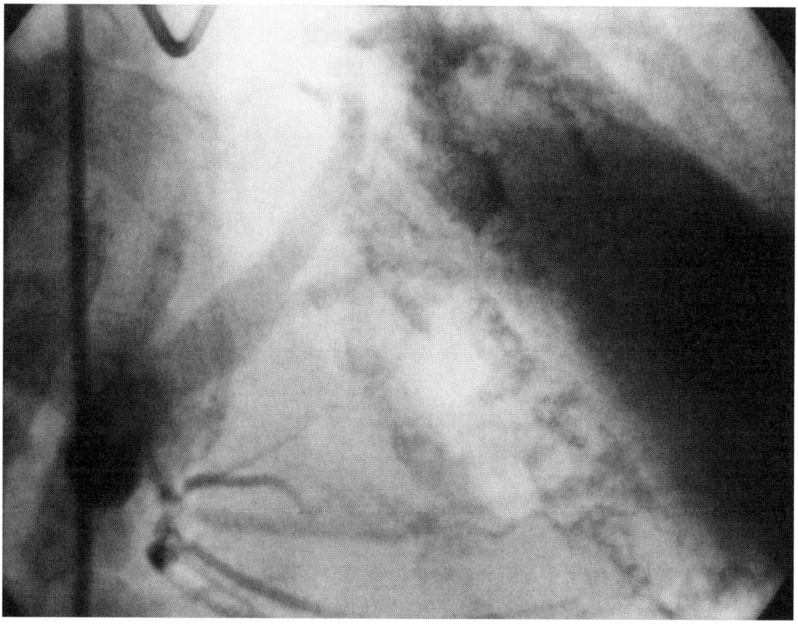

FIGURE 2.
Venous phase of a left anterior oblique angiogram demonstrating the coronary sinus. Note the proximity of the posterior interventricular vein to the coronary sinus ostia.

60% of the delivered cardioplegia dose is nutrient flow, and capillary flow is equivalent in the left and right ventricles.

TECHNIQUES FOR RETROGRADE CARDIOPLEGIA ADMINISTRATION

There are three general approaches to retrograde cardioplegia administration. The first is the uncommonly used "atrial isolation" or "right heart isolation" technique. For this approach, bicaval cannulation is used with caval snares. The pulmonary artery is cross-clamped and cardioplegia solution delivered directly into the right atrium. Because the technique is somewhat cumbersome, it is not widely used. However, in theory, excellent distribution should be obtained and good clinical results with its use have been reported.[39]

By far the most commonly used technique is transatrial cannulation of the coronary sinus. This is easily performed with either an auto-inflating or manually inflating cannula. The cannula is generally placed before initiation of cardiopulmonary bypass when the coronary sinus is full and distended. The final approach is direct coronary sinus cannulation via a right atriotomy. In such

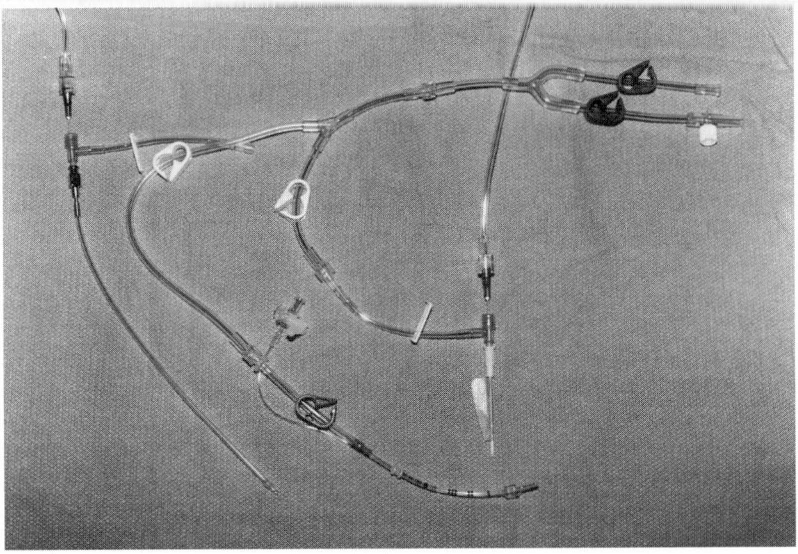

FIGURE 3.
Clinical setup for pediatric cardioplegia delivery. Cardioplegia inflow is circled to a vent line. Thus, once the cross-clamp is released, the aortic root may be vented through the same cardioplegia line. The cardioplegia inflow line is connected with a Y tube to the antegrade and retrograde lines. Antegrade cardioplegia is delivered through an IV cannula (the gauge is varied according to patient weight) that has a side port hole at its tip. Two retrograde cannulas are shown here: a standard pediatric retrograde cannula with a pressure port and a Spencer coronary perfusion cannula. Both the retrograde Spencer cannula and the antegrade IV cannula are connected to a T piece that allows a 22-gauge needle to directly measure cardioplegia line pressure.

cases a purse-string suture can be placed about the sinus ostium (care must be taken to avoid the atrioventricular node) to prevent regurgitation.

For pediatric patients, pediatric transatrial cannulas that are effective for patients around 20 kg and above are available. For pediatric patients less than 20 kg, we open the right atrium and directly cannulate the sinus. A purse-string suture is then applied. We have found that the Spencer coronary artery perfusion cannula work quite well for pediatric retroperfusion (Fig 3). A T piece should be added to allow pressure monitoring during cardioplegia delivery. This system has been used effectively in neonates 3 kg or larger. For pediatric patients 5 kg or less, we deliver the cardioplegia by hand through syringes.

The question of which approach to use, transatrial or direct with a purse-string suture, frequently arises. The answer is never absolute, however, and we individualize the decision according to the clinical situation. In general, the direct approach is used in (1) pediatric patients less than 20 kg, (2) any case in which the right atrium is to be opened, (3) any patient with significant right ventricular hypertrophy, and (4) cases in which cross-clamp times are expected to run 120 minutes or more.

CLINICAL APPROACHES TO MYOCARDIAL PROTECTION VIA RETROGRADE CARDIOPLEGIA

As was described earlier, we currently believe that the use of both antegrade and retrograde cardioplegia enhances overall microvascular distribution. This will be reflected later inasmuch as virtually all our clinical approaches to myocardial protection involve both antegrade and retrograde cardioplegia. Additionally, for most procedures both warm and cold cardioplegia is used. We and others call this "an integrated approach to myocardial protection." This generally involves a warm continuous cardioplegia dose for initiation of arrest, intermittent cold cardioplegia doses for maintenance, and warm continuous cardioplegia for reperfusion. The integrated warm-cold-warm strategy affords two theoretical advantages. First, a single cross-clamp technique is used. It is believed that both the location and the total number of times an aortic clamp is applied relate to the number of embolic complications associated with cardiac surgery.[40] Second, the cross-clamp is released only after the heart is beating regularly with the heart completely unloaded. In other techniques, the cross-clamp may be released before the heart is beating regularly. In such cases, if mild aortic insufficiency is present or if unloading of the heart is not complete, the heart will become distended. Distension is in effect an elevation of left ventricular end-diastolic pressure. When left ventricular end-diastolic pressure becomes close to extracorporeal perfusion pressure, coronary flow is seriously reduced. Under these circumstances, ventricular fibrillation frequently occurs. Distension and fibrillation occurring as a result of ischemia are particularly injurious near the time of reperfusion. Therefore, whenever possible we do not remove the cross-clamp until the heart is beating regularly. We use blood cardioplegia for all procedures in which diastolic arrest is induced and maintained. We use four basic crystalloid cardioplegic solutions, all of which contain four parts blood to one part crystalloid. These solutions are standard arrest, warm

TABLE 4.
Composition of Solutions Used for Cardioplegia (Four Parts Blood to One Part Crystalloid)

Solution	Composition
Standard arrest	500 mL 0.2 mol/L NS 200 mL 0.3 mol/L Tham 50 mL CPD* 60 mmol/L KCl
Warm arrest†	500 mL 0.2 mol/L NS 200 mL 0.3 mol/L Tham 50 mL CPD* 60 mmol/L KCl 250 mL 0.46 mol/L monosodium glutamate/aspartate
Standard maintenance	500 mL 0.2 mol/L NS 200 mL 0.3 mol/L Tham 50 mL CPD* 30 mmol/L KCl
Modified reperfusion†	500 mL 0.2 mol/L NS 200 mL 0.3 mol/L Tham 50 mL CPD* 30 mmol/L KCl 250 cm3 0.46 mol/L monosodium glutamate/aspartate

*Decreasing the CPD amount will result in increased ionized calcium levels.
†When appropriate, mechanical leukocyte filtering may be added (see the text).
Abbreviations: NS, normal saline; *Tham,* tromethamine; *CPD,* citrate/phosphate/dextrose.

arrest ("induction," "resuscitation," or "hot shot"), standard maintenance, and modified reperfusion (Table 4). When completed, these cardioplegic solutions have a pH of 7.6–7.7, an osmolality of approximately 320 mOsm, an ionized calcium content of 0.6–0.8 mmol/L, and a potassium level of 8–10 or 16–20 mmol/L. Calcium levels are adjusted by adding or reducing citrate-phosphate-dextrose. One may also use cardioplegia solutions depleted of leukocytes by leukocyte filtering. We have used this process clinically for cardiac transplantation and neonatal heart surgery.

CORONARY ARTERY SURGERY

When we suspect that the myocardium is stressed or energy depleted, we begin coronary procedures with warm induction cardioplegia given antegradely and then retrogradely. The myocardium is then cooled with antegrade followed by retrograde cardioplegia. For elective procedures when normal ventricular function is present, warm induction is not required. Intermittent cold blood cardioplegia is used during distal anastomosis. If a right-sided graft is required, we perform this distal anastomosis first. Intermittent cold retrograde cardioplegia may then be delivered concurrently with antegrade right-graft perfusion in between distal anastomosis. We believe that this combination ensures good right ventricular and left ventricular capillary cardioplegic flow. Additional antegrade grafts may be perfused to left heart coronary vessels, but this not necessary. If no right-sided graft is needed, half-antegrade, half-retrograde intermittent cold doses may be delivered during distal construction.

We use a single cross-clamp technique for coronary surgery. During proximal construction an initial dose of retrograde warm reperfusion cardioplegia is given and followed by warm continuous retrograde cardioplegia with the aortic root actively vented. If a right-sided graft is present, this is simultaneously perfused with the retrograde cardioplegia. We perform the proximal anastomosis to the right-sided graft last. During construction of the final proximal anastomosis, warm unmodified pump blood is given. The pump blood washes out the cardioplegia solution, and the heart generally regains a sinus or junctional rhythm at this time. Once the final proximal anastomosis is complete, care should be taken to de-air the left ventricle and aortic root. The retrograde blood is stopped and antegrade blood given with the cross-clamp remaining on. The grafts are then de-aired by needle and the cross-clamp removed. The aortic root is then vented until the patient is weaned from bypass.

This approach is used for uncomplicated redo coronary procedures as well. On occasion, one may be operating when a fresh clot is present within a vein graft or the old vein graft is suspected of embolizing atherosclerotic material. In such cases, initial arrest may be better achieved with retrograde cardioplegia alone to prevent potential embolization. In such situations, antegrade cardioplegia is given only through constructed grafts and not the aortic root. If ventricular function is poor or if prolonged cross-clamp times are anticipated, we often use bicaval cannulation and directly cannulate the coronary sinus. This is done through an atriotomy and with a purse-string suture about the sinus.

AORTIC VALVE SURGERY

Coronary sinus perfusion for myocardial protection was initially introduced by Dr. Lillehei in 1956 for aortic procedures.[41] Coronary sinus perfusion remains extremely useful for aortic valve procedures. We begin these procedures with a warm arrest followed by a cold dose. For aortic stenosis, it is frequently possible to arrest the heart antegradely without ventricular distension occurring. If this is not possible or if aortic insufficiency is present, the heart may be arrested initially with retrograde cardioplegia. An interesting observation is nearly always noted during warm transatrial retrograde arrest of the heart: the left ventricle becomes electrically silent well before the right ventricle. Indeed, it is very common for the right ventricle to begin fibrillating while the left ventricle is fully arrested. Subsequently, the right ventricle will arrest, particularly when cold cardioplegia is begun. We believe that this is further clinical evidence that with transatrial coronary sinus perfusion, left ventricular capillary flow greatly exceeds right ventricular capillary flow. As such, if initial arrest must be undertaken retrogradely, we believe that the aorta should be opened quickly and individual right coronary ostial perfusion begun with a hand-held coronary perfusion cannula. Both retrograde and direct right coronary perfusion may be performed simultaneously.

We have used cold intermittent retrograde cardioplegia during the period that the aortic root is open. Every third dose, or approximately every 40 minutes, we add a simultaneous antegrade direct right coronary dose. During closure of the aortotomy, we begin continuous warm retrograde cardioplegia, first with a reperfusion dose. During the final few minutes of closure, this is changed to unmodified warm blood from the perfusion circuit. The heart then regains a rhythm, and after de-airing, warm blood is given antegradely as further de-airing is performed. The cross-clamp is then released with the heart beating. If the heart is believed to be energy depleted, the initial warm arrest cardioplegic dose may be substrate enhanced.

MITRAL VALVE SURGERY

We perform mitral valve procedures with bicaval cannulation. The mitral valve may then be approached through either the left or the right atrium with opening of the septum. For redo procedures, complex repairs, or procedures associated with coronary artery bypass, the right atrial approach allows for direct coronary sinus perfusion with purse-string suture placement. This ensures good retrograde cardioplegic distribution and allows for three or four retrograde doses to be given without a supplemental antegrade dose, which expedites the conduct of these operations and reduces cross-clamp time. The heart is initially arrested with warm and then cold antegrade and retrograde cardioplegia. Cold intermittent doses are then given as stated earlier. Warm reperfusion cardioplegia followed by warm continuous cardioplegia is begun during atriotomy closure or proximal coronary completion, depending on the procedure. As with aortic procedures, warm unmodified blood is given during final de-airing and the heart allowed to regain a rhythm before cross-clamp removal.

ASCENDING OR ARCH AORTIC SURGERY

Retrograde cardioplegia greatly facilitates ascending and arch aortic operations. We use bicaval cannulation for these procedures to allow for direct coronary sinus cannulation with a purse-string suture through an atriotomy, as well as retrograde cerebral perfusion during circulatory arrest. We always vent the left ventricle through the left superior pulmonary vein shortly after initiation of cardiopulmonary bypass to ensure that no ventricular distension occurs. It is beyond the scope of this text to present all our techniques of myocardial protection for the many variants of aortic procedures. However, we will present some general approaches.

If the procedure is such that systemic hypothermia is not required or the initial arrest may be performed before systemic hypothermia is induced, a warm induction arrest is performed. If this is not possible, the heart will generally be bradycardiac and hypothermic at the time of initial arrest. As such, it is arrested with cold standard arrest cardioplegia. If the aortic valve is competent and a cardioplegia cannula can be safely placed in the ascending aorta, the initial arrest is performed antegradely. This is not generally the case, so the initial arrest is frequently performed retrogradely. This initial arrest is best performed by direct coronary sinus cannulation with purse-string suture placement. We believe that the coronary sinus should not be occluded until antegrade coronary flow is halted. Therefore, either pump flow should be discontinued (circulatory arrest cases) or a cross-clamp applied and then the purse-string suture placed and retrograde flow begun. Shortly after retrograde arrest the aorta is opened and the coronary ostia identified. Supplemental antegrade right coronary artery perfusion may then be given. Intermittent cold retrograde maintenance cardioplegia may be used during the procedure with a supplemental antegrade direct coronary artery dose given approximately every third dose or 40 minutes. If conduct of the operation permits, a warm continuous reperfusion approach should be used as described for aortic valve procedures. If this is not possible and coronary reperfusion must occur when the extracorporeal circuit perfusate is still hypothermic, it should be done with the left ventricle decompressed and the aorta, left ventricle, and left atrium carefully deaired.

PEDIATRIC SURGERY

Because the majority of pediatric procedures are intracardiac, retrograde cardioplegia may be easily and reliably used. With bicaval cannulation the coronary sinus may be directly cannulated and a purse-string suture applied for occlusion. As described earlier, commercially available pediatric cannulas are available and work well for patients 20 kg or greater. For patients 3 kg and above, Spencer coronary perfusion cannulas work well (see Fig 3). It is very important to directly measure retrograde pressure in pediatric patients. Small variations in flow can translate into large changes in pressure. For patients 5 kg and below, it is advisable to hand-deliver the cardioplegia solution to ensure appropriate pressure (i.e., 30–40 mm Hg).

For most procedures in which bicaval cannulation is used, myocardial protection can be performed as follows. The heart is initially arrested with warm blood cardioplegia and then cold blood cardioplegia delivered antegradely. Warm induction cardioplegia may be used if the heart is thought to be energy depleted. The right atrium is opened and a purse-string suture is placed about the coronary sinus and the cardioplegia cannula introduced. Subsequent intermittent cold cardioplegic doses are given retrogradely. Every third to fourth dose or every 35–50 minutes, an antegrade dose may be given. Just before an antegrade dose, it is important to de-air the aortic root. This prevents air being delivered down the coronary arteries, which leads to uneven and poor cardioplegic distribution. Air can be removed from the aortic root by submerging the heart in saline solution or blood, delivering retrograde cardioplegia, and gently pulling on the aortic root with a syringe attached to the antegrade cardioplegia cannula. When de-airing of the root is complete, the antegrade cannula may be reattached to the cardioplegia line and antegrade cardioplegia given. It is not necessary to release the coronary sinus purse-string suture during intermittent cold maintenance antegrade cardioplegia delivery inasmuch as the effluent drains through thebesian veins.

When the procedure is complete, an initial dose of reperfusion cardioplegia followed by warm continuous blood cardioplegia is given. During the final few minutes of the procedure, warm unmodified blood is started. This is generally done as the right atriotomy is closed around the cardioplegia cannula and purse-string snare. The heart then regains a rhythm and the aortic root is de-aired. Antegrade unmodified blood is then given and the retrograde cannula and purse-string snare removed. The left ventricle and left atrium are de-aired and the cross-clamp removed with the heart decompressed and beating. This approach is easily used for ventricular septal defect closure, repair of tetralogy of Fallot, repair of double-outlet right ventricle, etc. With modification, the retrograde approach may be used for the arterial switch operation, repair of truncus arteriosus, repair of anomalous coronary artery, and others. In neonates, we frequently add leukocyte depletion to the initial arrest induction cardioplegia and reperfusion cardioplegia.

TECHNICAL CONSIDERATIONS

During retrograde cardioplegic administration one should be certain that the cannula is well positioned and that the dose is being delivered to the myocardium. During transatrial cannulation, the catheter should be placed well into the sinus to prevent dislodgment upon positioning of the heart. By placing the left hand over the right ventricular outflow tract and then the left atrial appendage, the cannula's tip should be felt just below the left atrial appendage. During a cardioplegic dose, pressure should be monitored. A pressure of 30–40 mm Hg should typically be obtained with an infusion rate of 0.5 mL/g of myocardium per minute. Thus, a typical 300-g heart should have a retrograde flow of approximately 150 mL/min. If a low pressure is obtained, the cannula may lie in the right atrium, inferior vena cava, or right ventricle. If the cannula is placed too deep into the sinus, it may perforate the sinus into the pericardium or more commonly perforate the sinus into the left atrium. If good coronary sinus position is observed and low pressure continues, a persistent left superior vena cava may be present.

During retrograde perfusion, a crude assessment of the quality of perfusion can be made by observing the epicardium of the heart. The epicardial veins of both ventricles should be full. However, the LAD vein will typically be fuller than the PDA vein as described earlier. Smaller epicardial veins should be full with oxygenated cardioplegia flow on both the left and right ventricles. If the atria or ventricles have been opened, oxygenated blood should flow from their edges. If the heart is opened, its chambers should fill with bright red thebesian effluent. The aortic root effluent should be noted. If the aorta is open, at least one quarter the delivered cardioplegia dose should be seen exiting the two coronary ostia. If the aorta is closed, it should be vented so that at least one quarter of the administered dose will be found to be returned. If these conditions are not noted, cardioplegia delivery is likely to be inadequate.

At times, transatrial coronary sinus cannulation is difficult or impossible. This may be related to several factors such as a small coronary sinus, a prominent ostial valve, or even the lack of a coronary sinus. If the cannula cannot be introduced when the heart is full, cardiopulmonary bypass should be initiated. The apex of the heart can then be elevated and the origin of the coronary sinus inspected. An attempt to pass the catheter can be made under direct vision. If this is not successful, we then attempt to pass a pediatric retrograde cannula. If this is not possible, it is important to inspect the coronary sinus anatomically. If the sinus is not visualized in the atrioventricular groove with its PDA, middle cardiac, and LAD vein entering it, the sinus may not anatomically exist. If this is the case, further attempts at retrograde cannulation should be abandoned. If a normal-appearing sinus is present but still cannot be cannulated, one should assess the importance of retrograde cardioplegia in context of the overall procedure. If it is deemed mandatory, the technique can be converted to bicaval cannulation and the right atrium opened. Direct cannulation is nearly always possible when an epicardially normal-appearing coronary sinus is present. Frequently, upon opening the atria a prominent valve or membrane is present. Other times an atrial muscle bundle may straddle the orifice.

It is frequently possible to see the anatomy of the coronary sinus on preoperative angiograms. This is particularly true in the left anterior oblique view and with digital cineangiography. We now ask our cardiologists to obtain one left anterior oblique view of left main injection with venous follow-through. If a particularly small sinus is noted, we prepare to cannulate this with a pediatric retrograde cannula. If the sinus is short, we have found that with routine adult cannula placement the tip frequently dislodges into the right atrium upon positioning of the heart.[42] If retrograde use is deemed important, such procedures may be performed with bicaval cannulation and direct coronary sinus cannulation.

Retrograde cardioplegia may also be a useful approach to help in de-airing the heart. This is particularly true with less invasive approaches to valvular surgery in which elevation of the left ventricle and needle de-airing are impossible. Because some of the retrograde cardioplegia dose flows into the left atrium and ventricle through thebesian veins, air may be displaced with this cardioplegia solution if the aortic root or left ventricle is vented. When a good period of warm continuous retrograde cardioplegia is used with aortic root venting and intermittent ventilation, nearly all left-sided air can be removed without needling the left atrium or ventricle. Intraoperative transesophageal echocardiography is very helpful in ensuring adequate de-airing of the left-sided chambers when retrograde cardioplegia/blood is used during minimally invasive valvular procedures.

CLINICAL RESULTS WITH RETROGRADE CARDIOPLEGIA

Several institutions and authors have demonstrated the clinical efficacy of retrograde cardioplegia used alone or in combination with antegrade cardioplegia.[17, 43–46] Unfortunately, development of the antegrade and retrograde delivery approach as well as the warm and cold approach to myocardial protection has led to controversy regarding the optimum technique. Indeed, the merits of continuous or intermittent cold antegrade vs. warm antegrade vs. cold retrograde vs. warm retrograde are frequently debated in the literature.[47–50] Taken on the whole, there is little evidence to suggest that one technique is superior to any other when it is used universally for all procedures. Indeed, the advantages that warm continuous retrograde cardioplegia may have over intermittent cold antegrade cardioplegia in acute coronary occlusion cases may be negated by its disadvantages for mitral stenosis cases when pulmonary hypertension and right ventricular hypertrophy are present without coronary disease. If only one approach is used for all cases, mediocrity is ensured.

We believe that each procedure should be individualized and an "integrated approach to myocardial protection" used to take advantage of warm or cold, intermittent or continuous, retrograde or antegrade techniques for myocardial protection. Furthermore, the approach to myocardial protection should be planned so that overall short- and long-term results are optimized. In other words, in an octogenarian patient with a normal ejection fraction, the mortality risk of stroke is greater that the risk of myocardial failure. This suggests that a myocardial protection strategy should be planned in which a single cross-clamp technique is used. In a 40-year-old with a normal ejection fraction, the predicted mortality from all causes is near 1%. Mortality related to myocardial protection is well less than 1%. For such procedures, the mortality difference resulting from differing myocardial protection techniques must be very small. Indeed, the patient's 10-year survival is much more closely related to the quality of distal anastomosis than to the technique of myocardial protection. Does it make sense to perform this procedure with continuous cardioplegia or intermittent cardioplegia? An integrated approach to myocardial protection allows the surgeon the freedom to use retrograde cardioplegia to its full advantage within the context of the entire operation.

REFERENCES

1. Salerno TA, Houck JP, Barrozo CAM, et al: Retrograde continuous warm blood cardioplegia: A new concept in myocardial protection. *Ann Thorac Surg* 51:245, 1991.
2. Julia P, Kofsky ER, Buckberg GD, et al: Studies of myocardial protection in the immature heart: III. Models of ischemic and hypoxic/ischemic injury in the puppy heart. IV. Improved tolerance of immature myocardium to hypoxia and ischemia by intravenous support. *J Thorac Cardiovasc Surg* 101:14, 1991.
3. Rosenkranz E, Okamoto F, Buckberg GD, et al: Safety of prolonged aortic cross-clamping with blood cardioplegia. III. Aspartate enrichment of glutamate blood cardioplegia in energy-depleted hearts. *J Thorac Cardiovasc Surg* 91:428, 1986.
4. Lazar HL, Buckberg GD, Manganaro AM, et al: Myocardial energy replenishment and reversal of ischemic damage by substrate enhancement of secondary blood cardioplegia with amino-acids during reperfusion. *J Thorac Cardiovasc Surg* 80:350, 1980.
5. Allen BS, Okamoto F, Buckberg GD, et al: Studies of controlled reperfusion after ischemia. XIII. Reperfusate conditions: Critical importance of total ventricular decompression during regional reperfusion. *J Thorac Cardiovasc Surg* 92:605S, 1986.
6. Buckberg GD: Recent advances in myocardial protection using antegrade/retrograde blood cardioplegia. *Eur Heart J* 10:43, 1989.
7. Buckberg GD: Myocardial temperature management during aortic clamping for cardiac surgery. *J Thorac Cardiovasc Surg* 102:895, 1991.
8. Opie LH: Reperfusion injury and its pharmacologic modification. *Circulation* 80:1049, 1989.
9. Boli R: Mechanisms of myocardial "stunning." *Circulation* 82:723, 1990.
10. Allen BS, Okamoto F, Buckberg GD, et al: Studies of controlled reperfusion after ischemia: XVI. Early recovery of regional wall motion in patients following surgical revascularization after eight hours of acute coronary occlusion. *J Thorac Cardiovasc Surg* 92:636, 1998.
11. Foglia RP, Buckberg GD, Lazar HL: The effectiveness of mannitol after ischemic myocardial edema. *Surg Forum* 30:320, 1980.
12. Haan C, Lazar HL, Bernard S, et al: Superiority of retrograde cardioplegia after acute coronary artery occlusion. *Ann Thorac Surg* 51:408–412, 1991.

13. Gundry SR, Kirsh MM: A comparison of retrograde cardioplegia versus antegrade cardioplegia in the presence of coronary artery obstruction. *Ann Thorac Surg* 38:125, 1984.
14. Gates RN, Laks H, Drinkwater DC Jr, et al: Can improved microvascular perfusion be achieved using both antegrade and retrograde cardioplegia? *Ann Thorac Surg* 60:1308, 1995.
15. Gates RN, Lee J, Laks H, et al: Evidence of improved microvascular perfusion when using antegrade and retrograde cardioplegia. *Ann Thorac Surg* 62:1388, 1996.
16. Kaley G, Altura BM: In Kaley G (ed): *Microcirculation.* Baltimore, Md, University Park Press, 1977, p 121.
17. Drinkwater DC, Cushin C, Laks H, et al: The use of combined antegrade-retrograde cardioplegia in pediatric open-heart surgery. *J Thorac Cardiovasc Surg* 104:1349, 1992.
18. Allen BS, Murcia-Evans D, Hartz RS: Integrated cardioplegia allows complex valve repairs in all patients. *Ann Thorac Surg* 62:23, 1996.
19. Evans CL, Starling EH: The part played by the lungs in the oxidative processes of the body. *J Physiol* 46:413, 1913.
20. Gregg DE: *Coronary Circulation in Health and Disease.* Philadelphia, Lea & Febiger, 1953.
21. Thebesius AC: *Dissertatio Medica de Circulo Sanguinus in Corde.* Lugduni Batavorum, Elsevier, 1708.
22. Grant RT, Viko LE: Observations on the anatomy of the thebesian vessels of the heart. *Heart* 15:103, 1929.
23. Smith GT: The anatomy of the coronary circulation. *Am J Cardiol* 9:327, 1962.
24. Parsonnet V: The anatomy of the veins of the human heart with special reference to normal anastomotic channels. *J Med Soc N J* 50:446, 1953.
25. Thorton JJ, Gregg DE: Effect of chronic cardiac venous occlusion on coronary arterial and cardiac venous hemodynamics. *Am J Physiol* 128:179, 1939.
26. Lee J, Gates RN, Laks H, et al: A comparison of distribution between simultaneously or sequentially delivered antegrade/retrograde blood cardioplegia. *J Card Surg* 11:111, 1996.
27. Ihnken K, Morita K, Buckberg GD, et al: The safety of simultaneous arterial and coronary sinus perfusion: Experimental background and initial clinical results. *J Card Surg* 9:15, 1994.
28. Beck CS, Stanton E, Batinchok W, et al: Revascularization of the heart by graft of systemic artery into the coronary sinus. *JAMA* 137:436, 1948.
29. Eckstein RW, Hornberger JC, Sano T: Acute effects of elevation of coronary sinus pressure. *Circulation* 7:422, 1953.
30. Gates RN, Laks H, Drinkwater DC, et al: The microvascular distribution of cardioplegic solution in piglet hearts: Retrograde versus antegrade delivery. *J Thorac Cardiovasc Surg* 105:845–853, 1993.

31. Lolley DM, Hewitt RL: Myocardial distribution of asanguinous solutions retroperfused under low pressure through the coronary sinus. *J Cardiovasc Surg* 21:287, 1980.
32. Shiki K, Masuda M, Yoneenaga K, et al: Myocardial distribution of retrograde flow through the coronary sinus of the excised normal canine heart. *Ann Thorac Surg* 41:265, 1986.
33. Stirling MC, McClanahan TB, Schott RJ, et al: Distribution of cardioplegic solution infused antegradely and retrogradely in normal canine heart. *J Thorac Cardiovasc Surg* 98:1066–1076, 1989.
34. Gates RN, Laks H, Drinkwater DC, et al: Gross and microvascular distribution of retrograde cardioplegia in explanted human hearts. *Ann Thorac Surg* 56:410, 1993.
35. Ardehali A, Gates RN, Laks H, et al: The regional capillary distribution of retrograde blood cardioplegia in explanted human hearts. *J Thorac Cardiovasc Surg* 109:935, 1995.
36. Allen BS, Winkelman JW, Hanafy H, et al: Retrograde cardioplegia does not adequately perfuse the right ventricle. *J Thorac Cardiovasc Surg* 109:116, 1995.
37. Aronson S, Lee BK, Zaroff JG, et al: Myocardial distribution of cardioplegic solution after retrograde delivery in patients undergoing cardiac surgical procedures. *J Thorac Cardiovasc Surg* 105:214–221, 1993.
38. Rudis E, Gates RN, Laks H, et al: Coronary sinus ostial occlusion during retrograde delivery of cardioplegic solution significantly improves cardioplegic distribution and efficacy. *J Thorac Cardiovasc Surg* 109:941–947, 1995.
39. Menasche P, Kural S, Fauchet M: Retrograde coronary sinus perfusion: A safe alternative for ensuring cardioplegic delivery in aortic valve surgery. *Ann Thorac Surg* 34:647, 1982.
40. Wareing TH, Davila-Roman VG, Brarzilia B, et al: Management of the severely atherosclerotic ascending aorta during cardiac operations: A strategy for detection and treatment. *J Thorac Cardiovasc Surg* 103:453, 1992.
41. Lillehei CW: Direct vision correction of calcific aortic stenosis by means of a pump-oxygenator and retrograde coronary sinus perfusion. *Dis Chest* 30:123, 1956.
42. Author's unpublished data.
43. Menasche P, Subayi JB, Veyssie L, et al: Efficacy of coronary sinus cardioplegia in patients with complete coronary occlusion. *Ann Thorac Surg* 51:418, 1991.
44. Diehl JT, Eichhorn EJ, Konstam MA, et al: Efficacy of retrograde coronary sinus perfusion in patients undergoing myocardial revascularization: A prospective randomized trial. *Ann Thorac Surg* 45:595, 1988.
45. Arom KV, Emery RW: Coronary sinus cardioplegia: A clinical trial with only retrograde approach. *Ann Thorac Surg* 53:965, 1992.

46. Bhayana JN, Kalmbach T, Booth FV, et al: Combined antegrade/retrograde cardioplegia for myocardial protection: A clinical trial. *J Thorac Cardiovasc Surg* 98:956, 1989.
47. Carrier M, Pelletier LC, Searle NR: Does retrograde administration of blood cardioplegia improve myocardial protection during first operation for coronary bypass grafting? *Ann Thorac Surg* 64:1256, 1997.
48. Louagie YA, Gonzales E, Jamart J, et al: Assessment of continuous cold blood cardioplegia in coronary bypass grafting. *Ann Thorac Surg* 63:689, 1997.
49. Arom KV, Emery RW, Peterson RJ, et al: Evaluation of 7000+ patients with two different routes of cardioplegia. *Ann Thorac Surg* 63:1619, 1997.
50. Kamlot A, Bellows SD, Simkhovich BZ, et al: Is warm retrograde blood cardioplegia better than cold for myocardial protection? *Ann Thorac Surg* 63:98, 1997.

CHAPTER 6

Transmyocardial Laser Revascularization

Keith A. Horvath, M.D.
Assistant Professor of Surgery, Division of Cardiothoracic Surgery, Northwestern University Medical School, Chicago, Illinois

Transmyocardial laser revascularization (TMR) involves the use of laser energy to create a transmural channel through ischemic myocardium. Theoretically, blood within the ventricle can directly perfuse the heart via the laser channels, and the ensuing stimulation of angiogenesis causes an increase in collateral vessel development. At present, three different types of laser light are being used for this technique: CO_2, holmium:YAG, and excimer. The procedure has been performed via thoracotomy, via thoracoscopy, and percutaneously. The early results have been encouraging, the long-term results are pending, and the exact mechanism is unclear.

Attempts to revascularize the heart by direct perfusion were first described by Beck and later by Vineberg.[1, 2] The success of Vineberg's technique of internal mammary artery implantation demonstrated that direct perfusion was possible and, as evidenced by angiograms, even led to neovascularization and collateral formation. With these findings and an understanding of the reptilian heart, Sen and others performed direct perfusion by transmyocardial acupuncture.[3–10] The limited success of these procedures was overshadowed by the discovery of the ability to perform coronary artery bypass grafting (CABG). Interest in direct perfusion has resurfaced inasmuch as the number of patients who cannot be treated by either CABG or by percutaneous transluminal coronary angioplasty (PTCA) is growing. Transmyocardial laser revascularization has been developed to treat these patients. The mechanical trauma that resulted in poor long-term patency of transmyocardial acupuncture was overcome in theory by the use of a laser to create the channels. Laser energy ablates the tissue in a less traumatic fashion than can be accomplished by acupuncture. Mirohseini first used a laser to perform this type of revascularization, and it was used in combination with CABG in a number of patients in the early 1980s.[11–15] The CO_2 laser he used was relatively low powered and therefore required an arrested heart. Although his results seemed encouraging, it proved difficult to assess the contribution of laser revascularization when combined with CABG. With time, a laser was developed to perform the procedure on a beating heart and allowed the introduction of TMR as sole therapy for unreconstructable coronary artery disease.

CLINICAL EXPERIENCE

Three different wavelengths of laser light are being used clinically to perform TMR: holmium:YAG, excimer, and CO_2. The largest series with the longest follow-up has used the CO_2 laser. Since 1990, over 4,000 patients worldwide have been treated with this laser. After an initial study on 15 patients that established the safety of the procedure, a multicenter nonrandomized study was performed on 200 patients.[16] The entry criteria for this study were patients with severe angina that was refractory to medical therapy. They had to have evidence of reversible ischemia. Additionally, they could not be candidates for PTCA, CABG, or heart transplantation. Preoperatively, the patients' recent angiograms were reviewed to confirm that they were not candidates for conventional revascularization. Additionally, their anginal class was assessed and their antianginal medications were reviewed, as were their admissions to the hospital for angina in the year before the procedure. To evaluate the extent and severity of their ischemia, all patients underwent myocardial perfusion scans at rest and with stress. After documentation of a significant area of reversible ischemia, the patients were enrolled in the study. Eighty percent of the patients were men, and they had an average age of 63 years (range, 35–85 years). Eighty percent had had a previous CABG, and many had undergone two or three previous bypass operations. Likewise, 40% of the patients had had a prior PTCA and, in some cases, up to 11 previous angioplasties. Thirty-five percent had diabetes and 70% were hypertensive. The patients' average ejection fraction was 47% (range, 15% to 77%). All of the patients were in Canadian Cardiovascular Society anginal class III (20%) or IV (80%).

Intraoperatively, the patients had a transesophageal echocardiography (TEE) probe inserted. With the patients in a 45-degree right lateral decubitus position, an anterior thoracotomy was performed through the fifth intercostal space (Fig 1, A).

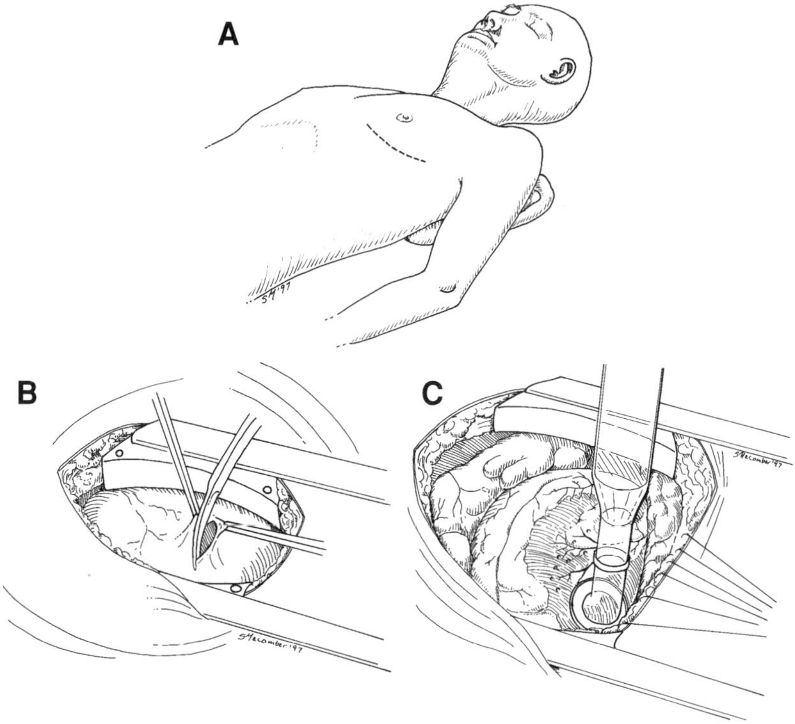

FIGURE 1.

A, operative positioning and incision for transmyocardial laser revascularization. **B,** pericardial opening via left anterior thoracotomy in the fifth intercostal space. **C,** laser handpiece against myocardium with typical placement and distribution of the laser channels.

The pericardium was then opened anteriorly to the left phrenic nerve, and the area of ischemic myocardium was exposed (Fig 1, B). The laser handpiece was then introduced through the chest wall and pericardium. With the aid of an HeNe aiming laser, the handpiece was positioned against the epicardium and the CO_2 laser was fired. In addition to the handpiece being at the end of an articulated arm, which allows easy positioning, a right-angle handpiece is available to treat the posterior and inferior regions (Fig 1, C). The pericardium can then be loosely reapproximated and the thoracotomy closed over one or two chest tubes. Single-lung ventilation is helpful intraoperatively, and thoracic epidural anesthesia can be beneficial for early postoperative pain control.

The patients received an average of 25 channels, which were confirmed to be transmural by TEE. The average laser pulse energy was 13 J with a pulse width of 50 msec. The average operative time was 2 hours with a laser time of 20 minutes. The 1-mm channels were created in a distribution of approximately $1/cm^2$. Hemorrhage from the channels was controlled by direct finger pressure or an epicardial suture if the finger pressure was inadequate. The majority of the patients were extubated in the operating room or within the first 18 hours postoperatively. The patients spent an average of 2 days in the ICU and 8 days in the hospital.

Although there were no intraoperative laser-induced arrhythmias, early morbidity included a 10% incidence of atrial fibrillation and a 2% incidence of myocardial infarction. Seven of the 200 patients had intra-aortic balloon pumps placed intraoperatively or in the initial postoperative period. The early mortality was 9% and the majority of these deaths were cardiac in nature. All of these patients who died early had unstable angina preoperatively, and 15 of the 18 had previously undergone a prior CABG. Additionally, patients with ejection fractions less than 40% and those older than 80 years were more likely to suffer perioperative mortality. Although it was not statistically significant, patients with unstable angina who received intravenous heparin and nitroglycerin en route to the operating room had a more complicated postoperative course. All of the patients were monitored for 1 year, and the late mortality was an additional 9%. Again, an ejection fraction less than 40% and age older than 80 years were independent risk factors for late mortality. There was a 4% reduction in perioperative mortality between the first 100 patients enrolled and the second 100 patients (11% to 7%). This reduction was undoubtedly caused by improved patient selection.

The patients returned for evaluation at 3, 6, and 12 months after the procedure. At these times they underwent repeat radionuclide perfusion scans, had their quality of life and angina class reassessed, and had their admissions for angina and antianginal medications reviewed. The overall survival rate was 83% at 1 year.

Preoperatively, the average angina class was 3.8. This improved to 1.46 at 3 months, 1.36 at 6 months, and 1.44 at 12 months. One hundred percent of the patients were in angina class III or IV preoperatively. Eighty percent of the patients dropped at least two angina classes, and 30% had no angina at each of the intervals postoperatively. Perfusion scans demonstrated a significant improvement in left ventricular perfusion at 6 and 12 months.[16] This decrease in the number of reversible defects was not accompanied by an increase in the number of fixed defects. In comparison, there

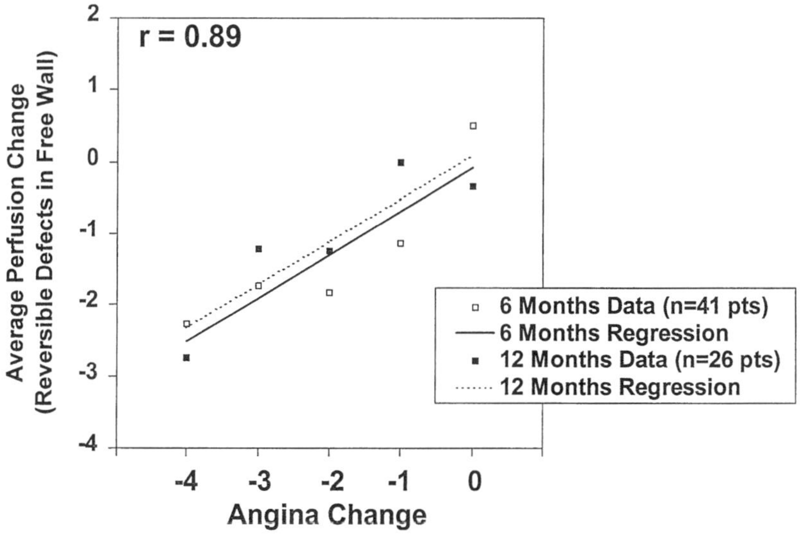

FIGURE 2.

Correlation of angina improvement and perfusion improvement for patients who underwent transmyocardial laser revascularization (phase II nonrandomized trial).

was no significant difference in the number of fixed or reversible defects in the untreated septum over the 12 months of follow-up. Again, when comparing the septum with the left ventricular free wall, there was no change in the resting perfusion of the septal region whereas there was an improvement in the resting perfusion in the left ventricular free wall. Additionally, there was a strong correlation between improvement in perfusion and a decrease in angina (Fig 2). The majority of the patients exhibited an improvement in perfusion and a corresponding improvement in angina class at 6 and 12 months.

At one institution, perfusion was studied by positron emission tomographic scanning.[17] In this study, subendocardial and subepicardial perfusion were compared. There was a significant improvement in perfusion overall, and this was most noticeable in the subendocardial region.

The patients' dosage and usage of nitrates, calcium channel blockers, and β-blockers were monitored throughout the study. All patients were initially restarted on their preoperative medications immediately after the procedure. At 1 year, 56% of the patients had decreased their usage of these cardioactive medications, and 19% had increased their medications.

Because of their end-stage coronary disease, these patients were frequently admitted to the hospital for angina. In the year before undergoing TMR, the patients averaged 2.5 admissions for angina. This average decreased to 0.5 admissions for angina after treatment ($P < 0.001$).

Of note, some patients (15) during the study as well as after the 1-year follow-up had undergone additional procedures such as PTCA, CABG, or cardiac transplantation. These patients underwent an additional intervention to treat progression of disease in their native vessels, in their previous bypass grafts, or as a result of progressive heart failure. Follow-up of patients longer than 1 year has been reported by individual institutions.[18] The results in these smaller groups of patients have been similar to those seen at the 1-year follow-up.

After reporting the results of this phase II nonrandomized study, a phase III trial was started with the same inclusion criteria, but the patients enrolled were randomized 1:1 to receive either TMR or continued maximal medical therapy. A total of 198 patients were enrolled in this multi-institutional study and were monitored for 1 year. The demographics for this study show no difference between patients randomized to laser treatment or those randomized to continue their medical management. Their average age was 62 years. Ninety percent had undergone a previous bypass operation, and 50% had undergone a previous angioplasty. Forty-five percent had diabetes and 60% had hypercholesterolemia. The average ejection fraction was 50% (range, 21% to 75%). All of the patients were in angina class III or IV at enrollment.

Intraoperatively, the patients received on average 30 channels confirmed by TEE. The median ICU stay was 2 days and the hospital stay was 8 days. At 12 months of follow-up, 70% of the patients treated with the laser showed a decrease of at least two angina classes whereas none of the medical management control group showed a significant improvement in angina class (Fig 3). Thirty percent of the control group had significant worsening of their angina over the period of follow-up.

Forty-eight percent of the laser group had a significant decrease in their use of β-blockers, calcium channel blockers, or nitrates over the period of follow-up. In contrast, only 11% of the control group had a significant decrease in their usage of these medications. Admission to a hospital ICU with administration of IV antianginal medications for at least 48 hours defined an unstable angina event. Figure 4 depicts the freedom from such episodes of unstable angina for both groups. As a result of few admissions for

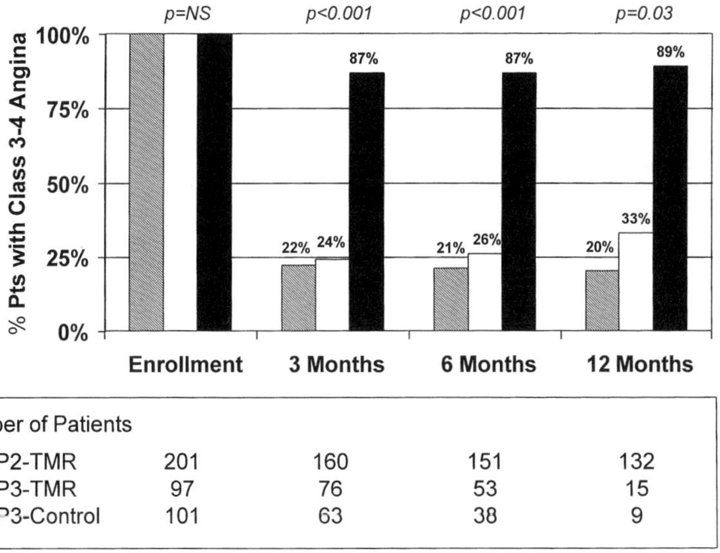

FIGURE 3.

Angina class distribution for phase II *(P2)* and phase III *(P3)* trials. *Abbreviations: TMR,* patients treated with transmyocardial CO_2 laser revascularization; *Control,* patients treated with medical therapy.

unstable angina, at our institution there was on average $4,700 savings over 6 months per patient treated with the laser as compared with the 6 months of medical treatment before TMR. Event-free survival for death, unstable angina, or class IV angina at 6 months was 77% for the TMR group vs. 22% for the medical management group ($P = 0.0001$). Quality-of-life indices increased an average of 130% for patients undergoing TMR as compared with no change in the medical management group. Final analysis of the 12-month single-proton emission CT perfusion data is pending, but preliminary results at 6 months indicate less ischemia in follow-up for patients treated with the laser as compared with those in the control group.

Mortality was 6% for the medical patients in the first 30 days of enrollment in the trial. After 6 months, patients in whom unstable angina developed were allowed to cross over from the medical group to the laser group. There was a 12% perioperative mortality for this crossover group as compared with a 4% perioperative mortality for patients having TMR initially. The crossover patients were, by definition, patients who had not only failed medical therapy but had also suffered an acute myocardial infarction and in whom postinfarction angina had developed or whose an-

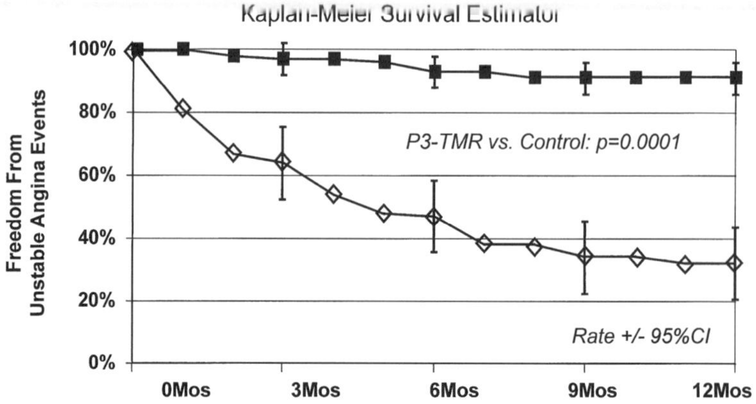

Number of Patients					
P3-TMR	97	95	73	47	47
P3-Control	101	68	33	21	18

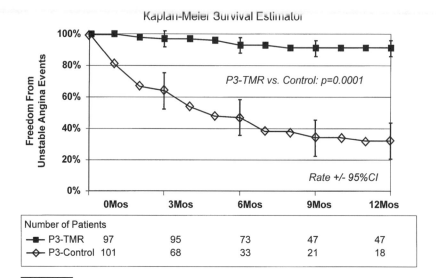

FIGURE 4.
Freedom from admissions for unstable angina in a prospective randomized phase III *(P3)* trial. *Abbreviations: TMR,* patients treated with transmyocardial CO_2 laser revascularization; *Control,* patients treated with medical therapy.

gina was unstable and only controllable by IV medications. This instability contributed to the higher perioperative mortality seen in the crossover group.

Final analysis and publication of these phase III data are forthcoming. At present, the Food and Drug Administration is allowing patients to be treated with TMR, and because 100 patients have been enrolled and are being monitored in the medical control group, the randomization has been stopped. Final review and approval of TMR based on these studies are pending.

In a retrospective analysis, patients with class III or IV angina who were either treated medically or underwent CABG, CABG with or without PTCA, or PTCA alone were compared with 100 patients from the same institution who underwent TMR with the CO_2 laser. Angina improvement was the same for TMR, CABG with or without PTCA, or PTCA alone. The degree of improvement with all of these therapies was significant when compared with patients treated by medical therapy alone ($P < 0.001$). Mortality at 6 and 12 months was less than 7% in patients treated with CABG with or without PTCA or treated with PTCA alone, but it was 12% for patients treated with TMR ($P < 0.001$). Mortality for the medical group was 14%. Although the mortality was the same for the laser-treated and medically treated groups, the patients treated with the laser had a significant reduction in angina.[19]

The results from a single institution have demonstrated similar improvement in angina status and, by serial dobutamine stress echocardiography, have documented an improvement in regional wall motion after TMR. Although there was no significant change at rest in global wall motion, there was a significant improvement in wall motion with dobutamine stress. These results were noted at 3 and 6 months after TMR.[20]

In addition to these clinical studies, autopsy studies have been performed on patients who have undergone TMR. One case report demonstrated patent channels in a patient 3 months after laser therapy.[21] Additional autopsy results from patients who died 3, 16, and 150 days after TMR have been described.[22] In these cases, 80% to 95% of the channels that had been created were found. In the early period after TMR, different stages of wound healing were noted in the laser channels.

At day 150 postoperatively, the laser-created channels showed scarring as well as an extensive capillary network. Patent or endothelialized channels were not demonstrated in this group of patients who were clinically noteworthy for their lack of response to TMR. The patients demonstrated no significant improvement in angina status in either the short term or the long term. This same group has demonstrated evidence of blood flow through the patent channels intraoperatively and up to 544 days postoperatively with the use of TEE. Again, patients who had evidence of Doppler blood flow through the channels were "*responders*" and had significant clinical improvement in their angina after TMR. Patients whose channels could not be identified were clinically "*nonresponders*" and did not have any improvement in their angina.

The aforementioned results were achieved with the use of a CO_2 laser. Early results with the use of a holmium:YAG laser have also been reported.[23, 24] Additionally, a few patients have been treated with an excimer laser.[25] Likewise, a few patients have been treated in the United States with a holmium:YAG laser delivered percutaneously via a catheter-based "inside-out" approach. This method creates 3-mm-deep partial channels into the endocardial surface of the left ventricle (unpublished). More patients have been treated percutaneously outside the United States, but the results have yet to be analyzed or published.

Ultimately, the potential largest use for this procedure is in combination with standard coronary artery bypass surgical revascularization—particularly in patients undergoing reoperative bypass surgery. Frequently there are vascular beds that can be bypassed and others that cannot in reoperative patients, and the use of TMR as an adjunct would be beneficial. Unfortunately, as was true of Mirhoseini's original clinical studies, the efficacy of the procedure needs to be shown when used as sole therapy before the use of it in combination with standard revascularization. An additional cohort of patients who may benefit from this procedure are cardiac transplant recipients in whom diffuse coronary disease has developed as a result of allograft rejection. Again, this application has been tried in a few cases, but significant numbers of patients with long-term results are pending.

MECHANISMS

Undoubtedly, the most interesting aspect of TMR is the potential mechanism or mechanisms of its effect. The possibility that these channels may improve perfusion and relieve angina has caused renewed interest in the study of chronic ischemia, the myocardial response to chronic ischemia, and the vascular remodeling of collateral formation. Proposed mechanisms include direct perfusion via patent channels, stimulation of angiogenesis, denervation, and the placebo effect.

Virtually every treatment for angina pectoris has been considered effective as a result of the placebo effect.[26] Surgical procedures in general carry the potential for a greater placebo effect because it is more difficult to eliminate bias on the part of the physician or the patient. Surgical procedures from ligation of the internal mammary artery to CABG have had their results ridiculed as being entirely due to placebo. Significant long-term improvement, objective measurements of results, and understanding of the mechanisms have led to the acceptance or rejection of surgical techniques. In the case of TMR, additional time and careful follow-up of patients will help determine the contribution of the placebo effect to the results.

Denervation has been suggested as a potential mechanism, and one animal study[27] has indicated that myocardium treated with the laser shows no response in mean arterial blood pressure in hearts treated with the laser and stimulated by bradykinin. This interesting result in a nonischemic canine model raises the question of denervation as a mechanism. The obvious concern is that TMR may create a situation in which patients' symptoms are improved because they cannot "feel" their angina as a result of denervation, and their symptomatic improvement may not be due to increased perfusion. Clinically, one would expect a significant increase in the number of adverse advents in patients treated with the laser as compared with matched patients continuing their medical therapy. This has not been observed. Additionally, the amount of myocardium that is ablated by the laser is less than 0.001% of the ventricle and is unlikely to completely or significantly denervate the heart. Furthermore, laser myocardial ablation (as used for the treatment of arrhythmias) eliminates similar or greater amounts of myocardium and has not been reported to change patients' anginal status or improve perfusion.

Angiogenesis is an obvious potential mechanism and would be the natural response to injury induced by the laser. The fact that the creation of new blood vessels or remodeling of existing blood vessels to improve collateral flow to ischemic myocardium treated with the laser is noted by perfusion scans that are significantly improved at 6 months supports the argument that angiogenesis is playing a role. Additional experimental work by several investigators has shown neovascularization and evidence of angiogenesis in and around the laser channels.[28] Enhancement of this response by the addition of angiogenic growth factors has also been shown experimentally.[29] The response of myocardium to chronic ischemia and the significant collateral formation that is frequently seen in these patients could be enhanced by the laser channels and the delivery of laser energy to the myocardium. Further investigation is being undertaken to determine whether there is significant upregulation of angiogenic growth factors in chronically ischemic laser-treated myocardium.

Direct channel patency early and endothelialization of these channels over time have also been proposed as a mechanism. The early clinical symptomatic improvement indicates that there may be improved perfusion immediately as a result of the channels. As mentioned, experimentally and clinically, channels have been found to be patent over time;[21, 30] however, several other reports have indicated that the channels have not remained patent.[22, 28]

Unfortunately, the majority of experimentation regarding mechanisms have used either nonischemic or acutely ischemic myocardium in animal models that are not analogous to the human coronary circulation or clinical scenario. Further experimental work in appropriate animal models is needed.

CONCLUSION

Transmyocardial laser revascularization has been shown to improve angina status in patients for whom no other option is available. Clinical studies—both nonrandomized and randomized—have yielded similar results regarding this angina class improvement. Perfusion scans have also demonstrated a decrease in the amount of ischemia in these patients. Although differences exist between the various wavelengths of light used, the amount of energy delivered, and the depth of penetration with different approaches, whether these differences will have an impact on the clinical results is unknown. Completion of the randomized controlled studies and further investigations are necessary to confirm these findings and to further elucidate the mechanism of TMR.

REFERENCES

1. Becks CS: The development of a new blood supply to the heart by operation. *Ann Surg* 102:801–813, 1935.
2. Vineberg A: Clinical and experimental studies in the treatment of coronary artery insufficiency by internal mammary artery implant. *J Int Coll Surg* 22:503–518, 1954.
3. Sen PK, Udwadia TE, Kinare SG, et al: Transmyocardial acupuncture: A new approach to myocardial revascularization. *J Thorac Cardiovasc Surg* 50:181–189, 1965.
4. Goldman A, Greenstone SM, Preuss FS: Experimental methods for producing a collateral circulation to the heart directly from the left ventricle. *J Thorac Surg* 31:364–374, 1956.
5. Massimo C, Boffi L: Myocardial revascularization by a new method of carrying blood directly from the left ventricular cavity into the coronary circulation. *J Thorac Surg* 34:257–264, 1957.
6. Khazei AH, Kime WP, Papadopoulos C, et al: Myocardial canalization: A new method of myocardial revascularization. *Ann Thorac Surg* 6:163–171, 1968.
7. Walter P, Hundeshagen H, Borst HG: Treatment of acute myocardial infarction by transmural blood supply from the ventricular cavity. *Eur Surg Res* 3:130–138, 1971.
8. Pifarré R, Jasuja ML, Lynch RD, et al: Myocardial revascularization by transmyocardial acupuncture: A physiologic impossibility. *J Thorac Cardiovasc Surg* 58:424–431, 1969.
9. Wakabayashi A, Little ST, Connoly JE: Myocardial boring for the ischemic heart. *Arch Surg* 95:743–752, 1967.
10. Anabtawi IN, Reigler HF, Ellison RG: Experimental evaluation of myocardial tunnelization as a method of myocardial revascularization. *J Thorac Cardiovasc Surg* 58:638–646, 1969.
11. Mirhoseini M, Cayton MM: Revascularization of the heart by laser. *J Microsurg* 2:253–260, 1981.

12. Mirhoseini M, Fisher JC, Cayton MM: Myocardial revascularization by laser: A clinical report. *Lasers Surg Med* 3:241–245, 1983.
13. Mirhoseini M, Shelgikar S, Cayton MM: New concepts in revascularization of the myocardium. *Ann Thorac Surg* 45:415–420, 1988.
14. Mirhoseini M, Muckerheide M, Cayton MM: Transventricular revascularization by laser. *Lasers Surg Med* 2:187–198, 1982.
15. Mirhoseini M, Cayton MM, Shelgikar S: Clinical report: Laser myocardial revascularization. *Lasers Surg Med* 6:459–461, 1986.
16. Horvath KA, Cohn LC, Cooley DA, et al: Transmyocardial revascularization: Results of a multi-center trial using TMR as sole therapy for end stage coronary artery disease. *J Thorac Cardiovasc Surg* 113:645–654, 1997.
17. Horvath KA, Mannting FR, Cummings N, et al: Transmyocardial laser revascularization. Operative techniques and clinical results at two years. *J Thorac Cardiovasc Surg* 111:1047–1053, 1996.
18. Frazier OH, Cooley DA, Kadipasaglu KA, et al: Myocardial revascularization with laser: Preliminary findings. *Circulation* 92:1158S–1165S, 1995.
19. Maisch B, Funck R, Herzum M, et al: Does transmyocardial laser revascularization influence prognosis in endstage coronary disease? *Circulation* 94:295S, 1996.
20. Donovan CL, Landolfo KP, Lowe JE, et al: Improvement in inducible ischemia during dobutamine stress echocardiography after transmyocardial laser revascularization in patients with refractory angina pectoris. *J Am Coll Cardiol* 30:607–612, 1997.
21. Cooley DA, Frazier OH, Kadipasaglu KA, et al: Transmyocardial laser revascularization: Anatomic evidence of long-term channel patency. *Tex Heart Inst J* 21:220–224, 1994.
22. Gassler N, Wintzer H, Stubbe H, et al: Transmyocardial laser revascularization: Histologic features in human non-responder myocardium. *Circulation* 95:371–375, 1997.
23. Allen KB, Fudge T, Selinger SL, et al: Prospective randomized multicenter trial of transmyocardial revascularization versus medical management in patients with class IV angina. *Circulation* 96:564S, 1997.
24. Sundt TM, Mohr FW, Seitelberger R, et al: Transmyocardial revascularization with a holmium:YAG laser: Results of three- and six-month follow-up. *Circulation* 96:564S, 1997.
25. Mack CA, Magovern CJ, Hann RT, et al: Channel patency and neovascularization after transmyocardial revascularization using an excimer laser: Results and comparisons to nonlased channels. *Circulation* 96:9S, 1997.
26. Benson H, McCallie DP: Angina pectoris and the placebo effect. *N Engl J Med* 300:1424–1429, 1979.
27. Kwong KF, Kanellopoulos GK, Nickols JC, et al: Transmyocardial laser treatment denervates canine myocardium. *J Thorac Cardiovasc Surg* 114:883–890, 1997.

28. Fisher PE, Khomoto T, DeRosa CM, et al. Histologic analysis of transmyocardial channels: Comparison of CO2 and Holmium:YAG lasers. *Ann Thorac Surg* 64:466–472, 1997.
29. Sayeed-Shah V, Mann MJ, Reul RM, et al: Gene transfer in porcine myocardium with transmyocardial laser revascularization. *Circulation* 96:483S, 1997.
30. Horvath KA, Smith WJ, Cohn LC, et al: Recovery and viability of an acute myocardial infarction after transmyocardial laser revascularization. *J Am Coll Cardiol* 25:258–263, 1995.

CHAPTER 7

Advances in Immunosuppression for Heart Transplantation

Jon A. Kobashigawa, M.D.
Associate Clinical Professor of Medicine, UCLA School of Medicine; Medical Director, UCLA Heart Transplant Program, University of California, Los Angeles, California

Heart transplantation is no longer experimental and is the therapy of choice for selected patients with end-stage heart disease. In the late 1960s and 1970s, the only immunosuppressive agents available for maintenance immunosuppression therapy were azathioprine and corticosteroids. These two drugs act indiscriminately, and consequently cells not involved in the rejection response are also destroyed, thereby leading to a high risk for infectious complications. Poor survival rates reflected the limitations of these agents. Cyclosporine was formally introduced in the United States in 1983 and resulted in a significant improvement in clinical outcome in transplantation. According to the International Society of Heart and Lung Transplantation (ISHLT) registry, the 3-year survival rate from 1975 to 1981 (precyclosporine era) was 40% as compared with 70% in the cyclosporine era from 1982 to 1994.[1] Some of the improvement may be related to the addition of azathioprine to cyclosporine and corticosteroids (known as triple-drug therapy) in the mid-1980s, which allowed a reduction in cyclosporine dosage to minimize adverse effects, especially renal dysfunction.[2] The overall improved survival in the cyclosporine era appears to be due to less rejection and fewer complications of rejection therapy. However, after this initial survival improvement in the cyclosporine era, there has not been an appreciable increase in survival over the past 10 years. In addition, cardiac allograft rejection remains one of the most prevalent causes of mortality—25% in the first year after heart transplantation. Therefore, there is still a need for newer immunosuppressive agents with greater selectivity in immunosuppression to improve survival and minimize inherent drug toxicities. This chapter reviews current immunosuppressive medications and newer immunosuppressive agents in clinical trials in heart transplantation.

MECHANISM OF ACTION OF IMMUNOSUPPRESSIVE DRUGS

Transplantation immunosuppression is based on an understanding of the immune response to drugs that are designed to block specific steps in the immune cascade. Classification of immunosuppressive drugs can then be organized by mechanism of action (Table 1).

Halloran and Miller[3] best simplify the immune response as three signals (Fig 1). Signal 1 is recognition of antigen, which by itself usually leads to anergy or apoptosis. Signal 2 is costimulation from the antigen-presenting cell, and signal 1 plus signal 2 causes T-cell activation, which leads to cytokine gene transcription and cytokine production. Cytokines engage their receptors to provide signal 3, which leads to cell division. Before dividing, lymphocytes must have de novo synthesis of purine and pyrimidine

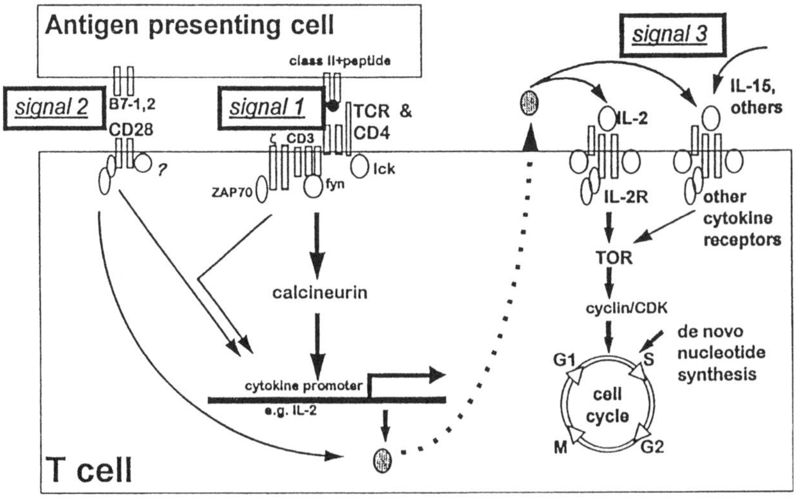

FIGURE 1.

Three signals for T-cell response. *Abbreviations: TCR,* T-cell receptor; *IL-2R,* interleukin-2 receptor; *TOR,* target of rapamycin. (Courtesy of Halloran PF: Immunosuppressive agents in clinical trials in transplantation. *Am J Med Sci* 313:283–288, 1997.)

TABLE 1.
Classification of Immunosuppressive Drugs

Non-protein "small-molecule" immunosuppressive drugs on the basis of their chemical nature and actions
1. Immunophilin-binding drugs that inhibit calcineurin: cyclosporine, tacrolimus, and their relatives
2. Immunophilin-binding drugs that inhibit the "target of rapamycin": rapamycin (sirolimus)
3. Inhibitors of de novo nucleotide synthesis
   - IMPDH inhibitors mycophenolate mofetil and mizoribine
   - DHODH inhibitors brequinar and leflunomide
4. 15-Deoxyspergualin
5. Peptides (e.g., "allotrap")
6. Polynucleotides (antisense)

Biological (protein-based) immunosuppressive drugs on the basis of their chemical nature and actions
1. Polyclonal antilymphocyte antibodies
   - Horse or rabbit antibodies created by immunizing animals in vivo
2. Monoclonal antibodies
   - Mouse monoclonals
   - Currently those being tested include anti-CD2, -CD3, -CD4, -CD5, -CD8, -CD11a/CD18 (LFA1), -CD25, -CD45, -CD54 (ICAM-1), -CD40
   - Humanized mouse monoclonals (e.g., CD25, CD4)
3. Cytokines and protein mediators
4. Soluble recombinant proteins and fusion proteins (e.g., CTLA4Ig)

Abbreviations: IMPDH, inosine monophosphate dehydrogenase; *DHODH,* dihydroorotate dehydrogenase; *ICAM,* intercellular adhesion molecule.
(Adapted from Halloran PF, Miller LV: In vivo immunosuppressive mechanisms. *J Heart Lung Transplant* 15:959–971, 1996.)

nucleotides. As the immunosuppressive agents are discussed, mechanism of action will be detailed according to Figure 2.

CYCLOSPORINE

Since the early 1980s, cyclosporine has been the mainstay of immunosuppression because of the initial improvement in cardiac transplant patient survival. Cyclosporine is isolated from the soil fungus *Tolypocladium inflatum Gams* (now renamed *Beauveria*

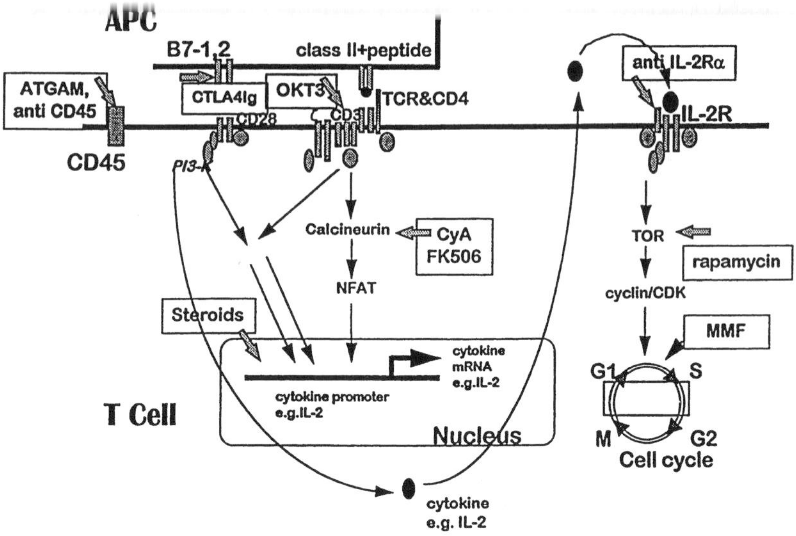

FIGURE 2.

Overview of the site and mechanism of action of immunosuppressive agents based on the three signals required for the immune response. *Abbreviations: APC,* antigen-presenting cell; *ATGAM,* antithymocyte γ-globulin; *TCR,* T-cell receptor; *IL-2R,* interleukin-2 receptor; *CyA,* cyclosporine; *FK506,* tacrolimus; *NFAT,* nuclear factor of activated T cells; *TOR,* target of rapamycin; *MMF,* mycophenolate mofetil. See the text for specific immunosuppression mechanisms of action. (Courtesy of Halloran PF, Miller LW: In vivo immunosuppressive mechanisms. *J Heart Lung Transplant* 15:959–971, 1996.)

nivea). It acts in two ways to specifically inhibit the activation and proliferation of cytotoxic T lymphocytes, the mediators of graft rejection. First, cyclosporine impedes the production and release of interleukin-2 (IL-2) by T-helper lymphocytes. At the molecular level, cyclosporine binds to cyclophilin (a member of the immunophilin-binding proteins), which leads to inhibition of *IL-2* gene transcription by blocking calcium-dependent signal transduction via calcineurin (see Fig 2). Second, cyclosporine inhibits IL-2 receptor expression on both T-helper and cytotoxic T lymphocytes. These two actions effectively and selectively limit the differentiation into and proliferation of cytotoxic T lymphocytes.

Cyclosporine is not the panacea drug despite its effectiveness in reducing rejection in comparison to previous therapies. Its major side effects include nephrotoxicity, neurotoxicity, hypertension, gingival hyperplasia, hirsutism, breast adenomas, seizures, osteoporosis, and hyperlipidemia. There has also been a question of whether cyclosporine increases the risk for development of transplant coronary artery disease, which is the major factor limiting long-term survival. This is suggested inasmuch as the incidence of transplant coronary artery disease has not decreased with the use of cyclosporine despite a lower rejection incidence. However, controversy exists because some animal data suggest that cyclosporine may in fact suppress the development of transplant coronary artery disease.

The most frequently occurring side effect associated with cyclosporine is renal dysfunction. The incidence of nephrotoxicity in cyclosporine-treated patients is 40% to 70%. Attempts to correlate cyclosporine toxicity with concentration have met with variable success. In a long-term study, postoperative renal function was assessed by serial determinations of serum creatinine with stabilization between 1 and 2 mg/dL.[4] Long-term cyclosporine use in heart transplant recipients has led to few patients progressing to end-stage renal disease. At the Texas Heart Institute, only 3 of 308 cardiac transplant recipients have progressed to end-stage renal disease, an incidence of approximately 1%.[5] Monitoring cyclosporine blood or plasma levels and adjusting the dosage have also been reported to be helpful in the management of other dose-dependent side effects, including hirsutism, tremor, hypertension, gingival hyperplasia, and hepatotoxicity.

Neoral is a new microemulsion formulation of cyclosporine. Pharmacokinetic studies in kidney, liver, and heart transplant recipients demonstrate an increased bioavailability of this formulation of cyclosporine. A recent heart transplant study has demonstrated that the cyclosporine area-under-the-curve concentration is increased by 24% in patients taking Neoral cyclosporine as compared with Sandimmune cyclosporine.[6] This more favorable pharmacokinetics of Neoral may result in improved clinical outcome. Kahan and colleagues have reported that a lower coefficient of variation (more constant cyclosporine pharmacokinetics) may result in less chronic rejection in renal transplant recipients.[7]

The advent of cyclosporine has revolutionized transplantation by improving survival and decreasing rejection. However, the toxicities of cyclosporine are significant and therefore the search for newer immunosuppressive medications continues.

TACROLIMUS

Tacrolimus (FK 506), a macrolide antibiotic isolated from *Streptomyces tsukubaensis,* shares many pharmacologic characteristics with cyclosporine. Tacrolimus exerts its immunosuppressive properties by engaging an FKBP and forms a complex that inhibits calcineurin[8, 9] (see Fig 2).

Initial studies performed at the University of Pittsburgh on liver and renal transplant patients found a favorable outcome with tacrolimus. This led to large-scale multicenter studies on liver transplant patients in the United States and Europe that were randomized between tacrolimus and cyclosporine. In the U.S. trial (n = 263 for tacrolimus, n = 266 for cyclosporine), patient survival rates were 88% for both groups, but graft survival was numerically superior for tacrolimus (82% vs. 79%).[10] There was less acute rejection in the tacrolimus group (P = 0.002) and less resistant and refractory rejection, but there were more adverse events (primarily nephrotoxicity and neurotoxicity) that necessitated withdrawal. The European Liver Transplant Study also showed less acute rejection (40.5% vs. 49.8%) and less refractory and chronic rejection.[11] In a combined analysis of the two studies at 2 years (527 tacrolimus patients vs. 531 cyclosporine patients), the tacrolimus group showed superior patient survival rates (83.5% vs. 78%, P = 0.03) and graft survival (77% vs. 72%, P = 0.057). Recent analysis suggests that the effects persist at 3 years. Overall, the tacrolimus group, however, had more nephrotoxicity than the cyclosporine group.

In renal transplantation, approximately 1,000 patients in the United States and Europe were enrolled in a randomized trial between tacrolimus and cyclosporine. In the U.S. study (205 tacrolimus patients vs. 207 cyclosporine patients), there was significantly less acute biopsy-proven rejection (30.7% vs. 46.4%) in the tacrolimus group and good graft survival (93% vs. 89%).[12] The European study results were similar, but graft survival was less in the tacrolimus group.[13] Again, nephrotoxicity and hyperglycemia were worse in the tacrolimus group. Thus, results in liver and kidney transplantation support the initial claims of tacrolimus having greater efficacy than cyclosporine, but it does have a tendency toward greater toxicity.

In heart transplantation, there have been two recent randomized trials of cyclosporine vs. tacrolimus for primary prevention. In the U.S. multicenter trial, 88 primary heart transplant patients were randomized to cyclosporine or tacrolimus in addition to azathioprine and corticosteroids.[14] Six-month follow-up revealed comparable survival rates, 91% in the cyclosporine group vs. 93% in the tacrolimus group. The probability or incidence of each grade of rejection as determined by endomyocardial biopsy whether treated or not and the types of treatment did not differ between groups. However, the tacrolimus group had a lower incidence of hypertension (52% vs. 79% in the cyclosporine group) and lower cholesterol levels at 6 months (181 mg/dL vs. 233 mg/dL in the cyclosporine group). There was no significant difference in renal function, hyperglycemia, hypomagnesemia, or hyperkalemia between the two groups during this 6-month study period. The authors concluded that tacrolimus appeared to be effective for early rejection prophylaxis.

The European multicenter study randomized 82 primary heart transplant patients to tacrolimus (2:1 ratio) vs. cyclosporine.[15] This resulted in 54 patients randomized to tacrolimus and 28 patients randomized to cyclosporine. Survival rates were higher in the cyclosporine group at 92.9% as compared with 79.6% in the tacrolimus group; however, this did not reach statistical significance ($P = 0.131$). The percentage of patients experiencing rejection was similar in the two groups (73.7% in the tacrolimus group vs. 81.5% in the cyclosporine group, $P = 0.444$). In this study, the tacrolimus group had more patients with abnormal renal function (61.1% vs. 49.3% in the cyclosporine patients), and more hyperglycemia was noted in the tacrolimus group (53.7% vs. 37.3% in the cyclosporine group). In the cyclosporine group, there was more hypercholesterolemia (25.0% vs. 9.3% in the tacrolimus group) and gum hyperplasia (10.7% vs. 0% in the tacrolimus group). The authors suggest that tacrolimus is comparable to cyclosporine in the first year.

A subgroup of the European tacrolimus vs. cyclosporine study was analyzed to assess those patients who received IV tacrolimus therapy ($n = 15$) in the immediate posttransplant period.[16] The authors found that the patients treated with IV tacrolimus had a reduced rejection rate in comparison to patients treated with cyclosporine (0.77 rejections per patient over the first 3 months vs. 1.48 rejections per patient over the first 3 months in the cyclosporine group). The average tacrolimus level for the tacrolimus group as a whole was 13.1 ng/mL at 12 months, whereas the average cyclosporine level was 166 ng/mL. This relatively low cyclosporine level may have been responsible for a slightly higher incidence of rejection. In a study by el-Gamel et al., patients with trough cyclosporine levels less than or equal to 200 ng/mL during the first 2 years posttransplant are reported to have more rejection than patients with levels greater than 200 ng/mL.[17] Therefore, the efficacy of early IV tacrolimus has not yet been established and needs to be further assessed in a prospective randomized trial.

Before the two randomized trials of tacrolimus vs. cyclosporine, uncontrolled studies suggested that tacrolimus may have a benefit over cyclosporine. Pham and colleagues at the University of Pittsburgh monitored 243 heart transplant recipients and reported that tacrolimus patients had more freedom from rejection than did cyclosporine-treated patients.[18] In addition, tacrolimus had a lower risk of hypertension and was associated with a lower dose of corticosteroids. However, this study was not randomized and the groups had baseline differences. Meiser and colleagues evaluated 25 heart transplant patients and reported that tacrolimus was superior to OKT3 monoclonal antibody in successfully treating persistent cardiac allograft rejection.[19] This study was also not randomized, and the patients were switched to tacrolimus therapy at a mean of 354 days postoperatively whereas the OKT3-treated patients were evaluated at a mean of 60 days after surgery. This difference in time posttransplant may have been responsible for the observed favorable outcome of tacrolimus. Sager and colleagues at the University of Wisconsin reported that 14 of 15 heart transplant patients and 14 of 15 lung transplant patients with persistent or refractory rejection improved their biopsy grade when switched from cyclosporine to tacrolimus therapy. However, again these are anecdotal reports and not randomized studies. It might be interesting to see whether patients with persistent or refractory rejection while receiving tacrolimus-based immunosuppression would respond to a switch to cyclosporine.

In the randomized heart transplant trials, tacrolimus appears to be comparable to cyclosporine in survival and rejection. However, its side effect profile may be worse in nephrotoxicity and hyperglycemia. There are problems with comparisons of tacrolimus and cyclosporine inasmuch as the optimal doses of both drugs are not known. It may be that the dose of tacrolimus was higher in these clinical trials than that used in practice and therefore toxicity tends to be higher. The use of different doses of tacrolimus and/or cyclosporine in clinical trials might even lead to different results and conclusions. Therefore, the relative role of tacrolimus vs. cyclosporine remains to be established.

MYCOPHENOLATE MOFETIL

Mycophenolic acid was originally discovered in 1896 from a *Penicillium* culture by Gosio.[20] Mycophenolic acid was eventually found to have antineoplastic, antibacterial, antifungal, antiviral, and most recently, immunosuppressive properties.[21–23] Mycophe-

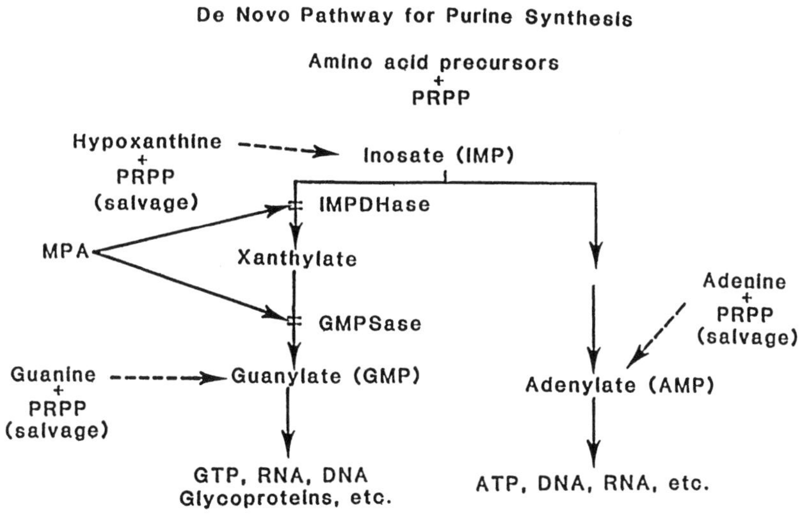

FIGURE 3.

Purine synthesis pathways. *Solid arrows* represent de novo pathways and *dashed arrows* represent salvage pathways. *Abbreviations: PRPP,* 5′-phosphoribosyl-1-pyrophosphate; *IMP,* inosine-5′-monophosphate; *MPA,* mycophenolic acid; *IMPDHase,* IMP dehydrogenase; *GMPSase,* guanylate synthetase; *GMP,* guanosine monophosphate; *AMP,* adenosine monophosphate; *GTP,* guanosine triphosphate; *ATP,* adenosine triphosphate. (Adapted from Taylor DO, Ensley RD, Olsen SL, et al: Mycophenolate mofetil [RS-61443]: Preclinical, clinical, and three-year experience in heart transplantation. *J Heart Lung Transplant* 13:571–582, 1994.)

nolate mofetil was developed at Syntex Corporation to be a more bioavailable form of mycophenolic acid. Previously, several animal studies have suggested beneficial effects of mycophenolate mofetil in solid-organ transplantation. In rat cardiac allografts, mycophenolate mofetil not only reduced rejection but also decreased the degree of allograft arteriopathy.[24–26] Subsequently, Sollinger et al. conducted the first human trials of mycophenolate mofetil in kidney transplant recipients.[27] Large, international randomized double-blind trials of mycophenolate mofetil in renal transplantation have demonstrated efficacy when compared with azathioprine or placebo in combination with cyclosporine. In these trials, acute rejection is prevented by approximately 50%.[28–30]

There are two major pathways for purine biosynthesis in T and B lymphocytes: the de novo pathway and the salvage pathway (see Fig 3).[31] However, the de novo pathway predominates in proliferating lymphocytes. In the de novo pathway, 5- phosphoribosyl-1-

pyrophosphate is converted to inosine monophosphate, which is further modified to guanosine monophosphate by the rate-limiting enzyme inosine monophosphate dehydrogenase (IMPDH). Guanosine triphosphate (GTP) is then produced and becomes involved in DNA synthesis. Mycophenolic acid is a selective, noncompetitive inhibitor of IMPDH and guanylate synthetase.[32] This results in inhibition of T- and B-lymphocyte proliferation. Lymphocytes that are depleted of guanine nucleotides become fixed in the S phase of the cell cycle.[33] In addition, inhibition of IMPDH results in the depletion of intercellular guanosine nucleotide pools. The reduction in GTP production slows the transfer of saccharide moieties to the glycoproteins expressed on some adhesion molecules, and therefore there is a reduction in the recruitment of monocytes and lymphocytes to sites of inflammation and graft rejection. Unlike cyclosporine, mycophenolic acid suppresses humoral immune responses (because it blocks B-cell proliferation) and does not inhibit cytokine (IL-1 and IL-2) production in humans.

Mycophenolate mofetil has been studied in refractory rejection in heart transplant patients. Ensley et al. first reported the use of mycophenolate mofetil in an 8-week, uncontrolled, nonrandomized, dose-response, pharmacokinetic and safety study involving 30 heart transplant patients with mild and moderate (ISHLT grades 1B, 2, and 3A) rejection.[34] Two of 6 (33%) patients receiving 500 mg/day of mycophenolate mofetil progressed to moderate (ISHLT grade 3A or 3B) rejection vs. 2 of 24 (8%) patients receiving between 1,000 and 3,000 mg/day of mycophenolate mofetil ($P = 0.10$). During this study there was no leukopenia or anemia noted, and 1 patient discontinued mycophenolate mofetil treatment because of gastrointestinal side effects. Our institution reported on 15 patients with refractory or persistent rejection (9 episodes of moderate rejection and 6 episodes of mild rejection).[35] All patients had undergone heart transplantation 1–20 months previously, and all 9 patients in the moderate rejection group had at least one previous moderate rejection episode treated with a course of cytolytic agents (OKT3 or antithymocyte γ-globulin). All study patients were treated with mycophenolate mofetil, 2–3 g/day, in place of azathioprine with no change in corticosteroids. The study duration was 56 days. The results revealed that all 9 patients with moderate rejection improved in their follow-up endomyocardial biopsy grade. Six of the 9 patients had complete resolution of rejection an average of 39 days after the start of mycophenolate mofetil. However, 3 of the 9 patients died, with these deaths occurring at 1.5, 3.5, and 4.5 months after the start of mycophenolate mofetil. All 3 patients had left ventricular ejection fractions of 40% or less at the start of therapy. All 6 patients with persistent mild rejection improved in their follow-up endomyocardial biopsy. Five of the 6 patients had complete resolution an average of 47 days after initiation of mycophenolate mofetil therapy. From this study, it was concluded that mycophenolate mofetil was capable of reversing persistent and refractory rejection. However, caution must be taken in patients with moderate rejection (ISHLT grade 3A) who have decreased left ventricular function. In these patients, concomitant augmentation with high-dose corticosteroids may be necessary with the start of mycophenolate mofetil. Two other single-center experiences in heart transplant patients also showed that mycophenolate mofetil is an effective adjunct in the treatment of recurrent or persistent rejection and has little discernible renal, hepatic, or bone marrow toxicity.[31, 36]

A large double-blind randomized trial of mycophenolate mofetil vs. azathioprine was reported in May 1997 at the American Society of Transplant Physicians.[37] In this double-blind, placebo-controlled trial, 28 centers randomized 650 patients to receive azathioprine (1.5–3 mg/kg/day) or mycophenolate mofetil (3,000 mg/day), in addition to cyclosporine and corticosteroids after primary cardiac transplantation. Rejection and survival data were obtained for 6 and 12 months, respectively. Quantitative angiography and intracoronary ultrasonography were performed at baseline and at 1 year. Because more than 10% of the patients withdrew before receiving the study drug, data were analyzed on randomized patients (intent to treat) and on patients who received study medications (treated patients). The results demonstrated that survival and rejection were similar in the randomized patients (mycophenolate mofetil, $n = 327$, and azathioprine, $n = 323$). In the treated patients (mycophenolate mofetil, $n = 289$, and azathioprine, $n = 289$), mortality was less at 1 year in the mycophenolate mofetil group (18 [6.2%] vs. 33 deaths [11.4%], $P = 0.033$), as was the requirement for any rejection treatment (65.7% vs. 73.7%, $P = 0.026$). Fewer mycophenolate mofetil–treated patients tended to have moderate rejection (ISHLT grade 3A or higher, $P = 0.055$) or require OKT3 or antithymocyte γ-globulin ($P = 0.061$). Although quantitative angiography results did not differ between groups, the change from baseline to 1 year in luminal area by intracoronary ultrasonography showed an increase in luminal area of 0.33 ± 0.30 mm^2 in the mycophenolate mofetil group as compared with a reduction in luminal area of 0.81 ± 0.29 mm^2 in the azathioprine group ($P = 0.007$).

Opportunistic infections and gastrointestinal symptoms were slightly more common but not significantly different in the mycophenolate mofetil group. It was concluded that the substitution of mycophenolate mofetil for azathioprine improves survival, decreases rejection, and is associated with a larger coronary artery luminal area at 1 year in cardiac transplant recipients receiving mycophenolate mofetil.

Mycophenolate is a new immunosuppressive agent with effects that appear to be additive to those of cyclosporine because it acts later in the lymphocyte activation pathway by an entirely different mechanism. Mycophenolate mofetil appears to be effective in the management of refractory or persistent biopsy-proven rejection in cardiac transplant patients receiving triple-drug immunosuppression (cyclosporine, prednisone, azathioprine). From the large multicenter trial, mycophenolate mofetil may be superior to azathioprine as primary immunosuppression in combination with cyclosporine and prednisone.

SIROLIMUS

Sirolimus (rapamycin) is an antibiotic similar to tacrolimus. It binds to the FKBP, but unlike the tacrolimus-FKBP complex, the sirolimus-FKBP complex does not inhibit calcineurin. It binds instead to the target of rapamycin, which interrupts the signaling pathway between cytokine receptors and cell cycling and causes cells to arrest at the G_1-to-S transition in their cell cycle (see Fig 2). In rat studies, sirolimus inhibits the vascular response to injury caused by allograft rejection. This antiproliferative effect may prevent the effect of arterial intimal thickening associated with chronic rejection.

In renal transplant patients, phase I and II trials suggest that sirolimus in combination with cyclosporine can reduce acute rejection by 10% to 25%. The principal toxicities include hypertriglyceridemia and thrombocytopenia without nephrotoxicity. Phase III randomized trials are under way, including studies to use sirolimus without cyclosporine. In heart transplantation, sirolimus was used in varying doses in a randomized trial for the treatment of acute moderate rejection.[38] Sixty recipients of primary heart transplants were enrolled in a multicenter, randomized, dose-ranging study of rapamycin as primary therapy for focal moderate (ISHLT grade 2, $n = 37$) or moderate (ISHLT grade 3A, $n = 23$) rejection. Because of increasing evidence that many grade 2 and some grade 3A rejections resolved without therapy, 18 patients were assigned to receive placebo (group I), whereas 12 received low-dose (group II), 15 received medium-dose (group III), and 15 received high-dose rapamycin (group IV). No other therapy was added and no changes were allowed in maintenance immunosuppression during the 14 days after enrollment. Repeat biopsy was obtained at 1, 2, 3, 4, 8, and 12 weeks after the diagnostic biopsy. Success was defined as reversal to mild rejection (ISHLT grade 1) or to no rejection (ISHLT grade 0). For grade 2 rejection at 14 days, treatment success was seen in 67% of group I, 87% of group II, 56% of group III, and 83% of group IV patients. For grade 3A rejection, treatment success was seen in 50% of group I, 80% of group II, 80% of group III, and 100% of group IV patients. There were 12 patients with adverse events requiring discontinuation of the study, including lack of efficacy (n = 4), thrombocytopenia (n = 4), infection (n = 2), and neutropenia and nausea/vomiting each in 1 patient. Adverse events were relatively common but reversed with cessation of drug treatment. The authors concluded that rapamycin appears to be effective in the treatment of acute cardiac rejection in a dose-dependent manner and adverse events are similarly dose related.

Sirolimus is currently in clinical trials as maintenance immunosuppression to be used with and without cyclosporine. Preclinical and phase I and II studies have been promising; however, the use of sirolimus in heart transplant patients remains to be established.

OTHER DRUGS

Several new immunosuppressive drugs show promise in in vitro and in vivo studies. However, these drugs have not been pursued in clinical trials for various reasons.

BREQUINAR

Brequinar is an agent that blocks de novo pyrimidine synthesis in lymphocytes and has shown considerable promise in animal studies. Unfortunately, side effects, including thrombocytopenia and gastrointestinal toxicities, have suspended its development.

DEOXYSPERGUALIN

Deoxyspergualin (gusperimus) is a new immunosuppressive agent with an unknown mechanism of action. This agent was used in Japan and administered parentally for the treatment of acute rejection; however, it produced severe leukopenia. It is unclear whether further clinical trials are planned.

MIZORIBINE

Mizoribine is a purine analogue that inhibits IMPDH. Unlike mycophenolate mofetil, it is a competitive inhibitor and must be phosphorylated to be active. There have been limited clinical trials, and its use has been as a substitute for azathioprine. Its future in human clinical trials is not known.

LEFLUNOMIDE

Leflunomide is a new immunomodulatory drug in phase II clinical trials. Its primary metabolite A77 1726 is a malononitrilamide that has been proposed to inhibit de novo pyrimidine biosynthesis and growth factor receptor–associated tyrosine kinase activity. This results in inhibition of T- and B-cell proliferation and suppression of immunoglobulin production and interferes with cell adhesion.[39] Its clinical use has not been established.

BIOLOGICALS

These protein-based immunosuppressive drugs are administered IV and have high specificity, selectivity, and potency. There are a variety of classes of biologicals that can be used in transplantation.

POLYCLONAL ANTILYMPHOCYTE GLOBULIN

Polyclonal antilymphocyte globulins are produced by the immune response of animals exposed to human T cells. The sera of these animals, which contain antibodies to the human T lymphocyte, are then removed. Polyclonal antilymphocyte globulins from the horse (equine) have been reported to be effective for steroid-resistant and severe rejection episodes and have been used as an induction agent (used immediately posttransplant to induce tolerance) in solid-organ transplantation. However, these agents have not been found to be of proven value as induction therapy in heart transplantation, and therefore their routine use has been limited. A new polyclonal rabbit antithymocyte globulin that is reported to be more effective is being studied in North America in clinical trials.

MONOCLONAL ANTIBODIES

The murine monoclonal antibody against the CD3 antigen (OKT3) is the treatment of choice for severe rejection and has also been used as induction therapy in solid-organ transplantation. It has occasional severe first effects because of rapid release of multiple cytokines secondary to T-lymphocyte cell lysis. OKT3 is highly effective in arresting T-cell–mediated rejection and suppressing allo-antibody responses, which are T cell dependent. Associated morbidity with OKT3 monoclonal antibody use (cytomegalovirus infection and lymphoproliferative disease) and lack of studies to substantiate its value in induction therapy have limited its routine use.

Other monoclonal antibodies are in development and are directed against various components of the immune system, including adhesion molecules, cytokine receptors, CD4 antigen, portions of the T-cell receptor, and other targets. Recent advancements include the development of humanized monoclonal antibodies, which allow use for long periods of time without inciting an antibody response against the monoclonal antibody. There have been recent clinical trials assessing monoclonal antibodies against IL-2 receptors (CD25). Dacliximab is such a humanized monoclonal antibody against the IL-2 receptor. Two randomized, double-blind, placebo-controlled trials using 1.0 mg/kg IV within 24 hours before kidney transplantation, followed by administration every 14 days for a total of five doses, were performed in Europe and in the United States. In the European trial, dacliximab was administered in combination with cyclosporine and corticosteroids to 116 patients vs. 111 patients who received placebo.[40] Biopsy-proven rejection at 6 months was reduced in the dacliximab patients (47% for placebo vs. 28% for dacliximab, $P = 0.001$). In the U.S. trial, dacliximab was given in combination with cyclosporine, corticosteroids, and azathioprine.[41] One hundred twenty-six patients were randomized to dacliximab vs. 134 patients randomized to placebo. Biopsy-proven rejection at 6 months was 35% in the placebo group vs. 22% in the dacliximab group ($P = 0.03$). Based on these clinical trials, dacliximab has now been approved in the United States for induction therapy in renal transplant patients. Its use in heart transplantation has not yet been studied.

Another novel monoclonal antibody technique is the use of a chimeric antibody. Basiliximab is a chimeric IL-2 receptor monoclonal antibody with a murine variable region and human constant region. This chimeric antibody was studied in a randomized trial in renal transplant patients.[42] Three hundred eighty renal transplant patients were randomized (double blind) to receive 20 mg of basiliximab on day 0 and day 4 ($n = 193$) or placebo ($n = 187$) in combination with cyclosporine and corticosteroids. The incidence of biopsy-confirmed acute rejection 6 months posttransplant was 29.8% in the basiliximab group vs. 44.0% in the placebo group ($P = 0.012$). Infection and other adverse events were similar in both groups. The authors concluded that prophylaxis with basiliximab significantly reduces the incidence of acute rejection episodes in renal transplant patients. Its use in heart transplant recipients is being planned.

OTHER BIOLOGICALS

CTLA4 is a regulatory molecule that blocks the CD28-B7 system (signal 2, see Fig 1). A CTLA4 immunoglobulin has been developed to effectively block this CD28-B7 system, and in animal trials this agent has promoted tolerance in organ transplantation. Renal transplant trials are currently under way. The combination of CD40 ligand plus CTLA4 immunoglogulin may be synergistic.[43]

Small peptides derived from class I major histocompatibility molecules have been evaluated in experimental animal models and have been suggested to be effective. Polynucleotides have also been used as antisense moieties in animal models with suggested immunosuppressive effects. Their use in human transplantation has not been established.

3-HYDROXY-3-METHYLGLUTARYL COENZYME A REDUCTASE INHIBITORS

Hypercholesterolemia is common after cardiac transplantation, and many studies have associated it with the development of cardiac allograft vasculopathy.[44] A study at our institution[45] evaluated the use of pravastatin, a 3-hydroxy-3-methylglutaryl coenzyme A (HMG-CoA) reductase inhibitor, in the primary prevention of hyperlipidemia in heart transplant recipients. Ninety-seven heart transplant patients were randomized to receive pravastatin or no HMG-CoA reductase inhibitor within 2 weeks posttransplant. Twelve months posttransplant, the pravastatin group had significantly lower mean cholesterol levels than did the control group (193 $\pm$ 36 vs. 248 $\pm$ 49 mg/dL), surprisingly less frequent cardiac rejection accompanied by hemodynamic compromise (3 vs. 14 patients), better survival rate (94% vs. 78%), and a lower incidence of cardiac allograft vasculopathy as determined by angiography and at autopsy (3 vs. 10 patients). In a subgroup of study patients, intravascular ultrasound measurements at baseline and 1 year after transplantation showed significantly less progression of intimal thickness in the pravastatin group than in the control group. In another subgroup of patients, the cytotoxicity of natural killer cells was significantly lower in the pravastatin group than in the control group (9.8% vs. 22.2% specific lysis). This study suggests that pravastatin may have an unexpected immunosuppressive effect in the presence of cyclosporine. Interestingly, inhibition of natural killer cells by other HMG-CoA reductase inhibitors has been demonstrated in vitro.[46]

CONCLUSION

Since the beginning of heart transplantation in the late 1960s, there have been many advances in immunosuppression. Foremost among them was the introduction of cyclosporine in the early 1980s, which has significantly improved heart transplant survival and quality of life. However, because of the toxicities of cyclosporine, other immunosuppressive agents have been developed with the intent of more effective and selective immunosuppression and less toxicity. These newer agents are targeted at very specific areas of the immune system and reflect our better understanding of the immune response during rejection. In the future, the drugs mentioned in this chapter may be used routinely in heart transplantation and result in improved survival and less toxicity.

REFERENCES

1. Hosenpud JD, Novick RJ, Breen TJ, et al: The registry of the International Society for Heart and Lung Transplantation: Twelfth official report—1995. *J Heart Lung Transplant* 14:805–815, 1995.
2. Oliveri D: Five year experience with triple-drug therapy. *Circulation* 82:276S–280S, 1990.
3. Halloran PF, Miller LW: In vivo immunosuppressive mechanisms. *J Heart Lung Transplant* 15:959–971, 1996.
4. Costanzo MR, Beto JA, Bansel BK, et al: Longitudinal effects of cyclosporine administration 0–60 months after heart transplantation. *Transplant Proc* 26:2704–2709, 1994.
5. Lewis RM, Van Buren CT, Radovancevic B, et al: Impact of long-term cyclosporine immunosuppressive therapy on native kidneys versus renal allografts: Serial renal function in heart and kidney transplant recipients. *J Heart Lung Transplant* 10:63–70, 1991.
6. White M, Pelletier GB, Tan A, et al: Pharmacokinetic, hemodynamic, and metabolic effects of cyclosporine Sandimmune versus the microemulsion Neoral in heart transplant recipients. *J Heart Lung Transplant* 16:787–794, 1997.
7. Kahan BD: Pharmacokinetic considerations in the therapeutic application of cyclosporine in renal transplantation. *Transplant Proc* 28:2143–2146, 1996.
8. Griffith JP, Kim JL, Kim EE, et al: X-ray structure of calcineurin inhibited by the immunophilin-immunosuppressant FKBP12-FK506 complex. *Cell* 82:507–522, 1995.

9. Kissinger CR, Parge HE, Knighton DR, et al. Crystal structure of human calcineurin and the human FKBP12-FK506-calcineurin complex. *Nature* 378:641–644, 1995.
10. The US Multicenter FK506 Liver Study Group: A comparison of tacrolimus (FK506) and cyclosporine for immunosuppression in liver transplantation. *N Engl J Med* 331:1110–1115, 1994.
11. European FK506 Mulicentre Liver Study Group: Randomised trial comparing tacrolimus (FK506) and cyclosporin in prevention of liver allograft rejection. *Lancet* 344:423–428, 1994.
12. Pirsch JD, Miller J, Deierhoi MH, et al: A comparison of tacrolimus (FK506) and cyclosporine for immunosuppression after cadaveric renal transplantation. *Transplantation* 63:977–983, 1997.
13. Mayer AD, Dmietrewski J, Squifflet JP, et al: Multicenter randomized trial comparing tacrolimus (FK506) and cyclosporine in the prevention of renal allograft rejection: A report of the European Tacrolimus Multicenter Renal Study Group. *Transplantation* 64:436–443, 1997.
14. Taylor DO, Barr ML, Radovancevic B, et al: A comparison of tacrolimus and cyclosporine based immunosuppression in cardiac transplantation. *J Heart Lung Transplant* 16:72A, 1997.
15. Reichart B, Meiser B, Vigano M, et al: Tacrolimus (FK506) versus cyclosporin in heart transplantation: Results from a randomized, European, mulicentre pilot study. *J Heart Lung Transplant* 16:43A, 1997.
16. Meiser BM, Überfuhr P, Martin S, et al: Initial intravenous administration of tacrolimus improves the long-term results after heart transplantation. *J Heart Lung Transplant* 16:45A, 1997.
17. el Gamel A, Keevil B, Rahman A, et al: Cardiac allograft rejection: Do trough cyclosporine levels correlate with grade of histologic rejection? *J Heart Lung Transplant* 16:268–274, 1997.
18. Pham SM, Kormos RL, Hattler BG, et al: A prospective trial of tacrolimus (FK506) in clinical heart transplantation: Intermediate-term results. *J Thorac Cardiovasc Surg* 111:764–772, 1996.
19. Meiser BM, Überfuhr P, Fuchs A, et al: Tacrolimus: A superior agent to OKT3 for treating cases of persistent rejection after intrathoracic transplantation. *J Heart Lung Transplant* 16:795–800, 1997.
20. Gosio B: Ricerche bacteriologiche e chimiche sulle alterazioni del mais. *Riv Igiene Sanita Publica* 7:825–868, 1896.
21. Williams RH, Lively DH, DeLong DC, et al: Mycophenolic acid: Antiviral and antitumor properties. *J Antibiot* 21:463–464, 1968.
22. Knudtzon S, Nissen NI: Clinical trial with mycophenolic acid (NSC-129185), a new antitumor agent. *Cancer Chemother Rep* 56:221–227, 1972.
23. Eugui EM, Mirkovich A, Allison AC: Lymphocyte-selective antiproliferative and immunosuppressive effects of mycophenolic acid in mice. *Scand J Immunol* 33:175–183, 1991.
24. Morris RE, Wang J, Blum JR, et al: Immunosuppressive effects of the morpholinoethyl ester of mycophenolic acid (RS-61443) in rat and

nonhuman primate recipients of heart allografts. *Transplant Proc* 23:19–25, 1991.

25. Steele DM, Hullett DA, Bechstein WO, et al: Effects of immunosuppressive therapy on the rat aortic allograft model. *Transplant Proc* 25:700–701, 1993.
26. Gregory C, Morris RE, Pratt R, et al: The use of the new antiproliferative immunosuppressants is a novel and highly effective strategy for the prevention of vascular occlusive disease. *J Heart Lung Transplant* 11:197A, 1992.
27. Sollinger HW, Deierhoi MH, Belzer FO, et al: RS-61443: A phase I clinical trial and pilot rescue study. *Transplantation* 53:428–432, 1992.
28. Tricontinental Mycophenolate Mofetil Renal Transplant Study Group: A blinded, randomized clinical trial of mycophenolate mofetil for the prevention of acute rejection in cadaveric renal transplantation. *Transplantation* 61:1029–1037, 1996.
29. U.S. Renal Transplant Mycophenolate Mofetil Study Group, Sollinger HW: Mycophenolate mofetil for the prevention of acute rejection in primary cadaveric renal allograft recipients. *Transplantation* 60:225–232, 1995.
30. European Mycophenolate Mofetil Study Group: Placebo-controlled study of mycophenolate mofetil combined with cyclosporin and corticosteroids for prevention of acute rejection. *Lancet* 345:1321–1325, 1995.
31. Taylor DO, Ensley RD, Olsen SL, et al: Mycophenolate mofetil (RS-61443): Preclinical, clinical, and three-year experience in heart transplantation. *J Heart Lung Transplant* 13:571–582, 1994.
32. Allison AC, Kowalski WJ, Muller CD, et al: Mechanism of action of mycophenolic acid. *Ann N Y Acad Sci* 696:63–87, 1990.
33. Lowe JK, Brox L, Henderson JF: Consequences of inhibition of guanine nucleotide synthesis by mycophenolic acid and virazole. *Cancer Res* 37:736–743, 1977.
34. Ensley RD, Bristow MR, Olsen SL, et al: The use of mycophenolate mofetil (RS-61443) in human heart transplant recipients. *Transplantation* 56:75–82, 1993.
35. Kobashigawa JA, Renlund DG, Olsen SL, et al: Initial results of RS-61443 for refractory cardiac rejection. *J Am Coll Cardiol* 19:203A, 1992.
36. Kirklin JK, Bourge RC, Naftel DC, et al: Treatment of recurrent heart rejection with mycophenolate mofetil (RS-61443): Initial clinical experience. *J Heart Lung Transplant* 13:444–450, 1994.
37. Costanzo MR, Mycophenolate Mofetil Study Investigators: Results of the randomized trial of mycophenolate mofetil vs azathioprine in heart transplantation (abstract). Presented at the 15th Annual Scientific Meeting of the American Society for Transplant Physicians, Chicago, May 10–14, 1997.

38. Miller L, Brozena S, Valantine H, et al: Treatment of acute cardiac allograft rejection with rapamycin: A multicenter dose ranging study. *J Heart Lung Transplant* 15:44A, 1997.
39. Silva HT Jr, Morris RE: Leflunomide and malononitrilamides. *Am J Med Sci* 313:289–301, 1997.
40. Hardie I, Nashan B, Johnson R, et al: Reduction of acute cellular rejection by HAT (Zenapax) in kidney transplant patients. Presented at the 8th Congress of the European Society for Organ Transplantation, Budapest, Hungary, Sept 2–6, 1997.
41. Vincenti F, Kirkman R, Light S, et al: Interleukin-2–receptor blockade with daclizumab to prevent acute rejection in renal transplantation. Daclizumab Triple Therapy Study Group. *N Engl J Med* 338:161–165, 1998.
42. Nashan B, Moore R, Amlot P, et al: Randomized trial of basiliximab versus placebo for the control of acute cellular rejection in renal allograft recipients. *Lancet* 350:1193–1198, 1997.
43. Larsen CP, Elwood ET, Alexander DZ, et al: Long-term acceptance of skin and cardiac allografts after blocking CD40 and CD28 pathways. *Nature* 381:434–438, 1996.
44. Johnson MR: Transplant coronary artery disease: Non-immunologic risk factors. *J Heart Lung Transplant* 11:124S–132S, 1992.
45. Kobashigawa JA, Katznelson A, Laks H, et al: Effect of pravastatin on outcomes after cardiac transplantation. *N Engl J Med* 333:621–627, 1995.
46. Cutts JL, Scallen TJ, Watson J, et al: Role of mevalonic acid in the regulation of natural killer cell cytotoxicity. *J Cell Physiol* 139:550–557, 1989.

CHAPTER 8

Management of Small Aortic Roots

John R. Doty, M.D.
Resident, Division of Cardiac Surgery, The Johns Hopkins Hospital, Baltimore, Maryland

Donald B. Doty, M.D.
Clinical Professor of Surgery, University of Utah School of Medicine; Chief, Department of Surgery, LDS Hospital, Salt Lake City, Utah

The collective experience with aortic valve replacement spans more than 35 years, yet there is not a single valve that is clearly superior for all patients. The surgeon is now faced with an array of choices, including mechanical prostheses, bioprosthetic xenografts, allografts, and autografts. A number of objective and subjective factors must be considered for proper valve selection, including device hemodynamic performance, risk of thromboembolism and infection, need for anticoagulation, long-term durability, and patient preference and reliability.

In patients with morphological narrowing of the aortic root, the choice of valve has greater implications. The surgeon is often limited in the size of the replacement device, and the obstructive nature of the various valves is compounded in small aortic roots. Aortic root enlargement procedures are a key component of the proper treatment of these patients, and the operative technique directly influences long-term results.

AORTIC ROOT ANATOMY

To properly treat pathology of the aortic root, a sound knowledge of the relevant anatomy is essential.[1] The aortic valve normally has a three-cusp architecture, and the leaflets coapt centrally to achieve competence. A trivial amount of incompetence may be present in a normal valve at this central coaptation point. The valve leaflets insert in a semilunar fashion to the aortic wall; this rim of dense fibrous connective tissue is the aortic annulus. The three highest points of attachment around the annulus are termed the commissures and are situated well above the ventriculoaortic junction. The lowest point of attachment for each leaflet, however, actually rests below the ventriculoaortic junction.

The triangular space directly inferior to each commissure is called the interleaflet triangle, and the tissue in this area is quite pliable and flexible. The posterior triangle, located between the left and noncoronary sinuses of Valsalva, is particularly important in patients with a small aortic root. The posterior commissure and triangle are aligned directly over the midpoint of the anterior leaflet of the mitral valve. The mitral annulus is not perfectly circular, but rather conforms to the shape of the aortic outflow tract. Because there are no chordae tendineae at the midportion of the anterior leaflet of the mitral valve, incisions can be safely made during posterior root enlargement.

The anterior relationships of the aortic valve are also important, particularly when removal of the pulmonary trunk for autografting is planned. Both the specialized conduction system and the first septal branch of the left anterior descending coronary artery lie in close proximity to the aortic annulus. The conduction system courses below the anterior commissure in the myocardium at the inferior rim of the membranous septum. The left bundle branch spreads out on the ventricular septum near the aortic annulus until the midpoint of the right coronary sinus and then travels down the ventricular septum on the left side. On the right side of the septum, the right bundle branch descends to the right of the septal papillary muscle. Anterior incision of the aortic root to the right of the septal papillary muscle, also known as the papillary muscle of the conus, can interrupt the conduction system.

The first septal branch of the left anterior descending coronary artery runs directly below the posterior cusp of the pulmonary valve, near the medial posterior commissure. The septal branch then crosses the infundibular septum toward the septal papillary muscle, often bringing blood supply to the His bundle or the bundle branches. Injury to the first septal branch can result in not only septal myocardial infarction but also heart block from interruption of the blood supply to the conduction system.

Several authors have studied the dimensions of the normal aortic root and determined ratios for measuring or calculating the diameter of the root at various levels. In general, most surgeons consider the aortic annulus to be at the level of the ventriculoaortic junction, which is the same diameter measured to determine the size of a prosthetic valve. The diameter of the sinotubular junction is normally about 90% of the diameter of the annulus, and this provides a useful rule of thumb for reconstructive operations on the aortic root.

The aortic root is considered small when the diameter of the aortic annulus measures 21 mm or less. Depending on the age and clinical status of the patient, the surgeon must then make the appropriate decisions during aortic valve replacement surgery regarding the type of valve for implantation and the need for aortic root enlargement. A wide range of valves are available, including mechanical prostheses, stented and nonstented bioprostheses, allografts, and autografts. Techniques for enlargement of the aortic root are also variable and must be tailored to the individual patient.

STRUCTURAL FACTORS TO CONSIDER WHEN CHOOSING A REPLACEMENT DEVICE

Mechanical prostheses and stented bioprostheses share a common problem because of the support frame and the sewing ring that are used in the construction of these types of prosthetic heart valves. The actual diameter of the orifice through which the blood will flow will be at least 5 mm smaller than the outside diameter of the device. This results in considerable reduction of the effective orifice of the valve. The problem is compounded as the valve diameter becomes smaller. Aortic allografts and stentless porcine bioprostheses, which are used as freehand subcoronary valve implants and enclosed within the patients' aorta, only reduce the size of the valve orifice about 2 mm, which is the thickness of the tissue being implanted. Because the pulmonary annulus is naturally 2 mm larger than a normal aortic annulus, the patient's own pulmonary valve (pulmonary autograft), when used to replace the aortic valve, will actually be an upsize and therefore achieve the most ideal hemodynamic performance of all available operations.

MECHANICAL PROSTHESES IN SMALL AORTIC ROOTS

Use of a prosthetic device to replace the aortic valve when the aortic root is small requires some special consideration. It is probably best to follow standard recommendations in this situation. Kirklin and Barratt-Boyes[2] have discussed this matter in their standard text on cardiac surgery:

> When a prosthesis is used, a size smaller than 23 mm often results in considerable obstruction, depending on the device and the patient's body surface area. Replacement device mismatch is a seri-

> ous iatrogenic disease that produces persisting or increasing left ventricular dysfunction, hemolysis, and a very difficult reoperation. Only in small and sedentary patients should a 19 mm device be used . . . . Similarly, a 21 mm . . . valve is acceptable only if the patient is small and sedentary. Otherwise, with aortic roots of this size . . . the aortic root must be enlarged.[2]

Replacement of the aortic valve with any modern mechanical valve that is 23 mm or larger will provide suitable hemodynamic performance for most patients. Mechanical valves that have a 21-mm orifice can create significant flow obstruction and should only be used for patients with a body surface area less than 1.5 m^2 and who are sedentary. Any mechanical valve that is 19 mm or smaller has a prohibitive pressure gradient across the valve and will result in severe outflow tract obstruction. This gradient should be considered relative to resolution of the left ventricular hypertrophy that results for aortic valve disorders. One recent study demonstrated that the left ventricular mass index was significantly reduced after replacement of the aortic valve with a mechanical valve measuring 23 mm or larger whereas the left ventricular mass index was not significantly reduced when 19-mm valves were used.[3] Sawant and associates,[4] however, reported that 19-mm St. Jude Medical prostheses were satisfactory irrespective of the body surface area in a study with follow-up extending to 16 years. It should be noted that the 10-year survival rate was 61.6%. In a related study including patients with 19- and 21-mm prostheses, they reported a 53.6% survival rate at 16 years. These studies are reminiscent of a study using small (17 and 19 mm) Starr-Edwards prostheses that was reported in 1986 by Foster and associates.[5] Although the patients were reported to have good functional capacity, there were resting pressure gradients as high as 50 mm Hg and only 60% were alive at 12 years. The question of persisting left ventricular outflow tract obstruction and its relation to survival was unanswered by these studies. Franzen and associates[6] measured the pressure gradient over 19- and 21-mm prostheses 1 week after implantation. They found that 5% of the patients had pressure gradients over 30 mm Hg.

In the United States, mechanical prostheses that have been designed for insertion in small aortic roots are currently available from three manufacturers. All of these valves require chronic anticoagulation and have equivalent performance regarding thromboembolic events, valve thrombosis, and anticoagulant-related hemorrhage.[7–10] All have excellent long-term durability. By the nature of the design, these prosthetic devices introduce some amount of turbulent flow. The sewing ring and support structure for each of these valves subtract from the effective orifice and create a fixed physical obstruction.

The Medtronic-Hall valve and the St. Jude Medical valve have some models with thinned sewing rings on small prostheses to allow the use of a slightly larger internal device in a smaller overall valve. The Medtronic-Hall valve is offered as an even-sized valve, so a 20-mm valve actually uses the valve mechanism of a standard 21-mm valve inside a thinner sewing ring, which allows implantation of this device in an annulus sized for a 19-mm standard prosthesis. The St. Jude Hemodynamic Plus (HP) valve retains the odd-sized device protocol within a thinner sewing ring, so a 19-mm HP valve actually uses the valve mechanism of a 21-mm standard valve and is sized for a 19-mm annulus. The Carbomedics Top Hat valve is intended for insertion in a supra-annular position to allow for the placement of valves that are 2 mm larger. Once these specifications are known, it can be seen that a Medtronic-Hall 20 mm, a St. Jude Medical 19 HP, and a Carbomedics Top Hat 21 have equivalent hemodynamic performance because the mechanisms within the sewing ring have equivalent diameters.

Thus, our opinion that a 19-mm mechanical prosthesis has a prohibitive pressure gradient refers to the standard prosthetic from each manufacturer. Rather than insert a 19-mm device, the aortic root should be enlarged in such patients to accommodate a larger prosthesis. The 21-mm valve should be reserved for small patients with a sedentary lifestyle; otherwise, the root should be enlarged. Insertion of a 23-mm or larger mechanical prosthesis should be satisfactory for any patient. This would include the Medtronic-Hall 22 mm, the St. Jude Medical 21 HP, and the Carbomedics 23-mm standard or Top Hat prostheses.

BIOPROSTHESES IN SMALL AORTIC ROOTS

An ever-widening range of bioprosthetic valves are available for aortic valve replacement, and some are very useful in patients with small aortic roots.[10] Several centers now have long-term experience with stent-mounted porcine aortic valves and bovine pericardial valves in the aortic position.[11–13] Bioprostheses have limited durability when compared with mechanical prostheses but do not require anticoagulation. Durability, however, is improving with better methods of valve preparation. The Medtronic Intact bioprosthesis, which consists of a porcine aortic valve fixed in glutaraldehyde at zero net pressure on the valve cusps with toluidine blue added

TABLE 1.
Hemodynamic Performance of the Carpentier-Edwards Pericardial Valve

Valve Size (mm)	Number	Gradient (mm Hg)	Orifice (cm^2)
19	8	18.8	1.08
21	14	13.4	1.3
23	13	11.3	1.4
25	12	13.8	1.5
27	3	9.0	2.2

(Adapted from Aupart MR, Sirinelli AL, Diemont FF, et al: The last generation of pericardial valves in the aortic position: Ten-year follow-up in 589 patients. *Ann Thorac Surg* 61:615–620, 1996.)

to retard calcification, has shown 100% freedom from explantation caused by structural deterioration at 8.5 years when used in the aortic position.[14] The Carpentier-Edwards bovine pericardial valve in particular has been shown to have good long-term hemodynamic performance in small aortic roots (Table 1)[12] and a 85% rate of freedom from explantation because of structural deterioration at 14 years.[15] The support structure and sewing ring of a stented bioprosthetic valve, however, will result in a 5-mm reduction of the effective orifice of the valve and a fixed obstruction in the outflow tract.

When same-size external bioprosthetic valves are compared, nonstented valves have a considerably larger internal diameter than stented valves. There are porcine aortic valves and bovine pericardial valves that have been developed for implantation without support stent; the patient's aorta is used to support the bioprosthesis. Only the Medtronic Freestyle bioprosthesis and the St. Jude Medical SPV Toronto bioprosthesis (both porcine aortic valves) have completed clinical trials and been released for general use in the United States by the Food and Drug Administration. Both devices have been extensively used in Europe. Nonstented valves are generally inserted by using a freehand subcoronary valve replacement technique, with the bioprosthesis attached directly to the aortic wall (Fig 1). These devices only reduce the size of the outflow tract by about 2 mm, or the thickness of the device aortic wall that supports the valve. The Medtronic Freestyle device is presented as a complete porcine aortic root, so it may also be inserted by in-

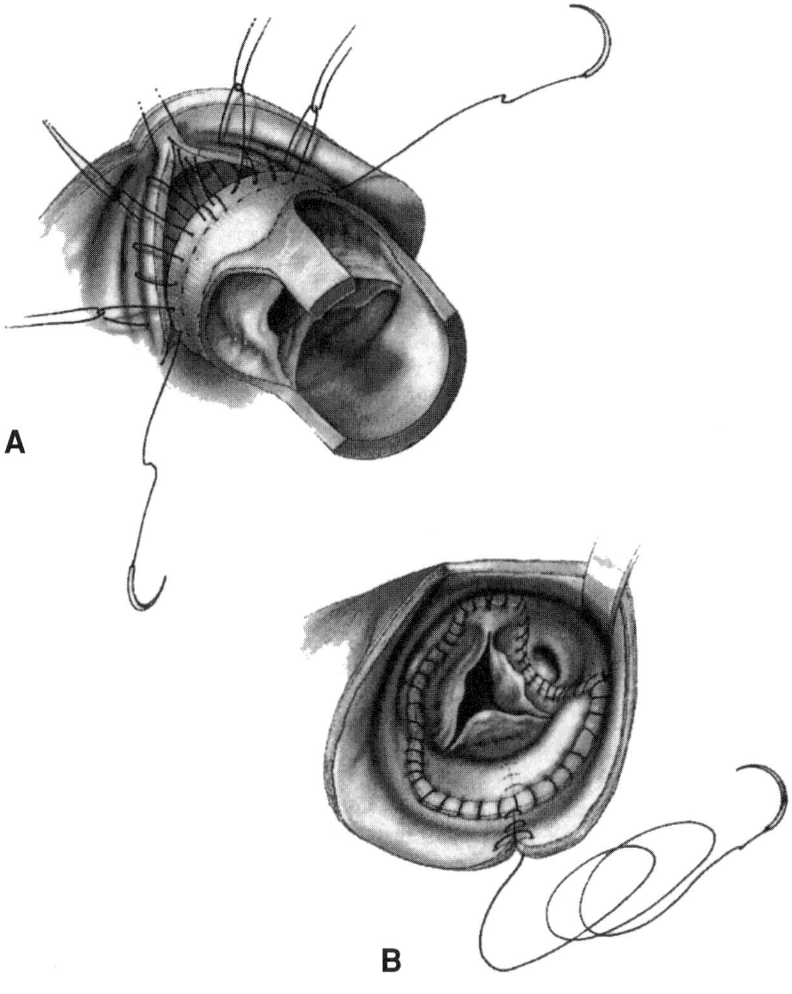

FIGURE 1.

A, Medtronic Freestyle bioprosthesis insertion by the freehand subcoronary valve replacement technique. The sinus aorta is removed from the right and left sinuses of Valsalva of the graft. Continuous sutures are used to attach the inflow end of the graft to the left ventricular outflow tract at the annulus. Multiple suture loops are placed with the valve held away from the annulus. Pulley strings aid in tightening the suture loops for tight approximation to the aorta. **B,** the sinus aorta of the graft is attached to the sinus aorta of the patient below the coronary ostia. The noncoronary sinus is left intact to fix the position of two of the three commissures for added accuracy and reproducibility of valve implantation. (Courtesy of Doty DB: *Cardiac Surgery: Operative Technique.* St Louis, Mosby, 1997.)

TABLE 2.
Hemodynamic Performance of the Medtronic Freestyle Bioprosthesis in Small Aortic Roots

Valve Size (mm)	Number	Gradient (mm Hg)	Orifice (cm^2)
19	7	12.9	1.29
21	20	8.0	1.56

(Adapted from Sintek CF, Fletcher AD, Khonsari S: Small aortic root in the elderly: Use of stentless bioprosthesis. *J Heart Value Dis* 5:308S–313S, 1996.)

clusion or freestanding root replacement techniques. Both the Medtronic Freestyle and the St. Jude SPV valve have proved to have excellent hemodynamic performance when used to replace the aortic valve, even in small sizes, including 19-mm prostheses (Table 2).[16] A recent study comparing nonstented bioprostheses, stented bioprostheses, and mechanical valves showed improved regression of left ventricular hypertrophy after aortic valve replacement with the nonstented valves.[17]

Our recommendation for stent-mounted bioprosthetic valves used for aortic valve replacement in small aortic roots is similar to that for mechanical valves: 19- and 21-mm valves should be avoided and the aortic root enlarged to accommodate a 23-mm prosthesis or larger. Nonstented porcine aortic valve bioprostheses, however, offer the advantage of good hemodynamic performance even in small sizes and may be implanted in any size aortic root.[18]

AORTIC ALLOGRAFT

Aortic allografts are versatile, flexible tissue and have excellent hemodynamic performance in the aortic position. The allograft can be preserved with various techniques; our longest experience has been with cryopreserved aortic allograft.[19–21] Cryopreservation achieves good structural integrity of the aortic leaflet tissue. The aortic wall is less well preserved and tends to calcify with time after implantation. Allografts are particularly well suited for use in small aortic annuli, often without root enlargement, but they can also be used to enlarge the root when necessary. These valves do

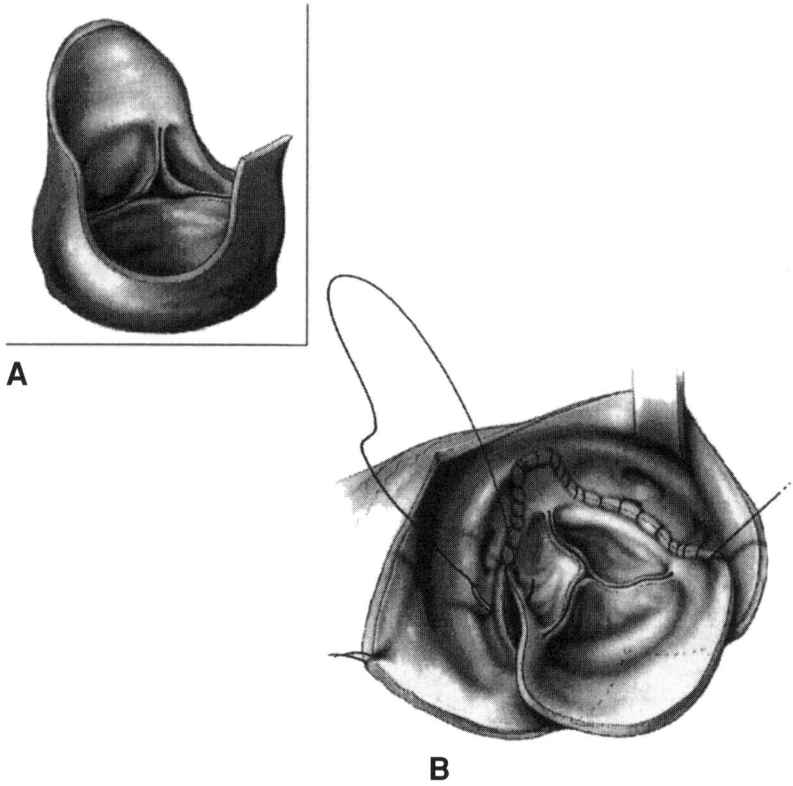

FIGURE 2.

A, an aortic allograft with an intact noncoronary sinus is implanted by the freehand subcoronary technique. The sinus aorta is removed from the right and left coronary sinuses of Valsalva. **B,** the sinus aorta of the graft is attached to the sinus aorta of the patient below the coronary artery ostia. Leaving the noncoronary sinus intact improves reproducibility of the operation by fixing the position of two of the three commissures. (Courtesy of Doty DB: *Cardiac Surgery: Operative Technique.* St Louis, Mosby, 1997.)

not require anticoagulation and are resistant to thromboembolism and endocarditis.[22–24]

Originally, aortic allografts were implanted in a subcoronary position after removal of the sinus aorta from all three sinuses of Valsalva. Retaining the noncoronary sinus, a technique described by Ross, ensures more reliable valve implantation by fixing the position of two of the three commissures (Fig 2, A). If the patient requires only valve replacement and has a normal aorta, the freehand subcoronary technique with the noncoronary sinus intact

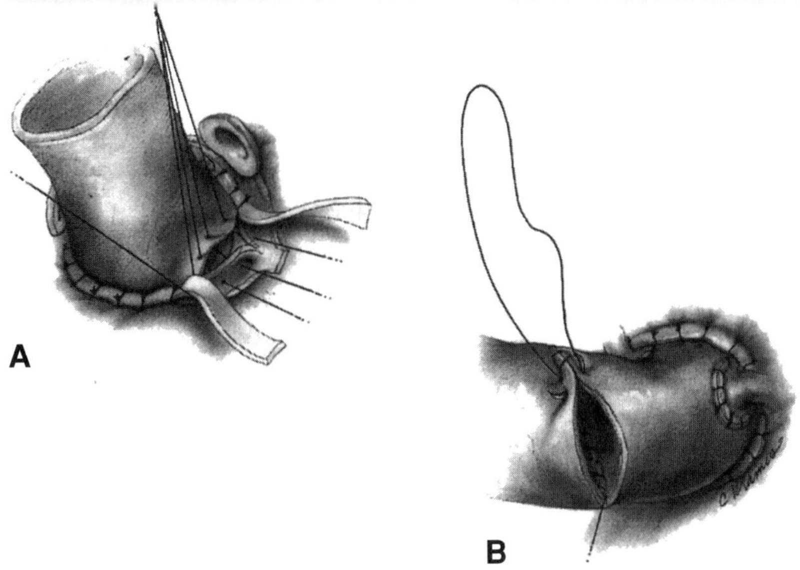

FIGURE 3.
A, aortic valve replacement using a complete root replacement technique with an aortic allograft. The entire aortic allograft root is attached to the aortic annulus by interrupted stitches with a Teflon felt strip incorporated within the suture loops for additional strength and hemostasis. **B,** the coronary arteries are anastomosed to the graft aortic root. An end-to-end anastomosis of the allograft to the ascending aorta is constructed. (Courtesy of Doty DB: *Cardiac Surgery: Operative Technique.* St Louis, Mosby, 1997.)

(Fig 2, B) provides a reproducible method of implantation of the allograft with smallest amount of allograft aorta included. The entire aortic root can also be replaced by using a freestanding root technique (Fig 3). More extensive root pathology, such as root abscess caused by endocarditis, poststenotic root dilation, or extensive aortic root destruction associated with complex congenital malformation or prior surgery, requires the freestanding allograft root technique. Full root replacement techniques have an additional advantage in small aortic roots in that there need not be even the minor downsize associated with subcoronary valve replacement techniques in which the allograft is inside the natural aorta. Miniroot or cylinder inclusion techniques are, in our opinion, a less desirable approach for allograft implantation. Inclusion techniques place the allograft inside the native aorta, where the allograft may be distorted by either redundant native aortic tissue or a root that is too small. The inclusion root technique has been promoted as a more reliable method than subcoronary freehand tech-

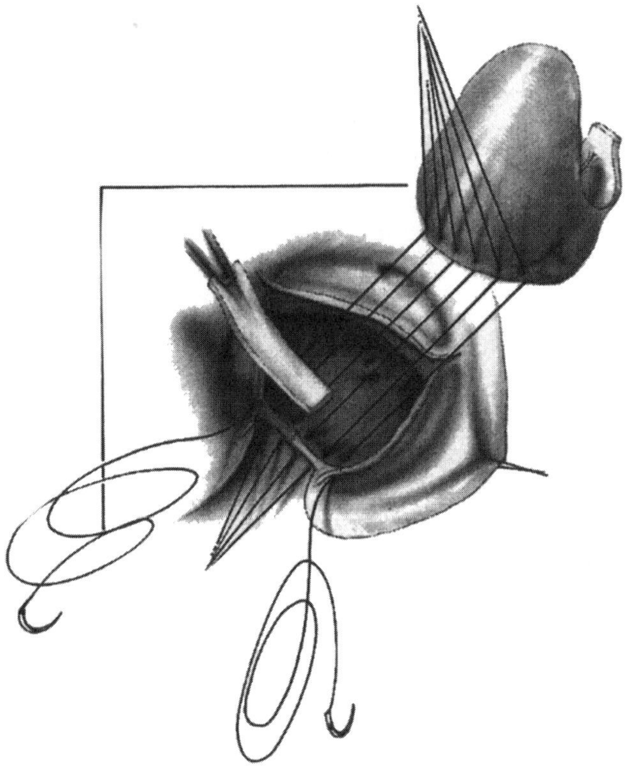

FIGURE 4.

An aortic allograft may be used to enlarge the aortic root by incision of the posterior commissure and interleaflet triangle and by removing the noncoronary sinus of Valsalva. An oversized allograft may be placed by expansion of the graft laterally onto the roof of the left atrium. A Teflon felt or pericardial strip is used to strengthen the proximal suture line and improve hemostasis. (Courtesy of Doty DB: *Cardiac Surgery: Operative Technique.* St Louis, Mosby, 1997.)

niques to achieve allograft valve competence and an easier operation. In our opinion, it is neither. Because the allograft aorta ultimately calcifies over time, the inclusion technique offers no advantage over the more reproducible and hemodynamically superior freestanding root replacement technique.

Root enlargement with aortic allograft is a useful technique that can be tailored to the severity of outflow tract obstruction. The posterior interleaflet triangle can be incised and a portion of the noncoronary sinus removed for isolated annular stenosis. A large allograft can then be used, with the proximal end attached to the mitral annulus and the roof of the left atrium (Fig 4). In patients with

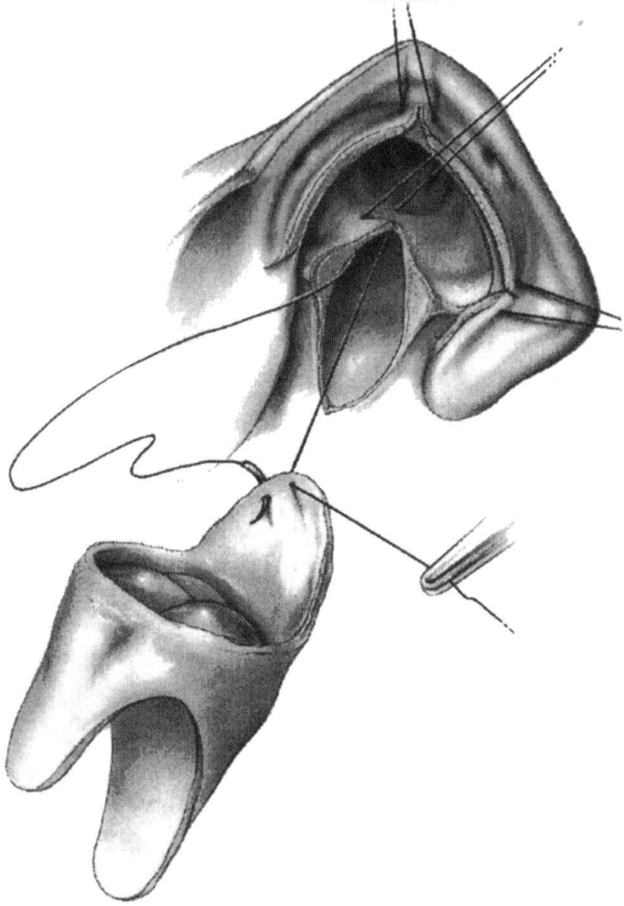

FIGURE 5.
The anterior leaflet of an aortic allograft may be used to widen the left ventricular outflow tract by incision into the anterior leaflet of the mitral valve. This is especially useful if there is subvalvular obstruction of the left ventricular outflow tract. (Courtesy of Doty DB: *Cardiac Surgery: Operative Technique.* St Louis, Mosby, 1997.)

subvalvular obstruction, the incision is carried down onto the mid-portion of the anterior leaflet of the mitral valve (Fig 5). The allograft mitral valve is then used to repair the defect in the recipient mitral valve, and the allograft noncoronary sinus is used to close the aorta after valve implantation.

Our experience with cryopreserved aortic allografts has shown excellent freedom from thromboembolism and endocarditis in long-term analysis, with 100% and 98% of patients free from these events at 10 years, respectively. Death from valve-related causes is also infrequent, with 93% of patients free from this event at 10 years. Cryopreserved allografts appear to have good long-term durability as well, with 92% of patients free from valve explantation at 10 years. The noncoronary sinus technique or its variant with root enlargement was superior to other methods in our experience in offering the best chance for freedom from valve explantation.

PULMONARY AUTOGRAFT

Regardless of the choice of valve replacement, all of the currently available valves carry an inherent risk of late failure and need for re-replacement. Mechanical prostheses may thrombose, become infected, or suffer excessive wear. Bioprosthetic and allograft tissues degenerate and calcify over time, thus rendering the valve either stenotic, incompetent, or both. Aortic valve re-replacement is associated with increased operative risk and represents a unique surgical challenge when required in a patient with a small aortic root.

The pulmonary autograft operation, or the Ross procedure, may offer the solution to long-term prosthetic valve failure.[25] It is particularly applicable to patients with small aortic roots inasmuch as the native pulmonary annulus is normally about 2 mm larger than the native aortic annulus, so when the pulmonary valve is used to replace the aortic valve, there may be a valve upsize. The autograft is the patient's own tissue, so the accelerated calcification and degeneration seen with allografts and porcine bioprostheses are unlikely. Ross reported long-term follow-up on patients who underwent aortic valve replacement with pulmonary autografts. Eighty-five percent of 339 patients were free from reoperation at 20 years. Most reoperations were for technical problems when the pulmonary autograft was used as a freehand subcoronary implant. Stelzer and associates[26] reported 131 patients who underwent aortic valve replacement using the total root replacement technique with a pulmonary autograft. The rate of freedom from reoperation for any cause was 88.6% at 10 years. Patients do not require anticoagulation, and studies using this procedure in the setting of endocarditis underscore the valve's resistance to infection.[27, 28]

In the operation, the aortic valve and root are excised; only the fibrous annulus and coronary ostia surrounded by sinus aortic buttons are retained (Fig 6, A). The patient's own pulmonary trunk is excised, including the pulmonary valve. Careful, shallow incision of the infundibular septum below the posterior cusp of the valve is required to protect the underlying first septal branch of the left anterior descending coronary artery (Fig 6, B). The pulmonary trunk is then attached to the fibrous annulus of the aortic root with interrupted stitches. A Teflon felt or pericardial strip is incorporated by tying the sutures around this strip (Fig 6, C). This is known as the supported root technique and will help prevent late dilation and valve incompetence by fixing the size of the outflow tract at the level of the pulmonary valve. The coronary arteries are anastomosed to the pulmonary trunk, which functions as the new aortic root, and the distal end of the pulmonary trunk is attached to the ascending aorta (Fig 6, D). The right ventricular outflow tract is reconstructed with an allograft pulmonary trunk.

Root enlargement techniques may be combined with the pulmonary autograft operation. It is our opinion that the left ventricular outflow tract should be altered and adjusted to match the size

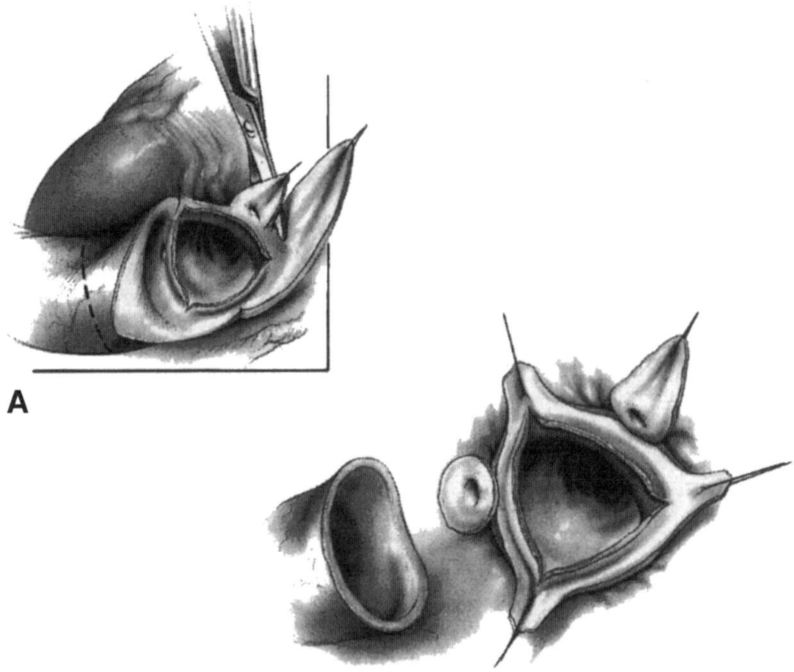

FIGURE 6.

A, aortic valve replacement with a pulmonary autograft (Ross procedure). the aortic root is excised with preservation of only the fibrous structure of the valve attachment and the coronary ostia surrounded by a rim of sinus aorta. *(continued)*

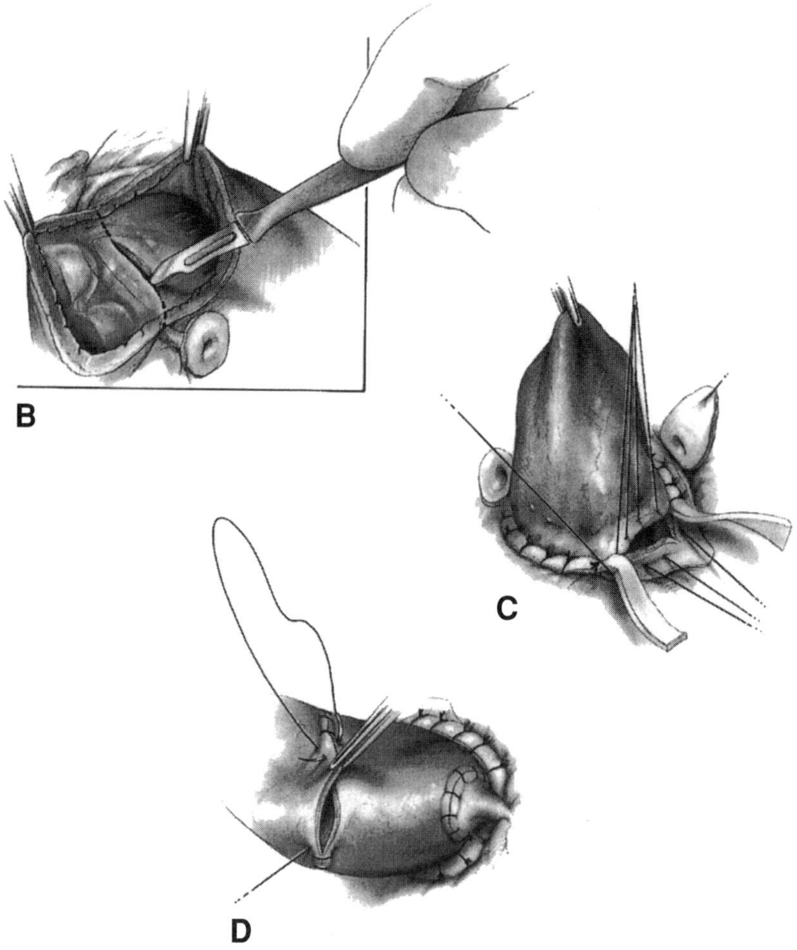

FIGURE 6. (continued)

B, the pulmonary trunk (autograft) is removed from the right ventricular outflow tract. A shallow incision of the infundibular septum below the posterior leaflet of the pulmonary autograft is required to prevent injury to the underlying first septal branch of the left anterior descending coronary artery. **C,** the pulmonary autograft is attached to the left ventricular outflow tract and the annulus of the aortic valve with interrupted stitches. A Teflon felt or pericardial strip is incorporated within the suture loops to fix the size of the left ventricular outflow tract at the level of the pulmonary autograft valve. **D,** the coronary arteries are anastomosed to the pulmonary autograft and an end-to-end anastomosis of the graft to the ascending aorta is constructed. (Courtesy of Doty DB: *Cardiac Surgery: Operative Technique.* St Louis, Mosby, 1997.)

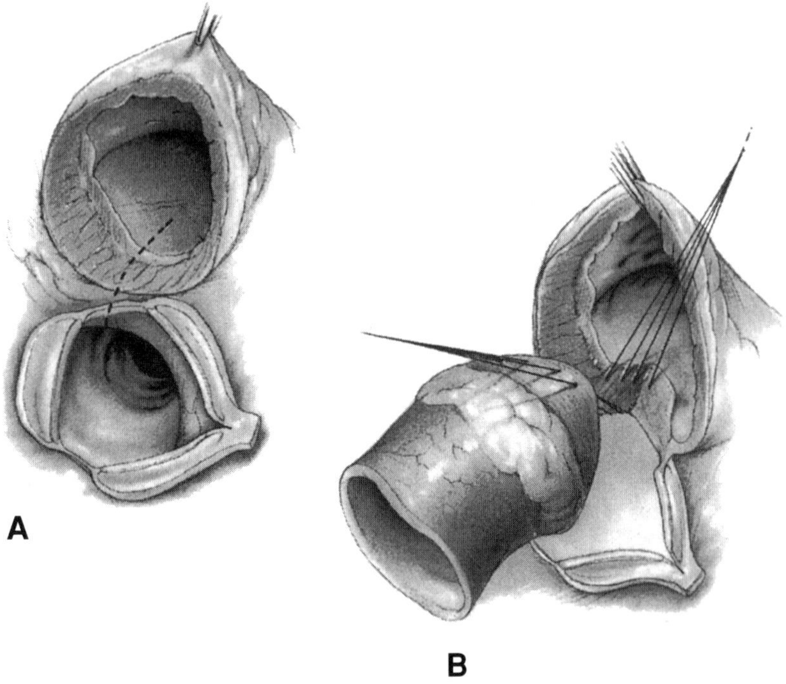

FIGURE 7.
A, a small left ventricular outflow tract may be enlarged to match the diameter of the pulmonary autograft by incision of the ventricular septum. This is called the Ross-Kunno procedure. **B,** the pulmonary autograft is seated lower in the left ventricular outflow tract. A large defect in the ventricular septum is filled in with right ventricular myocardium from below the valve of the pulmonary autograft. (Courtesy of Doty DB: *Cardiac Surgery: Operative Technique.* St Louis, Mosby, 1997.)

of the native pulmonary trunk in every Ross procedure. This opinion is shared by David and associates,[29] but not by Ross[30] or Botha and associates.[31] Attempting to place a large pulmonary trunk into a small aortic root may cause distortion or stenosis of the pulmonary valve. Stretching the flexible, compliant tissues of the pulmonary trunk to fit over a larger aortic root will ultimately result in valve failure because of incompetence. A small aortic root may be enlarged to match the size of the pulmonary trunk by established techniques.

After removal of the pulmonary trunk, the ventricular septum is incised to widen the left ventricular outflow tract (Fig 7, A). This maneuver is commonly known as the Ross-Konno operation. This

TABLE 3.
Exercise Performance After the Ross Procedure

Name	Heart Rate (bpm)	Gradient (mm Hg)	Max Work (watts)	Vo_2 (ml/kg/min)
M.D.	162	10	230	33.0
J.O.	181	14	261	44.0
L.G.	186	12	245	30.7
D.C.	181	10	321	45.1

(Courtesy of D.B. Doty and associates, unpublished data.)
Abbreviation: bpm, beats per minute.

incision is not as deep as the classic Konno operation and will prevent injury to the first septal branch of the left anterior descending coronary artery. Total relief of outflow tract obstruction can be achieved by progressive shaving of myocardium from the left side of the septum. The pulmonary autograft is seated deeply in the outflow tract by attaching it to the ventricular septum, and any defect in the septum may be filled with right ventricular myocardium on the autograft (Fig 7, B). This approach allows perfect matching of the diameter of the outflow tract to the diameter of the pulmonary autograft and complete relief of left ventricular outflow tract obstruction caused by the small aortic root.

The pulmonary autograft operation is more complex than simple aortic valve replacement and at this time is best applied to younger patients. Although the aortic valve disease may be permanently cured, the pulmonary allograft in the right ventricular outflow tract may require replacement. In our series of patients undergoing aortic valve replacement with pulmonary autografts, we have analyzed valve performance in a subgroup who were athletes (Table 3). During peak exercise, gradients over the left ventricular outflow tract and autograft valve were low while very high levels of work and oxygen consumption were obtained. The pulmonary autograft has excellent hemodynamic performance and is a good choice for valve replacement in young, athletic patients.

OPERATIONS FOR ENLARGEMENT OF THE AORTIC ROOT

Three techniques are generally used for enlargement of the left ventricular outflow tract: the Nicks-Nunez operation, the Rittenhouse-Manouguian operation, and the Konno-Rastan aortoventriculoplasty. A variant of the last operation, the Ross-Konno operation, has been described earlier. Most root enlargement operations in adult patients are best performed with a posterior approach.[32]

The Nicks-Nunez operation for posterior enlargement of the left ventricular outflow tract involves extension of the aortotomy incision into the posterior commissure and the underlying interleaflet triangle. This incision allows separation of the compliant tissues in the interleaflet triangle and enlarges the outflow tract by 2–3 mm. A prosthetic patch is then placed in the posterior commissure and a larger prosthetic valve can be inserted; the prosthetic patch is tapered to close the noncoronary sinus and aortotomy (Fig 8, A).

Additional enlargement of the aortic root can be obtained with the Nicks-Nunez operation by extending the incision across the annulus of the mitral valve and into the midportion of the anterior leaflet of the mitral valve. Enlargement of up to 4 or 5 mm can be achieved in this manner, and the defect in the anterior leaflet is repaired with a prosthetic patch (Fig 8, B). Interrupted stitches are preferable to prevent patch dehiscence and anterior leaflet distortion. The patch repair is continued across the defect in the roof of the left atrium. A larger prosthetic valve is then inserted and the noncoronary sinus and aortotomy reconstructed in a similar fashion.

The Rittenhouse-Manouguian operation, also for posterior enlargement, involves extension of the aortotomy into the noncoronary sinus. The left atrium is opened laterally to the aortic incision, and the aortotomy incision is then extended into the anterior leaflet of the mitral valve. This incision is slightly off center in the anterior leaflet and must be shifted to the exact midposition of the leaflet. A prosthetic patch is used to reconstruct the defect in the anterior leaflet of the mitral valve and the left atrium, and a larger prosthetic valve is inserted. Enlargement of 2–4 mm can be obtained by this operation.

The Konno-Rastan aortoventriculoplasty for anterior enlargement of the left ventricular outflow tract is used when extensive enlargement of more than 2–4 mm in diameter is required. Traditionally used in small children for placement of a large prosthesis to accommodate growth, this aortoventriculoplasty can be also useful in patients with subaortic tunnel stenosis. A vertical incision is made in the aorta into the right coronary sinus and extended into the right ventricular outflow tract anteriorly. The ventricular septum is then incised beginning at the aortic annulus and extending to the left of the conduction system. Division of the first septal branch is a risk during this portion of the procedure. The annulus of the aortic valve is thus greatly widened and the valve cusps are

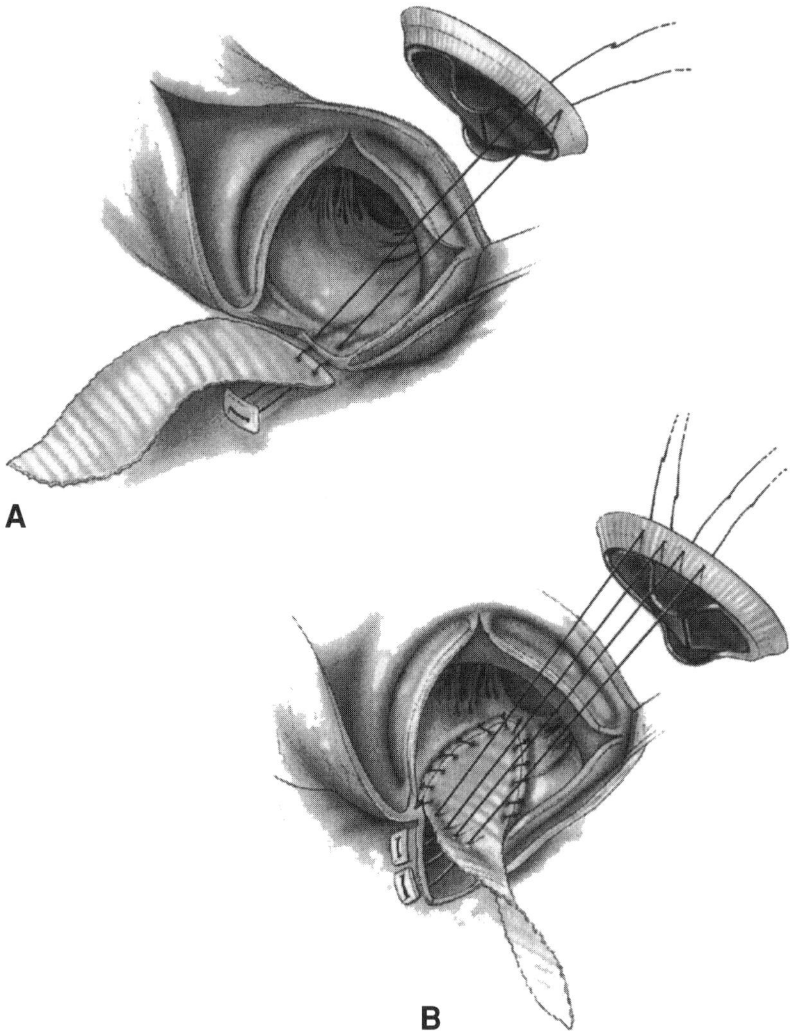

FIGURE 8.

A, Nicks-Nunez operation. The posterior commissure is incised into the interleaflet triangle to the level of the mitral annulus. The defect is filled in with a prosthetic patch to allow a larger prosthetic valve to be inserted. **B,** when added dimension of the left ventricular outflow tract is required, the incision is extended into the anterior leaflet of the mitral valve and the roof of the left atrium. The defect is filled in with a prosthetic patch to allow an even larger prosthetic valve to be inserted. (Courtesy of Doty DB: *Cardiac Surgery: Operative Technique.* St Louis, Mosby, 1997.)

TABLE 4.
Recommendations for Valve Replacement in Small Aortic Root

Valve	Age Group	Comment
Mechanical prosthesis	55–70 years	Enlarge root to accomodate a 23-mm prosthesis
Bioprosthesis	Greater than 70 years	Stentless xenograft has best hemodynamic profile
Pulmonary autograft	Less than 55 years	Well-suited for young, athletic patients
Aortic allograft	Any	Reserve for infection, associated coronary artery, or other valve disease

removed. A diamond-shaped patch is used to repair the defect in the ventricular septum to the level of the annulus and a large prosthetic valve inserted. The patch repair is then continued to close the aortotomy, and a second patch is used to repair the right ventricular outflow tract. The classic Konno-Rastan operation has largely given way to the Konno modification of the Ross procedure, and the former is seldom performed at present.

CONCLUSION

In summary, the surgeon must be prepared to use a variety of valve replacement devices in combination with aortic root enlargement techniques for patients with small aortic roots. Our current recommendations for selection of valve prostheses in this patient population are primarily based on patient age and activity and are listed in Table 4.

For patients younger than age 55, we prefer the pulmonary autograft operation with root enlargement as necessary to perfectly match the left ventricular outflow tract to the pulmonary trunk. Mechanical prostheses are generally used for patients age 55–70 years, and the root is enlarged to accommodate at least a 23-mm prosthesis. A 21-mm prosthesis may be used in a small (less than 1.5 m^2), sedentary patient. In patients over the age of 70, we prefer to use a stentless bioprosthesis because these valves appear to have the best hemodynamic performance of the xenografts in the smaller sizes. Aortic allografts are reserved for patients with active infection, for patients with associated coronary artery disease requiring multiple coronary artery bypass grafts or patients with disease of other heart valves requiring repair, and for younger patients with contraindications to anticoagulation.

REFERENCES

1. Anderson RH, Lal M, Ho SY: Anatomy of the aortic root with particular emphasis on option for its surgical enlargement. *J Heart Valve Dis* 5:249S–257S, 1996.
2. Kirklin JW, Barratt-Boyes BG: *Cardiac Surgery,* ed 2. New York, Churchill Livingstone, 1993, p 554.
3. Gonzalez-Juanatey JR, Garcia-Acuna JM, Vega Fernandez M, et al: Influence of the size of aortic valve prostheses on hemodynamics and change in left ventricular mass: Implications for the surgical management of aortic stenosis. *J Thorac Cardiovasc Surg* 112:273–280, 1996.
4. Sawant D, Singh AK, Feng WC, et al: Nineteen-millimeter aortic St. Jude Medical heart valve prosthesis: Up to sixteen years' follow-up. *Ann Thorac Surg* 63:964–970, 1997.
5. Foster AH, Tracy CM, Greenberg GJ, et al: Valve replacement in narrow aortic roots: Serial hemodynamics and long-term clinical outcome. *Ann Thorac Surg* 42:506–516, 1986.
6. Franzen SF, Hulfebrant IE, Konstantinov IE, et al: Aortic valve replacement for aortic stenosis in patients with small aortic root. *J Heart Valve Dis* 5:284S–288S, 1996.
7. Barner HB, Labovitz AJ, Fiore AC: Prosthetic valves for the small aortic root. *J Card Surg* 9:154S–157S, 1994.
8. Akins CW: Long-term results with the Medtronic-Hall valvular prosthesis. *Ann Thorac Surg* 61:806–813, 1996.
9. Roedler S, Moritz A, Wutte M, et al: The CarboMedics "top hat" supraannular prosthesis in the small aortic root. *J Card Surg* 10:198–204, 1995.
10. Barratt-Boyes BG, Christie GW: What is the best bioprosthetic operation for the small aortic root? Allograft, autograft, porcine, pericardial? Stented or unstented? *J Card Surg* 9:185S–164S, 1994.
11. Jamieson WR, Munro AI, Miyagishima RT, et al: Carpentier-Edwards standard porcine bioprosthesis: Clinical performance to seventeen years. *Ann Thorac Surg* 60:999–1006, 1995.
12. Aupart MR, Sirinelli AL, Diemont FF, et al: The last generation of pericardial valves in the aortic position: Ten-year follow-up in 589 patients. *Ann Thorac Surg* 61:615–620, 1996.
13. Pellerin M, Mihaileanu S, Couetil JP, et al: Carpentier-Edwards pericardial bioprosthesis in aortic position: Long-term follow-up 1980 to 1994. *Ann Thorac Surg* 60:292S–296S, 1995.
14. Barratt-Boyes GB, Jaffe WM, Ko PH: The zero pressure fixed Medtronic Intact porcine valve: An 8.5 year review. *J Heart Valve Dis* 2:604–611, 1993.
15. Baxter Healthcare Corporation, Edwards CVS Division, 1996 Post Approval Report, US IDE Cohort.

16. Sintek CF, Fletcher AD, Khonsari S: Small aortic root in the elderly: Use of stentless bioprosthesis. *J Heart Valve Dis* 5:308S–313S, 1996.
17. Walther T, Falk V, Diegeler A, et al: Stentless valve replacement in the small aortic root. *Cardiovasc Surg* 5:229–234, 1997.
18. Gross C, Harringer W, Mair R, et al: Aortic valve replacement: Is the stentless xenograft an alternative to the homograft? Early results of a randomized study. *Ann Thorac Surg* 60:418S–421S, 1995.
19. Doty DB: Replacement of the aortic valve with cryopreserved aortic allograft: The procedure of choice for young patients. *J Card Surg* 9:192S–195S, 1994.
20. Kirklin JK, Smith D, Novick W, et al: Long-term function of cryopreserved aortic homografts: A ten-year study. *J Thorac Cardiovasc Surg* 106:154–166, 1993.
21. O'Brien MF, Stafford EG, Gardner MAH, et al: Allograft aortic valve replacement: Long-term follow-up. *Ann Thorac Surg* 60:65S–70S, 1995.
22. Dossche KM, Defauw JJ, Ernst SM, et al: Allograft aortic root replacement in prosthetic valve endocarditis: A review of 32 patients. *Ann Thorac Surg* 63:1644–1649, 1997.
23. Doty DB: Aortic valve replacement with homograft and autograft. *Semin Thorac Cardiovasc Surg* 8:249–258, 1996.
24. Santini F, Dyke C, Edwards S, et al: Pulmonary autograft versus homograft replacement of the aortic valve: A prospective randomized trial. *J Thorac Cardiovasc Surg* 113:894–899, 1997.
25. Ross D, Jackson M, Davies J: The pulmonary autograft: A permanent aortic valve. *Eur J Cardiothorac Surg* 6:113–117, 1992.
26. Stelzer P, Weinrauch S, Tranbaugh R: Ten year experience with modified Ross procedure (total root replacement). *J Thorac Cardiovasc Surg,* in press.
27. Oswalt JD, Dewan SJ: Aortic infective endocarditis managed by the Ross procedure. *J Heart Valve Dis* 2:380–384, 1993.
28. Joyce F, Tingleff J, Pettersson G: Expanding indications for the Ross operation. *J Heart Valve Dis* 4:352–363, 1995.
29. David TE, Omran A, Webb G, et al: Geometric mismatch of the aortic and pulmonary roots causes aortic insufficiency after the Ross procedure. *J Thorac Cardiovasc Surg* 112:1231–1237, 1996.
30. Ross DN: Pulmonary autografts: The unresolved issues. *J Heart Valve Dis* 6:330–332, 1997.
31. Botha CA, Roser D, Rupp W, et al: The influence of geometric mismatch between the native aortic, native pulmonary and homograft pulmonary valve on the results of the pulmonary autograft operation. *J Heart Valve Dis* 6:355–360, 1997.
32. Sommers KE, David TE: Aortic valve replacement with patch enlargement of the aortic annulus. *Ann Thorac Surg* 63:1608–1612, 1997.

CHAPTER 9

Coronary Endarterectomy: Surgical Techniques for Patients With Extensive Distal Atherosclerotic Coronary Disease

Noel L. Mills, M.D.
Clinical Professor, Department of Surgery, Tulane University School of Medicine, New Orleans, Louisiana

Surgeons are now performing coronary artery bypass grafting on patients with more extensive coronary artery disease because of (1) improved drugs for medical management of coronary artery disease, (2) percutaneous coronary angioplasty and stent limits being extended to include multiple vessels, and (3) the realization that coronary artery bypass grafting is safer than had previously been appreciated in the older age groups.

PATHOLOGY OF ATHEROSCLEROTIC HEART DISEASE RELATED TO CORONARY ENDARTERECTOMY

A study of adult coronary artery disease over the course of 15 years led to a classification of coronary artery disease into distinct patterns. This has been helpful from several standpoints, especially when extensive distal disease is present. A more realistic expectation of the outcome of the operation can be offered when discussing the risk-benefit ratio with patients and cardiologists. Second, it affords the surgeon tangible guidelines for planning and performing an operation from a technical standpoint. In relation to coronary endarterectomy, it is evident that surface coronary artery disease, no matter how extensive, is more often associated with only minor, if any extension into the smaller coronary branches (less than 0.5 mm in internal diameter) as they perforate into the myocardium. This is clearly demonstrated by Vlodaver and Edwards on photomicrography.[1] Surgeons are therefore challenged to meticulously surgically attack extensively diseased coronary arteries in a way that is not too time consuming during cardioplegic arrest and that proves nonobstructive to those small myocardial branches.

Ten patterns of coronary artery disease have been derived from a combination of angiographic appearance, operative observations, and autopsy studies. Only the cardiovascular surgeon has the unique opportunity to observe the disease from these three aspects.

The ten patterns and their relative incidence are as follows (Fig 1):

Type I. Proximal discrete lesions (55%). Such lesions are found in the upper half of the left anterior descending (LAD) and circumflex arteries. The right coronary artery (RCA) is affected in its conduit portion, with the posterior descending and the inferior ventricular branches spared. Treatment of this pattern has changed radically from coronary artery bypass grafting to percutaneous coronary angioplasty over the last 10 years.

Type II. Severe multivessel distal disease (23%). This pattern is seen in diabetics and certain ethnic groups and involves disease down into the distal branches, even including arteries in myocardial tunnels. Often the surgeon has difficulty in finding an area free of disease to perform an arteriotomy.

Type III. Posterior plaque disease (7%). This pattern likewise involves the distal arteries but is the great deceiver angiographically in spite of multiple views. To the consternation of the surgeon, a bulging, diseased posterior wall is found after the arteriotomy is made through a normal wall anteriorly. The appropriate calibrated probe cannot be introduced without plaque damage, and an effective anastomosis with good runoff is more difficult to achieve.

Type IV. Ulcerative disease (3%). Overt ulcerations in the proximal arteries (especially the RCA) lead to multiple embolic scars within the left ventricular myocardium with varying degrees of left ventricular dysfunction depending on the age of the lesions.[2] Varying degrees of distal disease are found in this pattern.

Type V. Smoker's small-vessel syndrome (5%). This sometimes striking pattern is characterized by myointimal hyperplasia of the vessel wall in heavy smokers. More often than not, no coronary artery is larger than 1.5 mm in internal diameter in the

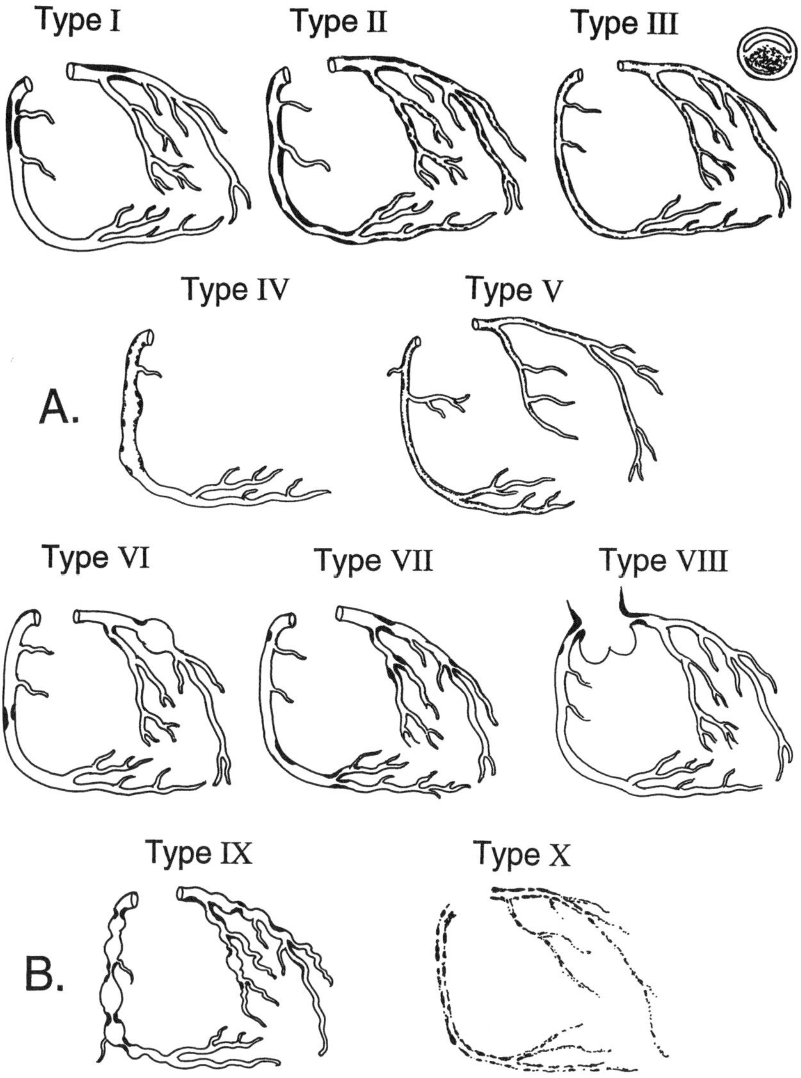

FIGURE 1.

Patterns of coronary disease. **A,** type I, proximal discrete lesions; II, severe multivessel distal disease; III, posterior plaque disease; IV, ulcerative disease; V, smoker's small-vessel syndrome. **B,** type VI, aneurysm disease; VII, multiple bifurcation stenosis; VIII, Ectasia-stenosis pattern; IX, ostial stenosis; X, distal calcification. Types I and X are amenable to standard coronary bypass. Type II is the usual pattern for extensive coronary endarterectomy. Types III and VII may have skip lesions and the specimen may break off and leave retained plaque that must be retrieved. Types IV and VIII often have liquid debris in the wall of the coronary artery. Technical difficulty is associated with type V, so endarterectomy is contraindicated. The coronary arteriotomy should be remote from aneurysm disease in the type VI pattern.

usual locations for performing an anastomosis. The arteries may be "silver wire" in appearance and are affected by disease distally.

Type VI. Aneurysm disease (1%). This type is associated with multiple stenosis and is not a poststenotic dilation. It is more commonly found in the proximal LAD coronary artery.

Type VII. Multiple bifurcation stenosis (fork-in-the-road syndrome) (3%). There is significant atherosclerosis at each bifurcation of the coronary arterial tree in vessels 1.5 mm or larger. In a patient with this pattern, hypertension may be diagnosed from only the angiogram. It is always associated with years of elevated blood pressure. Not infrequently, the distal vessels may be free of disease except when accordinization of the arteries is present, whereupon a buildup of atherosclerosis is found in the outer convex side of the vessel wall.

Type VIII. Ectasia-stenosis pattern (1%). Multiple areas of dilatations and intermittent stenoses are found. Not infrequently, there are embolic scars with associated regional left ventricular dysfunction from intermittent platelet emboli. Histologically, there is loss of arterial wall elastic tissue. The RCA is most often involved. Although the disease may be present in all of the coronary arteries, the very distal arteries are often normal, and the pattern is associated with aneurysms of other arteries (i.e., abdominal aorta).

Type IX. Ostial stenosis (1%). Characteristically, the lesions are found in females, may be missed by the angiographer, and are associated with varying degrees of calcification of the aortic sinuses and aortic valve.

Type X. Distal calcification (1%). This disease pattern may be diagnosed on fluoroscopy before dye injection because the coronary arteries are calcified down into distal branches. Piercing the vessel wall with the needle is often difficult. Conventional bypass is hazardous because of the difficulty of anastomosing a graft into the arterial lumen as a result of the calcium and intimal flaps from inadvertent dissection.

SELECTION OF THE APPROPRIATE CORONARY ARTERY FOR ENDARTERECTOMY

Planning which coronary arteries may be endarterectomized by analyzing the pattern of coronary disease is definitely helpful. Type II and III patterns are classic examples in which endarterectomy may be more prudent than performing an arteriotomy into thickened vessels and attempting bypass into disease-ridden areas. The ulcerative pattern (IV) may be associated with liquid debris, and care must be taken to avoid embolization if such is encountered during arteriotomy. In the type V pattern, although sometimes amenable to endarterectomy, it may be difficult to effect a good plaque-artery end point; a distal arteriotomy may become necessary and will present a meticulous technical challenge because of the small artery. Coronary endarterectomy should be avoided in an area of aneurysm (pattern VI). Coronary endarterectomy may be necessary at times in the type VII pattern, and arteriotomy is best performed at a bifurcation. Technically this pattern is more difficult because all larger branches may need to be endarterectomized. However, sequential coronary grafting beyond the diseased bifurcations is more often the technique of choice for this type when the coronary arteries are of sufficient size. The type VIII (ectasia-stenosis) pattern warrants a word of caution. When such vessels are endarterectomized, the remaining wall is very thin and easily subject to perforation. It is more difficult to suture after endarterectomy and to effect a leak-proof anastomosis. Also, a large-diameter vessel is left with sluggish flow. The long-term effects of the immediate response of laying down of platelets along the vessel wall and the formation of late aneurysms are unknown. Fortunately, the very distal vessels in this pattern are often free of disease, and bypass with or without sequential anastomosis when possible is a more logical approach. Types I and IX have distal vessels free of disease and represent the more "ideal" vessels for standard coronary bypass. A good long-term result is anticipated barring conduit availability problems. The type X pattern often represents end-stage "burned-out" atherosclerosis, and the vessel wall is generally of poor substance. The calcium must be fractured at the arteriotomy side to deliver this specimen from within the coronary artery (Fig 2). Patients with this pattern of disease usually have multiple atherosclerotic problems and are high risk for coronary bypass.

Distal disease with or without adequate visualization of the arteries on preoperative cineangiography is therefore an indication for coronary endarterectomy, especially in the presence of adequate left ventricular function. Problems arise, however, in patients with diffuse distal disease and an ejection fraction below 20%. The presence of angina, studies that predict live functioning muscle, and the absence of widespread Q waves separate this group into those who will benefit from endarterectomy and bypass and those who are transplantation candidates.

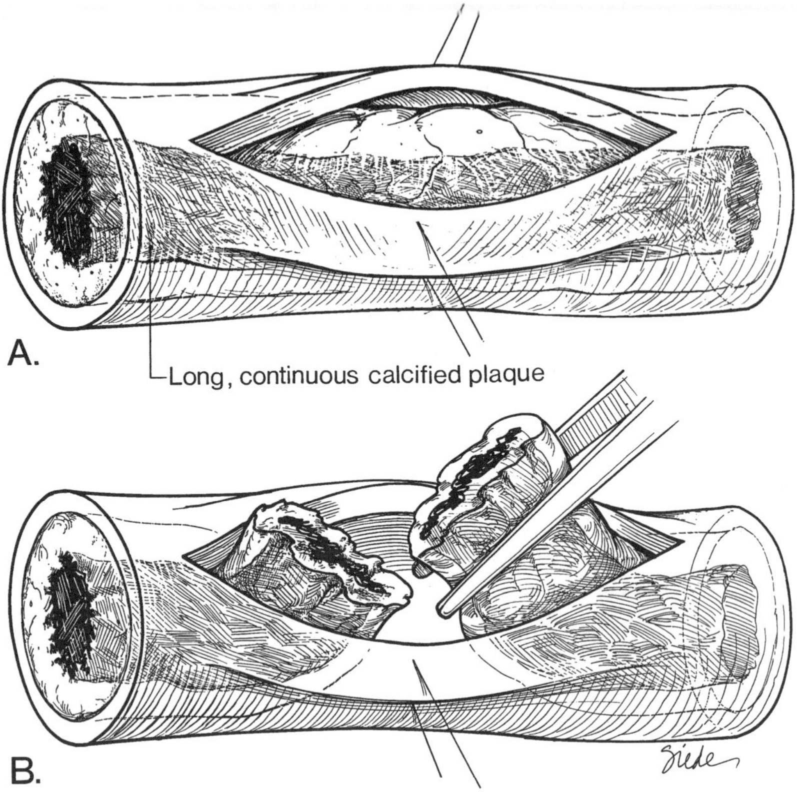

FIGURE 2.
The type X pattern is associated with vessels that are easily perforated **(A)**. Because of linear calcification **(B)**, the plaque must be fractured so that both ends may be retrieved as separate halves from the arteriotomy.

Selection of arteries and the relative technical ease of coronary endarterectomy is further delineated in Table 1. The RCA has been the classic artery for coronary endarterectomy in most previous reports because of its rather long conduit portion and accessible posterior descending branch. The distal branches beyond the crux of the heart have not been given special attention, perhaps as a result of poor visualization because they are covered by coronary sinus, veins, and epicardial fat in the groove.

True skip lesions perhaps represent the single biggest challenge whether in the right or left coronary artery system. Total endarterectomy through a single arteriotomy in this setting is difficult and may necessitate extensive time-consuming arteriotomies with long patches as advocated by Johnson et al.[3]

TABLE 1.
Selection of Arteries for Coronary Endarterectomy

Good	Average	Difficult
RCA	LAD	CFX marginal
Short lesions	Bifurcations	Trifurcations
Plaque continuity	—	Skip lesions
Fibrous and calcium plaque	Soft plaque	Ectasia
Visible artery distally	—	Vessel covered by epicardium and fat
Proximal occlusions (collateral circulation)	—	Proximal 50% stenosis (no collateral)

Abbreviations: RCA, right coronary artery; *LAD,* left anterior descending artery; *CFX,* circumflex coronary artery.

Attempts to endarterectomize vessels in myocardial tunnels is hazardous and should be avoided if at all possible. Overt tears of the coronary artery may occur because of the thin vessel wall.

Endarterectomy at trifurcations is time consuming and requires more patience to obtain an intact specimen. Soft plaque without continuity and fibrosis tend to break off at an inopportune point, even with only slight traction. Visible vessels always make for quicker endarterectomy and avoid the question of a distal flap, such as may occur with distal RCA plaque beyond the crux of the heart. Extremely tight stenoses or proximal occlusion of the coronary artery being endarterectomized offers less chance of myocardial damage as opposed to vessels with lesions only in the range of 50% to 75%. The former have usually developed protecting collaterals.

Early coronary experience with endarterectomy received a "bad name" for a number of reasons. First, no coronary bypass was done, distal arteriotomy for retained fragments was not performed, and no antiplatelet treatment was used postoperatively. Refined techniques with magnification and specific coronary artery surgical instruments were not available. Finally, no concentrated effort on educating patients about risk factor modification was undertaken. More often than not, patients returned to the use of tobacco. Hypercoagulable states went undiagnosed, lipid control was lacking, and hypertension and overweight were allowed to persist. It is the author's contention that active control of the aforementioned factors postoperatively is just as important as good technical performance of an endarterectomy.

TECHNIQUE FOR EXTENSIVE CORONARY ENDARTERECTOMY

"Extensive" endarterectomy in this chapter is defined as removal of coronary plaque 6 cm or greater. The endarterectomy is carried out through a small coronary arteriotomy. The key issue in obtaining a perfect endarterectomy is dissection in the correct plane, which is immediately below the external elastic membrane (Fig 3). This avoids leaving media, which is more thrombogenic, in contact with the bloodstream. Whenever possible, the initial arteriotomy should be made directly over calcification because it is easier to get into the correct plane of dissection. A characteristic pinkish color and slick appearance is observed as opposed to the lighter-colored irregular media.

GAS ENDARTERECTOMY

Gas endarterectomy, which originated in 1967, has been used with some limited success but has lost favor because of the lack of precise control of termination of the endarterectomy. Proximally, this may result in extensive dissection into the aortic root before such as appreciated. Distally, the dissection may go far beyond the diseased segment.[4]

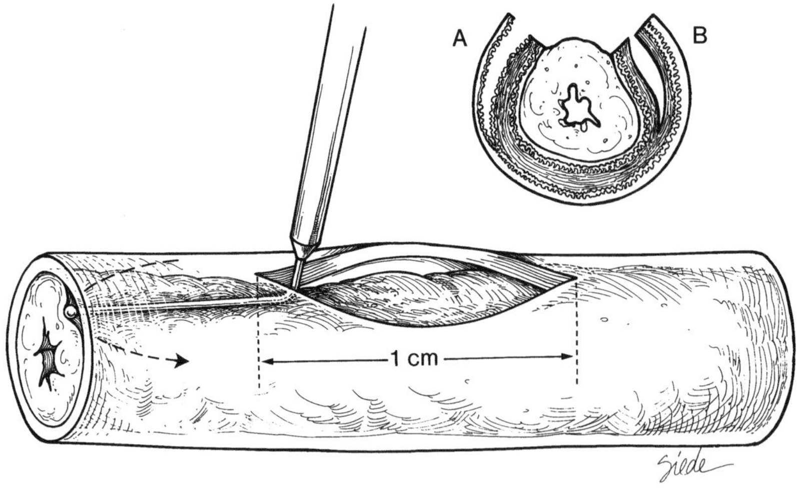

FIGURE 3.

A, a successful coronary endarterectomy is made in the plane immediately under the external elastic membrane with a ball nerve hook. **B,** media left behind is not only thrombogenic but leaves smooth muscle cells capable of becoming atherophils.

TOTAL OPEN ENDARTERECTOMY

Total open endarterectomy has the advantage of allowing the surgeon to directly visualize the endarterectomized vessel to avoid flaps, fragments, etc. However, suturing of the graft-patch is extremely time consuming, with significantly longer pump times needed. Also, a large vessel results from such a patch. Such may result in sluggish flow with laying down of platelets, fibrin, etc., on the walls of the endarterectomized vessel, which may lead to failure in the relatively early postoperative period. Bleeding from overlying severed veins is a nuisance with this technique.

ULTRASONIC CORONARY ENDARTERECTOMY

Myocardial revascularization using an ultrasonic probe was reported by Lane and Minot[5] in 1965. The ultrasonic hollow waveguide was demonstrated on cadaver coronary arteries. A problem of loss of energy from the generator to the working tip caused inadequate control of the power. The effect of the ultrasonic impulses on living coronary arteries was not determined. Although clinical studies were performed in larger arteries in the peripheral vascular circuit, there has been no reported use of US on coronary arteries for endarterectomy in humans.

MANUAL CORE TECHNIQUE

The manual core technique is advocated as being the most consistent way of obtaining the most precise "feathering" of the distal specimen. The arteriotomy is limited in length to an average of 10–12 mm, depending on the size of the coronary artery and the degree of compliance of the specimen.

SITE FOR CORONARY ARTERIOTOMY AND SUBSEQUENT GRAFT ANASTOMOSIS

The usual site on the LAD for coronary arteriotomy is near the junction of the upper and middle thirds of that vessel. The right coronary is opened most often at the crux of heart, thereby giving access to both the distal RCA and the posterior descending branch. The circumflex marginal arteriotomy is located distal to atrioventricular (AV) groove and just proximal to any major branch. If there is rock-hard calcium in an artery, that site is chosen over softer areas because it is easier to enter the correct endarterectomy plane immediately after opening the arterial wall. If there is a sizable branch with disease in the area to be endarterectomized (i.e., diagonal branch from the LAD), the arteriotomy is always performed adjacent to but not across the branch. This affords easy access to branches and their disease and makes for easier "feathering" of the specimen in both the branch and distal parent artery.

INSTRUMENTS AND MANUAL CORE TECHNIQUE

An appropriate rounded blade is used to perform a 6- to 8-mm arteriotomy. There is a tendency to cut too deeply with a pointed knife blade. A distinct attempt is made to *not* enter the lumen (see

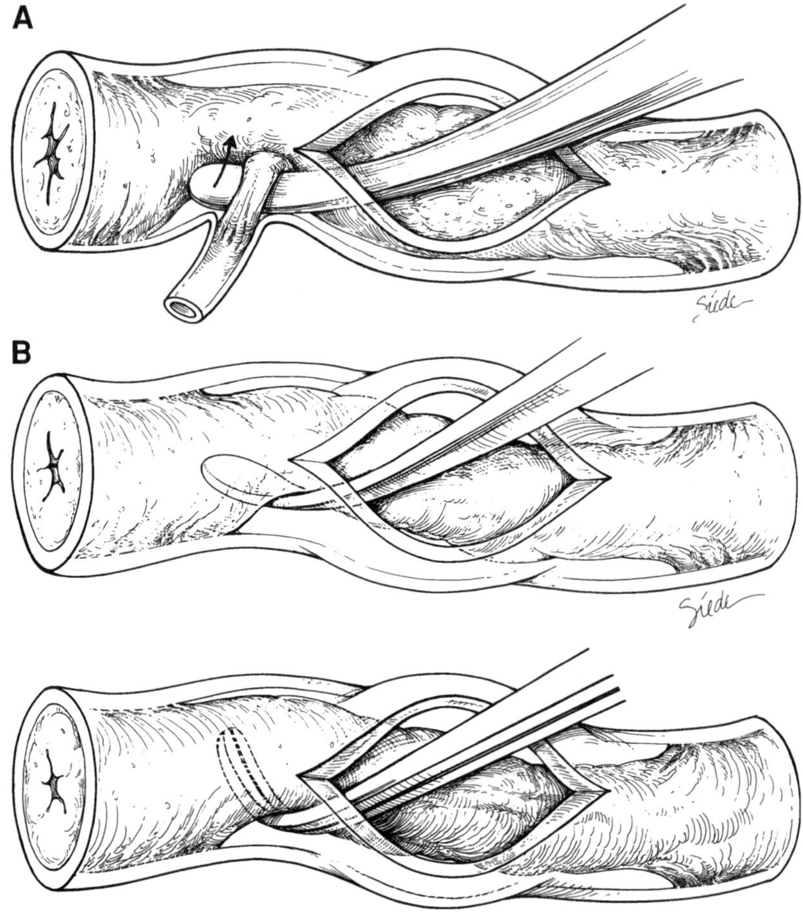

FIGURE 4.

A, a spatula is used to extend the separation of the external elastic membrane from the plaque superiorly, inferiorly, anteriorly, and posteriorly. The spatula is useful to "flip out" nearby septal perforator branches. **B,** a mini–right-angle clamp is useful to safely completely surround the plaque posteriorly.

Fig 3). The external elastic membrane is easily lifted with a short ball nerve hook, and 7-0 polypropylene stay sutures are used superficially on each side of the arteriotomy. The dissection plane is continued radially from the arteriotomy with the ball nerve hook. A spatula is then used to free the sides and the proximal part of the back wall rather than the ball nerve hook because of ease of perforation with the latter instrument (Fig 4, A). A short right-angle endarterectomy clamp is useful to completely surround the plaque posteriorly (Fig 4, B).

Wire loop instruments are the "workhorses" of the manual core technique for coronary endarterectomy. Sizes range from 20-gauge for larger vessels to 28-gauge for smaller coronary terminal branches. The diameter across the distal loop at the end of the wire may be changed during the course of endarterectomy in accordance with the inherent artery size (Fig 5). A 2-mm-diameter coronary artery will require a slightly larger (2.25 mm) diameter of wire loop at the distal end to obtain circumferential separation of the external elastic membrane and media.

As the wire is advanced distally, advantage is taken of the pathologic fact[1] that small (less than 1 mm) branches are free of atherosclerosis and "feather" off at the entrance into the myocardium. With proximal fixation *(not traction)* of the plaque with forceps, the loop serves as a forward separator as opposed to causing any so-called snowplow effect.

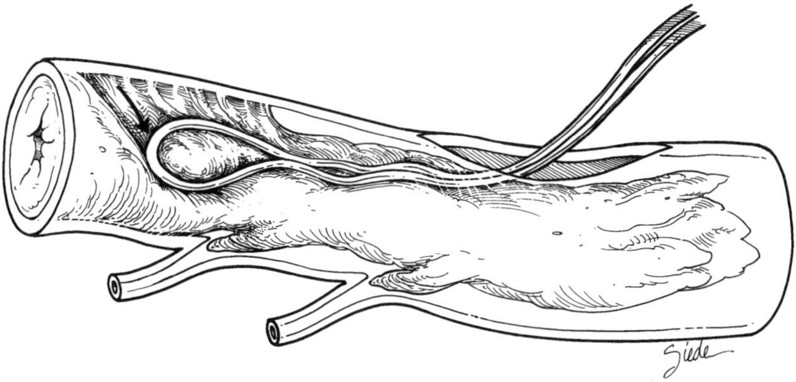

FIGURE 5.

Wire loops are the "workhorses" of manual endarterectomy. The diameter of the loop may be bent either larger or smaller to accommodate the size of the coronary artery. The tip should be kept rounded and smooth at all costs. A 2-mm-diameter coronary artery will require a slightly larger diameter of wire loop (2.25 mm) at the distal end to obtain circumferential separation of the external elastic membrane and media.

PROXIMAL EXTRACTION OF THE SPECIMEN

Before proceeding distally, the specimen is grasped with a "mini–plaque extractor." With the wire loops, separation is carried out proximally by "circular motion" with the curved end of the wire on first the anterior, next the sides, and finally the posterior interface of the external elastic membrane and the remaining plaque. The amount of pressure needed for separation varies, and with experience one can easily avoid damage. The wire loop is then used in a spiral motion circumferentially around the specimen. The extent or length of proximal endarterectomy varies with the specific artery being endarterectomized. The final step in proximal extraction is pulling the specimen out of the proximal coronary artery. This is begun by using steady traction on the plaque wall and alternately "walking" two tissue forceps up the specimen while providing countertraction on areas of unopened epicardium that show wrinkling or puckering. Wrinkling is an indication that the plaque remaining is stuck to the external elastic membrane (Fig 6). The specimen eventually breaks off proximally. At times, considerable force is necessary. If there is an obvious large retained fragment, it may be retrieved by using a long-bladed right-angle plaque retriever. After the proximal specimen is removed, cardioplegia is given for a short period by way of the aortic root to remove any possible retained debris.

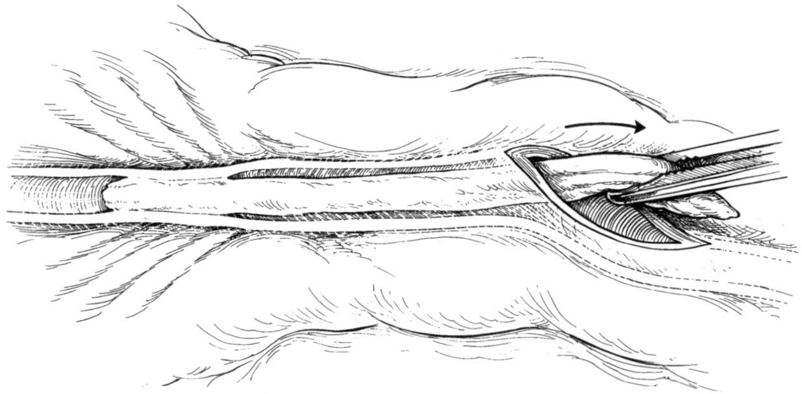

FIGURE 6.

Gentle traction on the plaque causes wrinkling and puckering of the overlying epicardium at points of persistent attachment of the external elastic membrane to the media. Often this is at a coronary artery branch.

RIGHT CORONARY ARTERY—PROXIMAL ENDARTERECTOMY

The proximal plaque is endarterectomized as far as possible, especially if there is total RCA occlusion. With 50% to 75% stenosis and no collateral noted on angiography, more care is taken to cleanly break the plaque off proximally. Plaque from the proximal RCA may often be retrieved to the level of the coronary ostia.

LEFT ANTERIOR DESCENDING—PROXIMAL ENDARTERECTOMY

The level of proximal endarterectomy is terminated at the arteriotomy and at a point that one may conveniently perform a bypass and completely remove the plaque distally. This is usually at the junction of the upper and middle thirds of the LAD. The point of fracture of a LAD atherosclerotic plaque is not as reliable as that of the RCA. One must therefore avoid leaving plaque within the LAD lumen adjacent to an endarterectomized septal perforator or diagonal branches. A clot may form between any retained endarterectomized plaque and the vessel wall and occlude those arteries (Fig

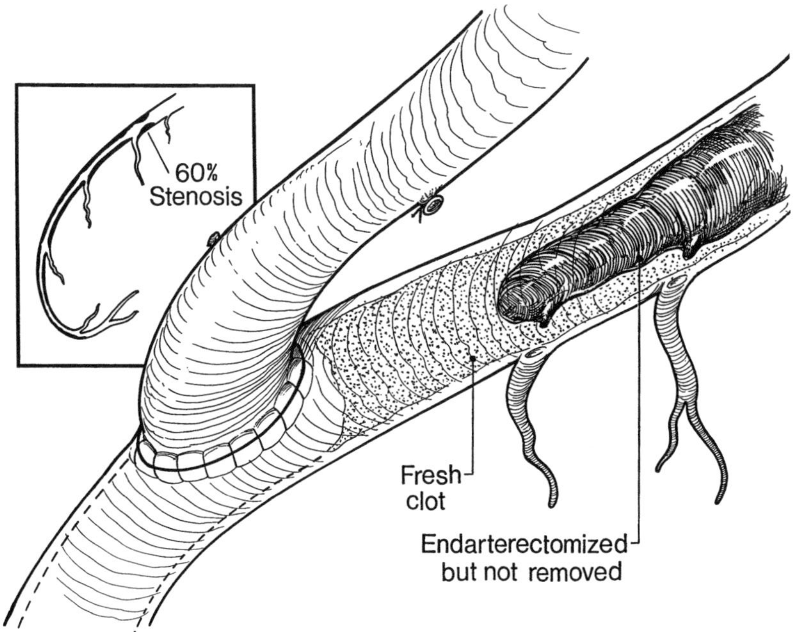

FIGURE 7.

If the proximal left anterior descending artery plaque is broken off inadvertently and endarterectomized plaque is left adjacent to a septal perforator or diagonal branches, thrombosis between the plaque and branches with resulting myocardial infarction may occur.

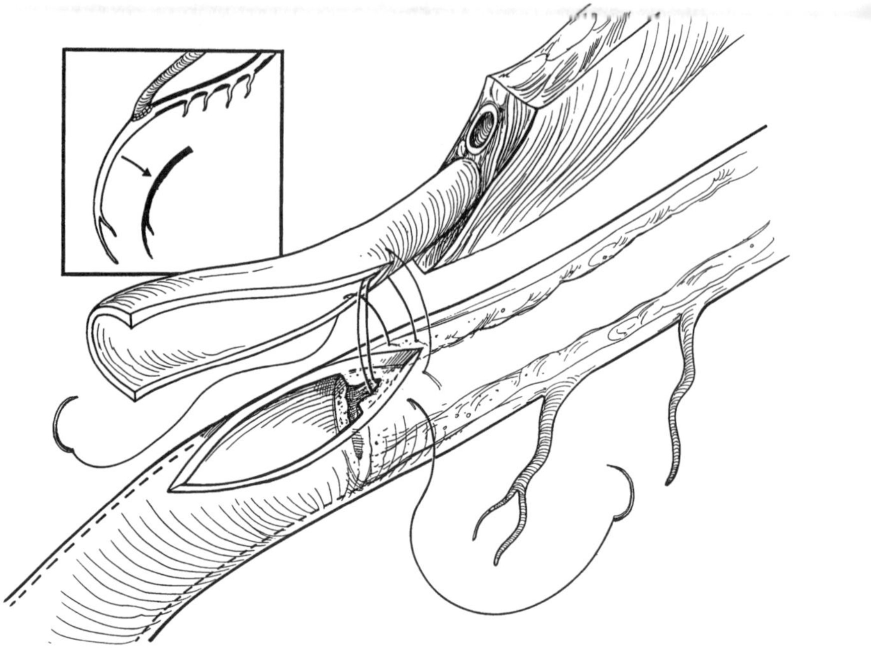

FIGURE 8.
Selected transection of the plaque at the site of anastomosis is preferred in the proximal left anterior descending artery. This is mandatory if there are no extremely tight stenoses or occlusion proximally.

7). Therefore, selected transection (usually at the site of anastomosis) of the proximal specimen to avoid the problem is preferred (Fig 8). In certain settings, a proximal retained plaque in the LAD can be removed by a wire snare technique (Fig 9).

CIRCUMFLEX MARGINAL BRANCHES—PROXIMAL ENDARTERECTOMY

Because of the paucity of left ventricular branches arising from the proximal end of the circumflex marginal coronary artery before it reaches the left ventricle, proximal endarterectomy is usually carried out from the coronary arteriotomy to the AV groove, where more often than not the proximal specimen easily breaks off.

RIGHT POSTERIOR DESCENDING—PROXIMAL ENDARTERECTOMY

If the arteriotomy is made in the posterior descending artery itself and the right system is open, the endarterectomy should not be carried proximally past the posterior descending–RCA junction for

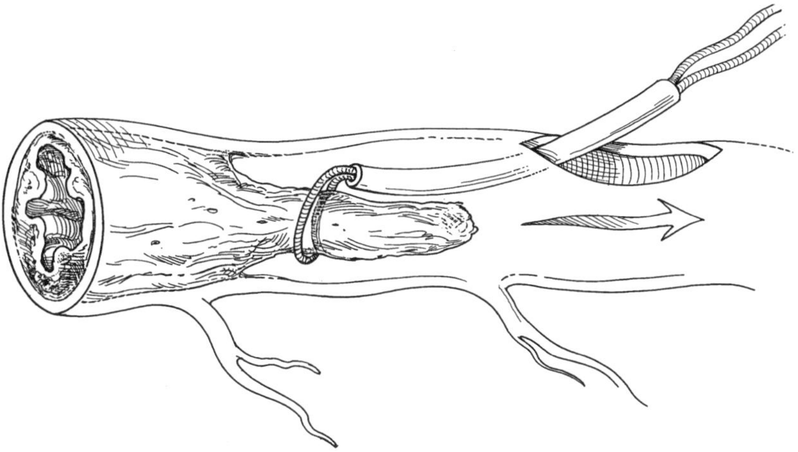

FIGURE 9.
A wire (30-gauge) snare technique may be used to retrieve proximal left anterior descending artery plaque that has been endarterectomized and inadvertently broken off.

fear of damaging that area and setting up a distal right coronary thrombosis. If the plaque in the right coronary is disturbed and separated, another arteriotomy in the RCA is performed to retrieve that distal disease.

LINEAR CALCIFICATION

In most instances the atherosclerotic plaque is flexible enough to remove as one would remove a 1-inch rope from within a same-size pipe. On occasion, pressure on the specimen with grasping forceps will cause the extrusion of semisolid atheromatous material, which must be sucked away. Less frequently and especially when dealing with the circumflex coronary artery, the lesions may have long areas of linear calcification. Calcium continuity is identified by moving the specimen at the anastomosis and finding that the entire atheromatous plaque moves as a whole. The plaque cannot be flexed to deliver it out of the 1-cm arteriotomy, so it must be fractured, divided, and removed as separate halves (see Fig 2).

DISTAL PLAQUE DISSECTION AND REMOVAL

RIGHT CORONARY ARTERY—DISTAL ENDARTERECTOMY

If both the posterior descending and the distal right coronary branches are to be endarterectomized, the distal right coronary is endarterectomized first. The arteriotomy is made close to the ori-

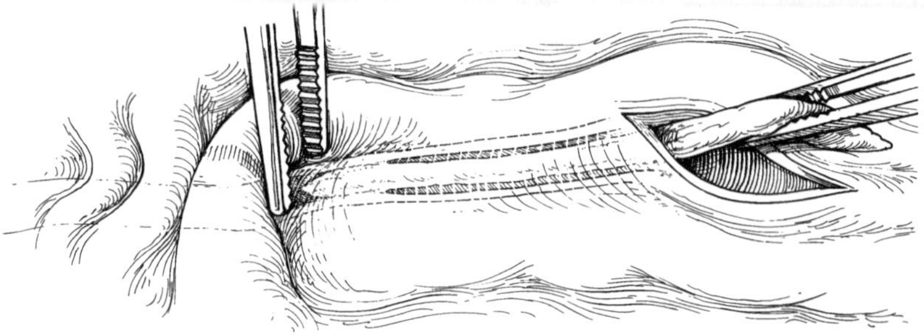

FIGURE 10.
The specimen is held firmly and the distal epicardium pulled away and stripped to "feather" the specimen at an appropriate point where the disease has played out. Release can be easily felt and the plaque withdrawn.

gin of the posterior descending branch. The wire loops are bent to conform to the gentle curve of the takeoff of the inferior ventricular branches from the RCA. Smaller wires are used to separate the core from each of the various branches. This may have to be done blindly with feel because of the overlying vein, fat, etc. With traction on the specimen, puckering can be identified as the point of persistent attachment of the plaque media and external elastic membrane. The tissue forceps technique of stripping is used to free the distal core and remove the specimen. The RCA proximal retrieved plaque is used as a handle. Distal dissection allows some of the proximal posterior descending artery to come into view, and dissection with the spatula is begun in that plane. Posteriorly, the AV nodal artery may be felt to still be attached, and that short core may be swept out near its origin with the spatula. An appropriately sized wire is advanced in the posterior descending artery under direct vision until the disease has terminated. With gentle traction on the specimen, puckering and/or wrinkling is seen at any spot where the core is still attached. If this occurs, patience is mandatory, and graded wires are reintroduced to free the area. Finally, when there is external wrinkling distally in the posterior descending artery in the area where the disease has terminated, separation with good feathering may be achieved with the tissue forceps by straddling the vessel at that distal point and gently stripping distally while the specimen is fixed with tissue forceps (Fig 10). External stripping distally is much more productive because traction on the plaque will result in the specimen breaking. The plaque will be felt to release and "feather," and the specimen can be withdrawn. The graft is then anastomosed to the arteriotomy with 7-0

(8-0 for extremely thin arterial walls) suture using a standard technique. Care is taken distally to use very close sutures inasmuch as anastomoses to endarterectomized vessels tend to be stenotic at the "toe" unless great care is taken.

MARGINAL BRANCHES OF THE CIRCUMFLEX—DISTAL ENDARTERECTOMY

Distal plaque removal of marginal branches is carried out after proximal withdrawal of the specimen. Plaque separation is started with the ball nerve hook distally for a short distance and continued with the spatula. Significant branches must be identified, entered, and endarterectomized separately if they are diseased. With plaque traction posteriorly toward the spine while the heart is held up, wrinkling again pinpoints areas of plaque attachment. When the disease terminates, the core is removed by constant mild traction from the proximal specimen, and the epicardium is gently "stripped" to separate the specimen and obtain good distal "feathering." If the specimen breaks off before termination of the disease, distal arteriotomy(s) is performed and the remainder of the plaque removed. Distal arteriotomies are always closed with a patch (Fig 11). The circumflex in the AV groove is very difficult to endarterectomize. There is difficulty in making the turn up into the origin of the marginal branches when the circumflex is opened in the AV groove. Perforations in that area are difficult to close. At this time, except in rare circumstances, endarterectomy is performed only on marginal branches. Other technical problems that could occur would be difficult to handle because of less accessibility to that coronary artery.

LEFT ANTERIOR DESCENDING AND ITS BRANCHES—DISTAL ENDARTERECTOMY

A left anterior descending artery that has small branches is relatively easy to endarterectomize. If it is 100% occluded, there is little risk. It becomes more difficult when multiple large diseased branches are present. At times it is wise to endarterectomize the LAD in its distal half and separately endarterectomize the high diagonal branches. After performing the arteriotomy and proximally retrieving the plaque, distal dissection is carried out anteriorly as far as possible to get to the distal extent of the disease even if it is around the apex. This is done with graded wires, with the smaller wires used for the apical area and care taken to keep the distal wire loop size in accordance with the inherent size of the LAD vessel itself (Fig 12).

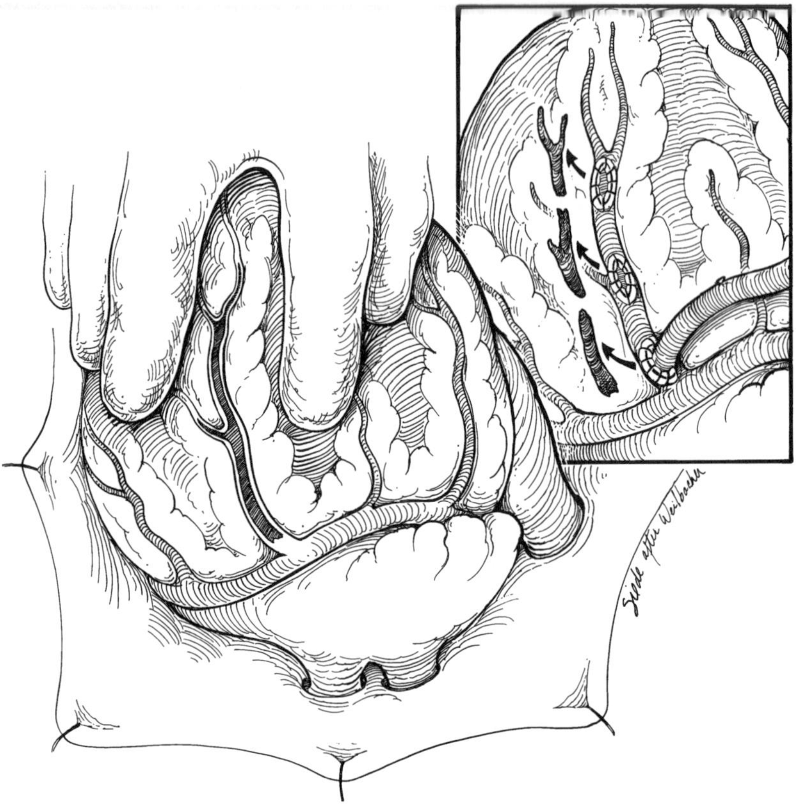

FIGURE 11.
Endarterectomy of a circumflex marginal branch may result in plaque breaking off at a branch before termination of the disease. A distal arteriotomy (3–4 mm) is performed, the remaining plaque is removed, and the arteriotomy is closed with a saphenous vein graft or preferably an internal mammary artery patch. The circumflex marginal with branches is one of the harder vessels to endarterectomize because of the awkward position needed to introduce endarterectomy instruments.

If the arteriotomy is near a diagonal, that branch is endarterectomized anteriorly. Wire separation is then carried out posteriorly on the LAD by first separating the sides and then proceeding distally. If unusual resistance is met from the large septal perforator, a side motion is carried out by twisting the wire loop to dislodge that core. Occasionally the spatula is helpful if the perforating vessel is close enough to the arteriotomy for direct visualization. Posterior separation of distal diagonal branches is not particularly difficult because there are no large posterior perforating branches in

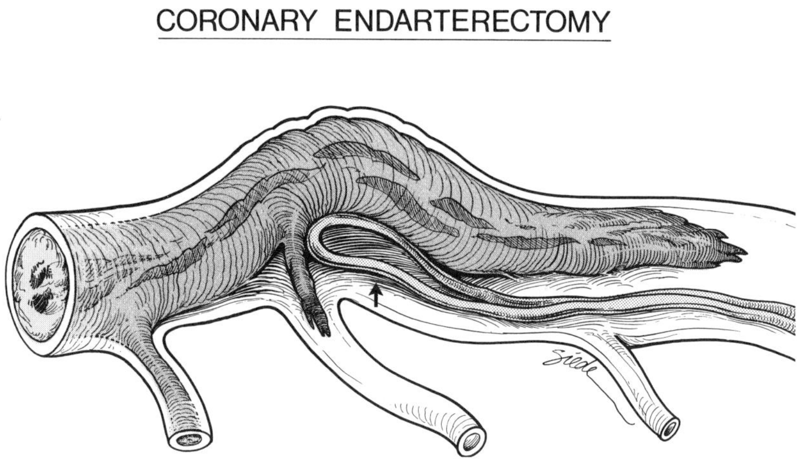

FIGURE 12.
Endarterectomy of the left anterior descending artery by using graded wire loops. Progressively smaller diameter loops are used distally.

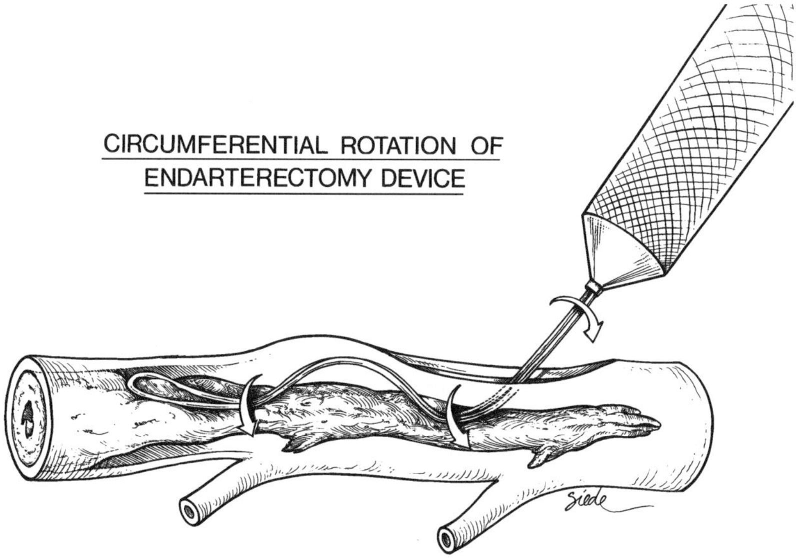

FIGURE 13.
Circumferential rotation of the wire loops is particularly helpful to release tiny branches.

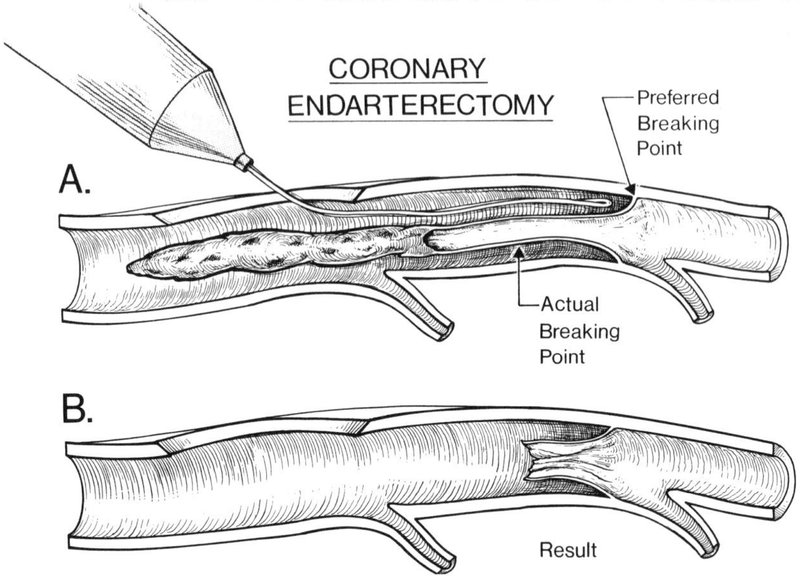

FIGURE 14.
A, with impatience and traction on the proximal specimen, a separation may occur remote from the preferred breaking point. **B,** this may result in distal occlusion of the coronary. Traction on the epicardium with tissue forceps will effect a separation at the exact preferred breaking point.

these arteries. Back-and-forth rotation of the wires more than 360 degrees is particularly helpful to release tiny branches (Fig 13). Separation of the apical bifurcation of the LAD or the so-called foot may be difficult and require opening of the epicardium to allow direct inspection of the wire advancing to each segment if both are diseased and arise at right angles. After the posterior wall as well as the diagonal branches have been separated, the specimen is withdrawn until wrinkling of the epicardium reveals any residual areas that are not separated. These are freed with wire loops if they are along the midportion of the core. If there is only distal attachment beyond the point where the atherosclerosis ends, tissue forceps are used to "strip" the overlying epicardium and free the core for extraction. *Caution:* The tissue forceps should not be used against bare distal vessel in which the epicardium has been opened because of the possibility of severe damage to the coronary artery. Also, traction should *not* be put on the specimen because it will tend to fracture at a point remote from the preferred breaking point (Fig 14).

ASSESSMENT OF ADEQUATE TERMINATION OF ENDARTERECTOMY—SPECIMEN "FEATHERING"

After removal of the core, the vessel is carefully inspected and palpated. Comparison of plaque anatomy with that of the preoperative angiogram may be helpful. Residual plaque can be seen and easily palpated in the majority of cases. Cardiogreen dye (10 mg/10 mL diluted in 50 mL of solvent) may be injected in the arteriotomy to determine areas of absent perfusion in the peripheral vascular bed. Injection of blood from the pump into the endarterectomized coronary artery in hearts protected by crystalloid cardioplegia can reveal a zone of no perfusion if there is distally occluding plaque. This is our preferred technique. Probes may be used but are generally withheld if good "feathering" was achieved because more harm than good might be done. If a definite retained plaque problem is suspected but not palpated, a calibrated probe should be tried. The exact location of the plaque can be pinpointed. The angioscope may also be used. Operative angiography is time consuming and somewhat cumbersome, but with frequent use it would perhaps offer the best method of assessing the immediate technical effect of the endarterectomy.

PROBLEMS

PERFORATION

Perforation can occur and most commonly is secondary to use of the ball nerve hook posteriorly. The most common location is on the underside of the RCA near the takeoff of the posterior descending artery. After the distal anastomosis is performed, perforation and anastomotic leaks should be sought by gently flushing pump blood through the bypass graft before removing the cross-clamp and performing the proximal anastomosis. Distal perforations covered by epicardium more than 3 cm from the anastomotic site are best left alone and cause no complications. Perforations accessible by way of the dissected area in the region of the anastomosis should be closed with 8-0 polypropylene suture.

BROKEN PLAQUE

Plaque that breaks prematurely results in obstruction to distal flow and must be addressed. A 3- to 4-mm arteriotomy is made directly over the remaining plaque as far distal as is convenient. The endarterectomy is then completed with good distal plaque termination and is surprisingly easy. This most often occurs in the distal third of the LAD near the takeoff of a small diagonal branch or in a skip zone. The arteriotomy is kept as small as possible and is closed by using four 8-0 polypropylene quadrant stitches and a small vein or preferably an internal mammary artery patch (Fig 15). The sutures are run from the ends to the middle and tied over a probe introduced from the proximal anastomosis to ensure against any technical mishap. Broken plaque in an artery 1-mm or smaller in diameter is probably best left alone.

INTRACORONARY DEBRIS

Irrigation with cardioplegia is carried out before performing the distal anastomosis. If known debris is thought to be inadvertently left in the distal coronary artery, forceful irrigation using a 10-mL syringe and a tiny catheter introduced through the arteriotomy as distal as possible may be carried out. More voluminous irrigation may be administered by way of a balloon catheter in the coronary sinus to remove distal debris. This has not been necessary in this author's experience.

ARRHYTHMIA

Arrhythmias from a ventricular focus were noted on occasion during early experience with extensive right coronary endarterectomy, but in more recent years, with experience it has become rare. Standard drug treatment has been successful, and no deaths secondary to arrhythmias have occurred.

PERIOPERATIVE MYOCARDIAL INFARCTION

The occurrence of perioperative myocardial infarction is 4% after standard coronary artery bypass and 8% with extended coronary endarterectomy when creatine phosphokinase (MB Fraction) and ECG changes are used to detect myocardial damage. If basic principles are used in the selection of arteries to be endarterectomized and the operation is technically correct, myocardial damage should be minimal and death rare.

SPECIAL PROBLEMS

Coronary artery bypass reoperation for extensive disease across a distal anastomosis presents a special problem. If the arteriotomy is made proximal or distal to an old anastomosis, the specimen cannot be endarterectomized safely across that anastomosis because sutures have been placed full thickness through the external elastic membrane. The old anastomosis therefore has to be opened and endarterectomy must be performed under direct vision if *more* than a distal endarterectomy is indicated.

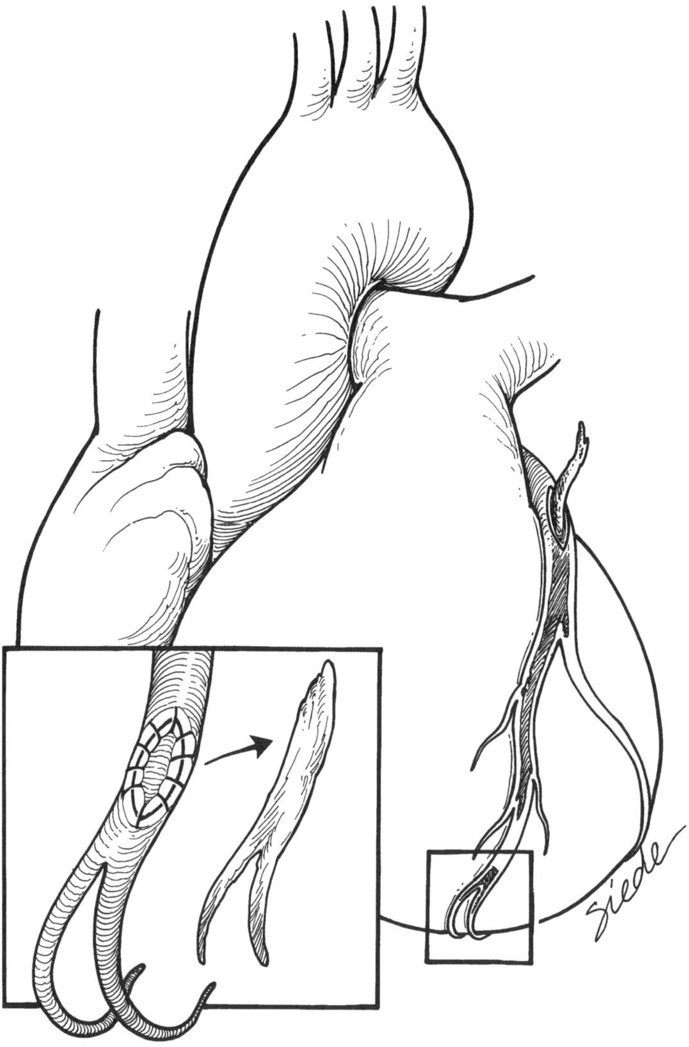

FIGURE 15.
A distal retained plaque occurs in the endarterectomized left anterior descending artery in 15% to 20% of cases. A 3- to 4-mm arteriotomy is made to retrieve the plaque. It is closed with a saphenous vein graft or internal mammary artery (preferable) patch over an appropriate-sized metal probe with 8-0 polypropylene suture.

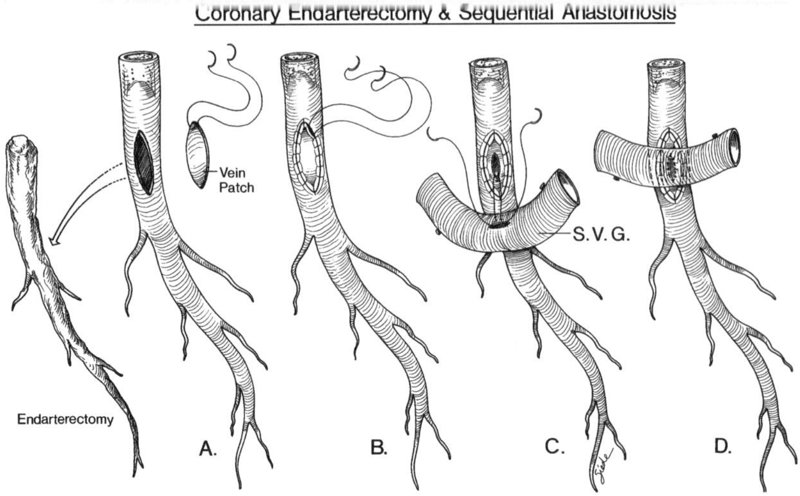

FIGURE 16.
When a sequential anastomosis is necessary over an endarterectomized vessel with a long arteriotomy, a special technique to address this problem is indicated. A vein patch (saphenous vein graft *[S.V.G]*) is sutured to the coronary arteriotomy and then a sequential anastomosis is performed to that patch.

On occasion an endarterectomy arteriotomy site will have to be opened 15 mm or more to effect an adequate endarterectomy. If a sequential anastomosis is planned in such a way that the graft crosses the coronary artery at a right angle, a problem occurs because of the long coronary arteriotomy. This can be managed by sewing a narrow vein patch to the arteriotomy and then making an appropriately sized veinotomy in the center of the vein patch for a sequential anastomosis to the saphenous graft (Fig 16).

On rare occasion, the proximal disease is bulbous and has expanded beyond the size of the native coronary even after that artery has been endarterectomized. Attempts to pull such a large plaque distally through the smaller coronary artery may cause stretching and tearing of the coronary artery proximal to the arteriotomy. This is analogous to trying to deliver a baby through too narrow a pelvis. Such damage that is not evident as immediate tearing could result in late aneurysm formation in the proximal coronary artery. When the problem is identified, it is solved by extending the arteriotomy proximally to avoid coronary artery damage. This is rarely necessary.

CLINICAL DATA

The author's initial experience with 245 patients having extensive (greater than 6 cm long) single or multiple coronary artery endarterectomies in association with coronary artery bypass over a 6-year period has produced good results that are an impetus to continue its use. Patient ages ranged from 32 to 79 (mean, 61), and 25% of the patients were females. An average of 4.4 bypasses per patient were performed. The most common artery endarterectomized was the RCA (50%), followed next by the left anterior descending, diagonal, and marginal. One to four arteries were endarterectomized (Fig 17). There were 6 hospital deaths (2.4%), but only 1 was related to endarterectomy. That patient suffered a perioperative myocardial infarction in the region of the endarterectomized LAD. An internal mammary graft with a free flow of 120 mL/min anastomosed to a 3-cm-long vein patch on the LAD was used in that patient. Anecdotal similar cases from other surgeons have led to abandonment of that technique. The mortality rate of 1,225 concomitant nonendarterectomy coronary artery bypass patients during the same period was 2.0%. The specimen lengths in the endarterectomy patients ranged from 6 to 15 cm. Coronary arteriotomy size rarely exceeded 10 mm (12 patients). A distal arteriotomy to retrieve retained plaque was necessary in 31 instances (LAD, 23; circumflex marginal coronary artery, 5; RCA, 2; diagonal, 1). Cross-clamp times averaged an extra 18 minutes per vessel endarterectomized. Low–molecular weight dextran was begun in the operating room after the administration of Promit to avoid an allergic reaction from the dextran. It was maintained postoperatively for 36–48 hours. All coronary bypass patients are given preoperative dipyridamole, and aspirin is started in the ICU. Sodium warfarin in minidosage (1–2 mg orally per day) is begun on postoperative day 1 and continued for a minimum of 6 months. Restudy of these patients has been difficult because of reluctance stemming from the absence of symptoms and spiraling medical costs. However, the incidence of perioperative myocardial infarction, operative mortality, and late morbidity with recurrence of symptoms has supported the expanded use of extensive coronary endarterectomy with the saphenous vein or internal mammary artery as grafts to the endarterectomized vessels in patients who previously may have been deemed inoperable.

A vignette of clinical experience has been noted in four patients who have had extensive coronary endarterectomy and have undergone reoperations or have come to postmortem exami-

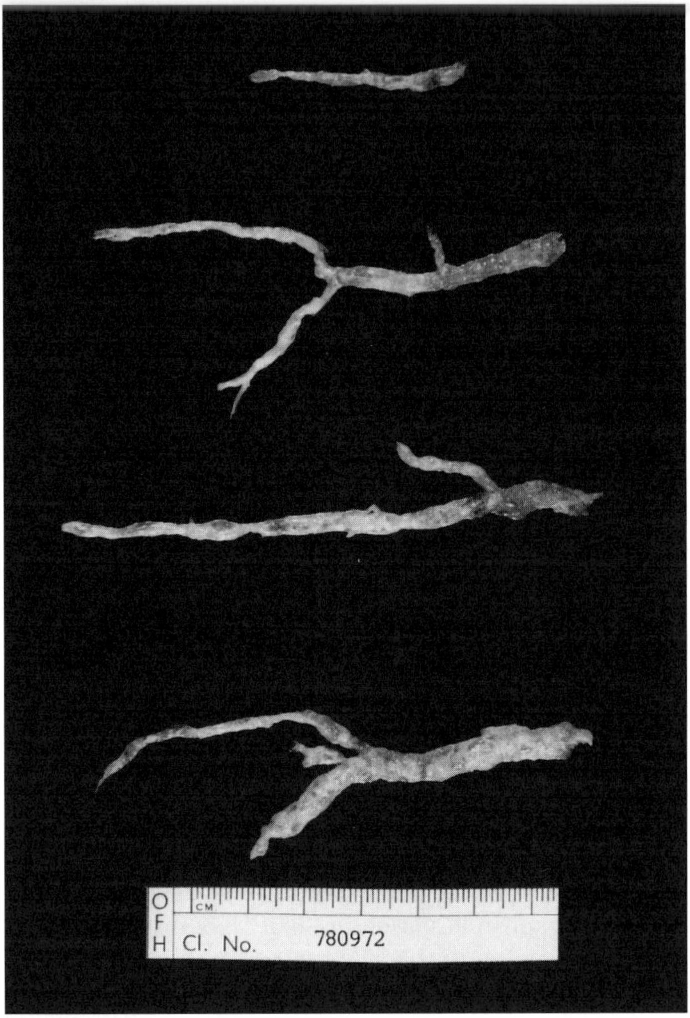

FIGURE 17.

Endarterectomy specimens of the left anterior descending, diagonal, circumflex marginal, and right coronary artery from a 65-year-old male patient. Angiography 6 years postoperatively revealed patency of all grafts and endarterectomized vessels. The patient expired 10 years postoperatively of noncardiac causes.

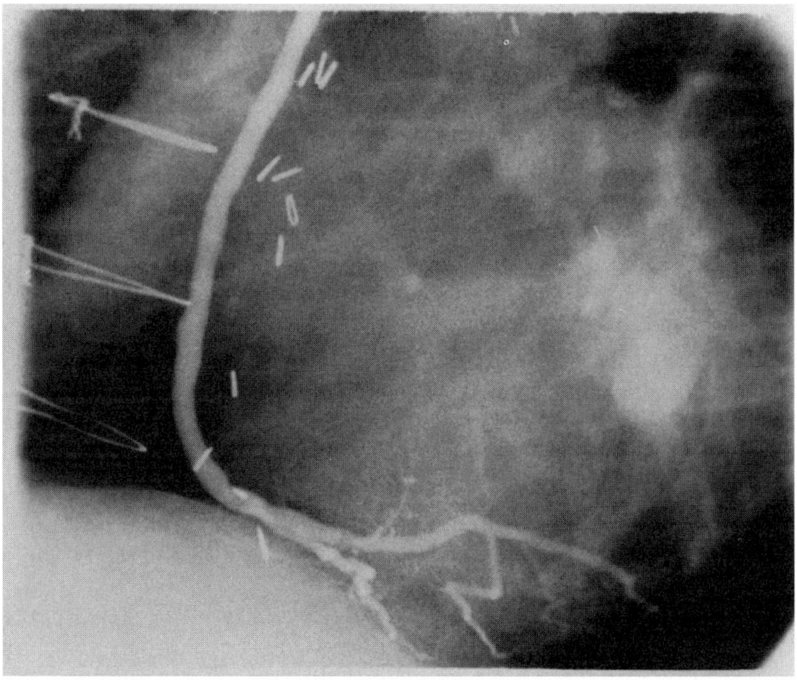

FIGURE 18.
Postoperative angiogram of a diabetic male patient $7\frac{1}{2}$ years after extensive endarterectomy of the right coronary artery. There was progression of atherosclerosis in all native coronary arteries and in all vein grafts, but the endarterectomized vessel was soft and disease free at reoperation.

nation 5–10 years after the original coronary artery bypass grafting. All had diabetes. There was significant progression of native disease and vein graft disease but no atherosclerosis in the endarterectomized arteries (RCA, 3; LAD, 1). It is interesting to theorize that in a subset of coronary atherosclerotic patients the disease is strictly a medial-layer entity (vascular smooth muscle cell proliferation and migration with subsequent atherosclerosis). When the media is removed (extensive coronary endarterectomy), the disease is arrested (Fig 18).

MAIN LEFT CORONARY ENDARTERECTOMY

On rare occasion, a main left coronary endarterectomy has been performed but is not classified as an "extensive" endarterectomy. The author's use of the endarterectomy technique for this subset of patients has been confined primarily to young patients with lo-

TABLE 2.
Summary of Technical Notes for Extensive Coronary Endarterectomy

1. Always perform a bypass.
2. Begin antiplatelet drugs in the operating room (low–molecular weight dextran after Promit).
3. Use atrial and ventricular pacer wires when dominant right posterior descending systems are endarterectomized.
4. Avoid opening the epicardium except at the point of anastomosis.
5. Inject blood or cardiogreen dye after completion of the anastomosis to detect leaks, perforations, and/or retained plaque.
6. Retrieve retained plaque with a 3-mm distal arteriotomy and close with an IMA or SVG patch using 8-0 suture *over a probe.*
7. Open near a bifurcation whenever possible.
8. Avoid retrograde endarterectomy (in the LAD and circumflex marginal) with non-100% occlusion of the coronary artery. Selectively cut the plaque with Potts' scissors at the arteriotomy site in those instances.
9. Avoid anastomosing an IMA to a thick area in the proximal LAD coronary artery (heel) anastomosis.
10. Use a wire snare technique to selectively cut off a specimen in the proximal coronary artery for the LAD and circumflex marginal arteries rather than set up a long blind endarterectomized area.
11. Note that an endarterectomy stops or tears at a previous anastomosis during reoperation.
12. A proximal arterial plaque (especially the RCA) may be larger than the coronary artery at the arteriotomy site and may damage the endarterectomized vessel if an attempt is made to pull it out of that opening.
13. Puckering or wrinkling along the course of the artery denotes where it is still attached.
14. Do not attempt to "feather" the distal plaque by pulling on the plaque.
15. External traction on the epicardium with the plaque held fixed at the arteriotomy is the best way to "feather" the plaque distally.
16. A flip-up motion with the spatula is the best way to retrieve short plaque extensions (septal perforator, diagonal) visualized near the arteriotomy.
17. Use of the IMA for the bypass graft works well even with long arteriotomies if the IMA free flow is good (>150 mL/min).
18. Use the IMA as a free graft after an extensive endarterectomy if the IMA pedicle graft free flow is less than 150 mL/min.
19. Avoid jeopardizing a distal vessel (i.e., second marginal) by chasing proximal plaque into the parent vessel (i.e., circumflex), unless the parent vessel has 100% occlusion.

(continued)

TABLE 2. (continued)

20. Have the assistant straighten the artery by traction on the heart when endarterectomizing tortuous arteries with the wire loop.
21. Rotate the wire loop 360 degrees back and forth on the anterior as well as the posterior side of the coronary artery.
22. It is convenient to mark the proposed external site of termination of the arteriotomy with a sterile marking pen.
23. Divide linear calcified plaque in the center of the arteriotomy. Endarterectomize each section separately as opposed to trying to pull the rigid, nongiving plaque through the arteriotomy and damaging the vessel.
24. Irrigation may begin distally through a 1-mm plastic catheter introduced through the arteriotomy before performing the anastomosis. Irrigation is carried out only as the catheter is withdrawn back through the arteriotomy.
25. A cardioplegia dose may be used to irrigate the proximal coronary artery before performing the anastomosis.
26. Avoid endarterectomy on vessels with ectasia or aneurysm or those within myocardial tunnels.
27. When distal branching with disease occurs, both branches must be entered and separately endarterectomized to avoid a retained fragment in one of the branches.
28. Perforations in very distal vessels with intact epicardium are best left alone. A perforation of the coronary artery adjacent to the arteriotomy must be dissected out and closed with 8-0 Prolene.
29. Bare distal vessel with epicardium removed should not be stripped with the tissue forceps for fear of severe damage to the coronary artery.
30. RGEA flow must be adequate (>150 mL/min, >1.5 mm ID) and spasm free for use with extensive endarterectomy.
31. Traction stitch at the toe of the anastomosis to prevent narowing of the anastomosis—very important!
32. An olive-tipped soft DLP (Medtronic, Grand Rapids, MI) needle may be used to instill low–molecular weight dextran into the endarterectomized coronary artery just before performing the graft coronary anastomosis when multiple endarterectomies are performed.
33. *Be patient!*

Abbreviations: IMA, internal mammary artery; *SVG,* saphenous vein graft; *LAD,* left anterior descending artery; *RCA,* right coronary artery; *RGEA,* right gastroepiploic artery; *ID,* internal diameter.

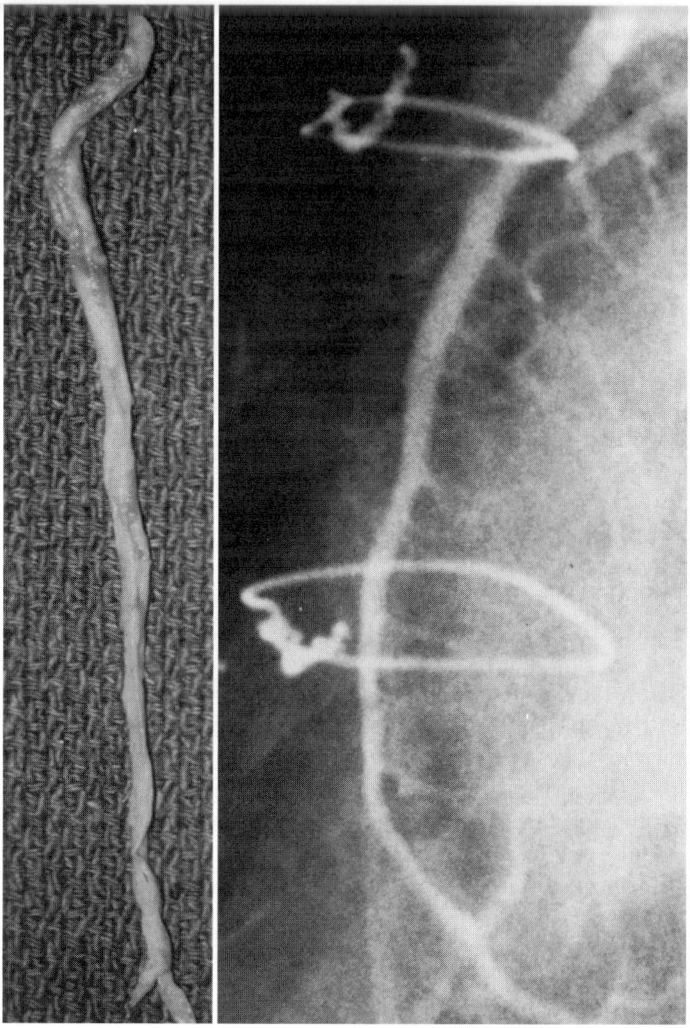

FIGURE 19.
Postoperative angiogram 10 years after left internal mammary–to–left anterior descending coronary artery bypass and extensive endarterectomy. The specimen retrieved at surgery is seen on the *left*.

calized disease. Extensive plaque is not removed. The pulmonary artery is dissected and retracted while on cardiopulmonary bypass in order to visualize the left coronary artery. The left coronary artery is endarterectomized by cutting down on it directly and extending the arteriotomy into the aorta. An open endarterectomy is performed, with "feathering" of the plaque ending in the main left coronary artery itself. The coronary artery is then closed with a saphenous vein or internal mammary patch that extends well into the aorta. The clinical results have been very rewarding, with total absence of symptoms in the five female patients. No reoperations have been necessary in the 2.5- to 10-year follow-up.

TECHNICAL NOTES

A summary of technical aspects of extensive coronary endarterectomy has been tabulated (Table 2).

CONCLUSIONS

Coronary endarterectomy is effective in bypassing coronary arteries that heretofore would have been classed as "inoperable due to distal disease." Early attempts at coronary endarterectomy, even though immediately successful, resulted in relatively early failure in most instances. Now, however, refined techniques using 4× loupe magnification and specialized instruments (Baxter V. Mueller Division, Deerfield, Ill) combined with cold cardioplegia protection of the myocardium and risk factor modification in the late follow-up period may offer such patients with severe distal disease an improved outlook (Fig 19). Most cardiac surgeons have had the unpleasant experience of finding "disease much worse than on the angiogram" and having to perform an anastomosis on fragmenting arterial walls in such vessels with poor runoff because of significant extensive distal disease. Properly performed coronary endarterectomy offers an alternative. With the increased popularity of percutaneous transluminal coronary angioplasty, patients will be seen in later stages of coronary artery disease and thus test the surgeon's skill and require the utilization of an ever-increasing armamentarium of technical advances.

REFERENCES

1. Vlodaver Z, Edwards J: The pathology of coronary disease. *J Thorac Cardiovasc Surg* 98:1392–1399, 1983.
2. Mills NL, Ochsner J: Distal thromboembolism and proximal coronary arteriosclerotic lesions. *Surgery* 72:1030–1036, 1972.
3. Johnson WD, Brenowitz JB, Kayser KL: Surgery for diffuse coronary disease. *Cardiology* 3:35–38, 1986.
4. Sawyer PN, Kaplitt M, Sobel S: Experimental and clinical experience with coronary gas endarterectomy. *Arch Surg* 95:736–742, 1967.
5. Lane WZ, Minot HD Jr: Ultrasonic coronary endarterectomy. *Ann Thorac Surg* 1:693–696, 1965.

CHAPTER 10

Genetically Engineered Organs

Ranjit John, M.D.
Research Fellow, Columbia University; Research Fellow, Department of Surgery, Columbia Presbyterian Medical Center, New York, New York

John H. Artrip, M.D.
Research Fellow, Columbia University; Research Fellow, Department of Surgery, Columbia Presbyterian Medical Center, New York, New York

Robert E. Michler, M.D.
Karl P. Klassen Professor of Surgery, Ohio State University; Chief, Cardiothoracic Surgery, Ohio State University Medical Center, Columbus, Ohio

Improvements in surgical technique and postoperative care and advances in immunosuppression have made solid-organ transplantation the procedure of choice for progressive and intractable organ failure. Unfortunately, the availability of donor organs has not kept pace with the increasing annual numbers of patients in need of organ transplants. According to the United Network for Organ Sharing scientific registry, over 67,000 patients were listed for transplantation during 1995, but only 20,000 received transplants.[1] The 5-year period between 1990 and 1995 witnessed over a 70% increase in the number of patients awaiting organ transplantation. Efforts to increase donation rates such as educational programs and "required request" legislation have not improved donation rates, as measured by a disappointing 28% increase in donors over the same 5-year period.[1, 2] Of Americans listed for heart transplantation, approximately 35% receive transplants during a given year and nearly 20% to 30% die before a donor is found.[3, 4] For certain populations of patients such as children, status II patients, or blood group O patients, the likelihood of receiving a transplant is even less. With 1-year heart transplant survival rates exceeding 90% at many centers, it is more likely for a patient to die while on the waiting list than to die within the first year after transplantation.[5] The severe shortage of donor organs together with the ability to genetically engineer organs has led to a resurgence of interest in the field of xenotransplantation.

Clinical advances in the field of xenotransplantation have been few when compared with the tremendous developments in allogeneic organ transplantation.[6, 7] In 1963, Reemtsma performed kidney xenotransplantation with chimpanzee donors. Kidney graft survival of up to 9 months was achieved with an immunosuppressive regimen consisting of actinomycin, azathioprine, and steroids.[6] A year later, Starzl reported six baboon-to-human renal transplants with azathioprine and steroids used for immunosuppression and achieved graft survival up to 2 months.[8] In the same year, Hardy performed the first clinical heart transplant with a chimpanzee donor and achieved graft survival of only 2 hours.[9] Subsequently, Cooley and Ross reported heart xenotransplants (sheep and pig, respectively); both grafts failed immediately upon reperfusion.[10, 11] More recently, in 1984 Bailey et al. performed a baboon-to-human heart transplant in an infant with cyclosporine-based immunosuppression. Despite ABO incompatibility, the cardiac xenograft survived for 20 days.[12] In 1993 and 1994, Starzl reported two baboon-to-human liver transplants with FK 506–based immunosuppression and achieved graft survival of 70 and 26 days in the setting of a difficult clinical course, including infection and stroke.[13, 14]

Owing to a combination of ethical, logistic, and molecular biological factors, the pig is presently considered the best potential donor for clinical xenotransplantation. It is believed that the pig also harbors relatively few infectious agents likely to be transmitted to humans. Nevertheless, the major barrier to successful organ transplantation between the pig and humans remains hyperacute rejection.[15, 16]

Hyperacute rejection of porcine organs results from the activation of complement initiated by the binding of naturally occurring recipient xenoreactive antibodies to donor vascular endothelium. This antibody and complement–mediated inflammatory response leads to endothelial cell activation, hemorrhage, edema, and vascular thrombosis with destruction and loss of graft function within minutes to hours.[17] Strategies to overcome hyperacute rejection have focused on inhibiting complement activation and the removal of xenoreactive antibody. Methods used to block complement include agents such as cobra venom factor and soluble complement receptor type 1 (CR1).[18, 19] Removal of xenoreactive antibodies has been achieved by column adsorption, extracorporeal organ perfusion, and inhibition of antibody binding with soluble carbohydrate therapy.[20, 21] Modest advances have been made in both organ function and survival with the use of these methods, but these advances remain unacceptable for clinical trials. The development of transgenic organs has added a new and promising modality in the prevention of hyperacute rejection. This review discusses the present status of genetically engineered organs with special emphasis on xenotransplantation.

TRANSGENIC ANIMALS

By definition, a transgenic animal is one that contains a segment of foreign genetic material within its own genome; the result is a new trait that can be transmitted to offspring. The technology to introduce genes into the germline of mammals was first reported by Jaenisch and Mintz in 1974.[22] Transgenic animals have been used to study mechanisms of gene regulation, mammalian development, and cardiovascular, renal, neurologic, and immune disease processes in humans.[23] In addition, transgenic technology has provided the ability to manipulate the genes of organ donor animals in the hope of preventing rejection in the recipient.

METHODS OF GENERATING TRANSGENIC ANIMALS

The first step in producing a transgenic animal is to identify the gene responsible for the trait to be transferred. This DNA segment is called the *transgene.* Typical transgenes also contain the DNA nucleotide sequences necessary for efficient transcription of the transgene. The efficiency of DNA integration into the host genome is influenced by DNA purity and concentration and the nucleotide sequence (promoter) used to "promote" gene insertion into the host genome.

Described in the following sections are the primary methods for introducing genes into animals.

Microinjection of DNA Transgene Into the Pronucleus of the Host

Transgene microinjection is the most commonly used method for creating transgenic animals, primarily because of its relative ease of performance. The major drawback with this technique is the randomness of transgene insertion into the host chromosomal DNA.[24] It is suspected that random chromosomal breaks in the host DNA serve as the site for integration of the injected foreign DNA. This random integration may result in position effects in which expression of the transgene is influenced by the specific site of integration and the surrounding DNA in the host chromosome. This effect could result in loss of cell specificity for expression of the transgene, an inappropriately high copy number of the transgene, or complete silencing of the transgene. Furthermore, a mutation could occur by random insertion of the transgene into the body of an essential gene.

Several groups have been successful in developing transgenic pigs that express human complement regulatory proteins by microinjection of minigene constructs.[25–27] Minigene constructs contain the gene of interest, transcription and translation initiation and termination sequences, and a promoter or regulatory region. Because of the problem of position effects with the microinjection of minigenes, Langford et al. used the technique of microinjection with a yeast artificial chromosome (YAC) that contained human membrane cofactor protein (MCP) along with flanking sequences to produce MCP transgenic pigs.[28] This technique of producing transgenic animals has two potential advantages. First, because the YAC contains the entire *MCP* gene and the 5′ and 3′ flanking sequences involved in the differential regulation of MCP, it is possible that the transgenic animals generated may produce all the different MCP mRNA slice variants seen in humans. Second, expression of MCP YAC may be independent of the site at which the YAC integrates into the porcine genome.

Retroviral Infection

Retroviral vectors are viral genomes that carry exogenous DNA into an early-stage embryo, for example, the use of a viral vector to transport the gene into an oocyte. In contrast to microinjected DNA, retroviruses integrate by a precisely defined mechanism into the genome of the infected cell. Only a single proviral copy is inserted at a particular chromosomal site, thereby decreasing the frequency of position effects. Also, no rearrangements of the host genome are induced, apart from a short duplication of host sequences at the site of integration.[22]

The main advantage of the use of retroviruses or retroviral vectors for gene transfer is the technical ease of introducing virus into embryos. In addition, it is easier to isolate the flanking host sequences of a proviral insert than those flanking a DNA insert derived from pronuclear injection. This fact is of considerable advantage when attempting to identify a host gene disrupted by insertion of the proviral DNA. However, the use of viral vectors limits the size of exogenous DNA that can be introduced into the host chromosome (inability to transfer transgenes larger than 10 kb).[23] At present, use of the retroviral technique is limited because of random integration.

Embryonic Stem Cell Technology

Embryonic stem cells are pluripotential stem cells isolated from the inner cell mass of a blastula-stage embryo. The major benefit of embryonic stem cells is that they remain pluripotent while continuing to multiply and divide. With the development of embryonic stem cell technology, genetic manipulations can be performed in cell culture. By using the technique of homologous recombination, one is able to inactivate, replace, or introduce subtle alterations into the endogenous gene of interest. After the intended genetic change has been verified, these embryonic stem cells can be injected into host blastocytes, where they can colonize the embryo and contribute to the germline of the resulting chimeric animal. The advantage of using embryonic stem cells is that in addition to performing conventional transfections like the addition of single-gene constructs, complex manipulations such as adding or deleting genes at specific sites can be accomplished.[29, 30]

Cloning

Several species, including mice, sheep, and monkeys, have been cloned by transferring nuclei from embryonic cells. It was previously believed that the DNA of older cells was irreversibly altered by maturation, chemical changes, and structural modifications and that these genomes were incapable of supporting development of the various early cell types needed to construct an animal.[31, 32] However, Wilmut and colleagues stunned the world by demonstrating that cell lines from an adult animal could be used to clone a lamb (Dolly), thereby showing that the DNA of an adult cell can no longer be viewed as maturing along an irreversible path of gene suppression during differentiation into a mature somatic cell.[33] Explanations for their achievement have been attributed to (1) the possibility that the nucleus used for transfer may have retained some stem cell characteristics, that is, an undifferentiated progenitor cell of many different tissue types, and (2) finding a method to make the donor nuclei more compatible with the cytoplasm of the recipient oocyte.

The major difficulty in nuclear transplantation studies has been obtaining cell cycle compatibility between the donor nucleus and recipient oocyte. In mammals, most of the early embryonic nuclei that are used as donors are either in the S or G_2 (nondiploid) phase of the cell cycle. When nuclei in these phases are introduced into metaphase II–arrested oocytes (the preferred recipient phase), they tend to undergo additional DNA duplication and premature chromosomal condensation with resultant aneuploidy and abnormal development. Wilmut et al. may have overcome this hurdle by transplanting nuclei from cells that had been arrested in the diploid G_0 phase of the cell cycle. This feat was accomplished by reducing the nutrient-laden serum supplied to the cells, thereby starving the cells into the dormant G_0 or G_1 stages of the cell cycle. Using cells from this stage of the cell cycle resulted in synchrony in the timing of DNA replication between the transplanted nucleus and the cytoplasm of the recipient oocyte and thus reduced the incidence of chromosomal abnormalities.[33] Amid all this excitement, it should be remembered that it took 277 attempts to produce Dolly from an adult cell and more than 50% of the cloned sheep pregnancies failed to develop to term.

An even more exciting development from the group led by Wilmut is the cloning of a group of lambs from fetal cells that were genetically manipulated in the laboratory to carry extra genes, including an undisclosed human gene that was introduced into the cells before they were cloned. To achieve this feat, they first exposed fetal fibroblasts to DNA that included both a human gene and a marker gene. A similar cloning strategy that was used to make Dolly was performed with these animals. All five of the newborn lambs carry the marker gene, and one named Polly has been shown to carry the human gene.[34] One important observation in these studies is that the presence of foreign DNA in the fibroblast genome did not disrupt the genetic development of the lamb. Also, an advantage to using fetal cells is that they are more efficient in achieving development than adult cells are, and one live birth is realized for every 60 nuclear transfers.

TRANSGENICALLY ENGINEERED ORGANS AND XENOTRANSPLANTATION

USE OF XENOANTIGEN IN XENOTRANSPLANTATION

The major xenoantigen recognized by human natural antibody is galactose-α-1,3-galactose (Gal epitope), a terminal disaccharide on glycoproteins.[35] This epitope is absent in humans, apes, and Old World monkeys because the enzyme responsible for this residue, α-1,3-galactosyltransferase (GalT), has been switched off during evolutionary development. Humans do not express the Gal epitope, and therefore human serum contains high-titer natural xenoreactive antibodies against the Gal epitope. These antibodies are barely detectable in the newborn period. Newborn primates are a "natural model" of xenoreactive IgM antibody depletion. In studies using newborn baboon recipients in the absence of immunosuppression, heterotopically transplanted porcine cardiac xenografts survived beyond the hyperacute period with a mean survival of 3.6 days. Histologic examination of the explanted xenografts demonstrated only minimal hemorrhage and thrombosis. Immunofluorescent examination failed to reveal IgM deposition and only trace deposition of IgG (maternal) and complement.[36, 37]

ROLE OF COMPLEMENT IN XENOTRANSPLANTATION

In the pig-to-primate model of xenotransplantation, complement activation by naturally occurring host xenoreactive antibodies results in hyperacute rejection within minutes to hours.[38] Antibodies serve as a binding site for complement protein 1q (C1q), which combines with C1r and C1s to form C1qrs. The latter catalyzes the cleavage of C4 to C4b, which in turn combines with C2a to form C4b2a. C4b2a is referred to as the classic-pathway convertase; it cleaves C3 and leads to amplification through the complement cascade. Activated complement induces various nonspecific effector mechanisms, including activation of platelets and neutrophils and production of vasoactive substances and other proinflammatory mediators. The immunochemistry of hyperacutely rejected porcine organs demonstrates the deposition of C3, C4, C5, membrane attack complex, fibrin, and platelets on endothelial cell surfaces with a distribution coinciding with xenoreactive antibody. Further evidence indicating the importance of the complement system has been shown by the absence of hyperacute rejection in complement-deficient animals.[39]

Although the alternative pathway may be important in rodent and other models of xenotransplantation, the classic pathway is of primary importance in primate xenotransplantation. Dalmasso et al. demonstrated this fact by using a simple model of porcine endothelial cell layers incubated with human serum as a source of human antibody and complement. Normal human serum was cytotoxic to porcine endothelial cells. The importance of the classic pathway was demonstrated by the inability of C2-deficient human serum to produce endothelial cell cytotoxicity. Cytotoxicity was restored by the addition of purified C2.[40]

Inappropriate activation of complement is prevented by a group of endothelial cell–associated proteins that are referred to as complement regulatory proteins. These proteins include decay-accelerating factor (DAF; CD55), MCP (CD46), and CR1 (CD35), which act on the C3 convertase stage, and homologous restriction factor (CD59), which acts on the membrane attack complex stage of the pathway. Because complement regulatory proteins are species specific, that is, they do not function against heterologous complement, xenografts are particularly susceptible to complement-mediated injury.[41] It is for this reason that the first transgenic pig organs to be developed contained human complement regulatory proteins.

TRANSGENIC TECHNOLOGY DIRECTED AT COMPLEMENT

The phenomenon of "homologous restriction" whereby complement is more efficient at lysing heterologous than homologous complement has led to a novel approach to the transplantation of organs across genetically disparate barriers. Transgenic pigs that express human, membrane-bound complement regulatory proteins on their tissues were produced to limit the effects of primate and human complement.[42, 43]

This approach has the added advantage of inhibiting complement activation only at the site of the transplanted organ, as opposed to the administration of systemic complement inhibitors such as cobra venom factor or soluble CR1, which interfere with overall host complement and thereby the host's immune response against infectious agents. Dalmasso et al. first tested this concept with porcine endothelial cells that expressed human DAF. These endothelial cells were not susceptible to complement-mediated lysis when exposed to human natural antibodies and complement.[40] Other in vitro studies with murine and porcine cell lines transfected with complement regulatory proteins showed significant protection of the transfected cells from the effects of human serum.[44–45]

Fodor et al. have engineered the production of transgenic mice and pigs that express the human terminal complement inhibitor CD59. To achieve expression of this protein, they used a murine major histocompatibility complex (MHC) class I gene. Class I MHC genes are ubiquitously expressed on most somatic cells and are a predominant endothelial cell surface antigen. Furthermore, the MHC class I promoter has the capacity to upregulate human CD59 expression in response to inflammatory cytokines. High-level cell surface expression of CD59 was achieved, especially on endothelial tissue. Porcine cells expressing CD59 were resistant to lysis when challenged with high-titer antiporcine antibody and human complement.[42]

In ex vivo xenogeneic perfusion models, the use of porcine organs transgenic for human DAF and CD59 has prevented the development of hyperacute rejection and increased organ survival for several hours. In contrast, ex vivo perfusion of nontransgenic hearts and kidneys with human blood resulted in complement-mediated destruction within minutes to an hour. After cessation of organ function, immunochemistry of transgenic porcine organs revealed only minimal deposition of C3b and C9 in vascular endothelium expressing DAF and CD59.[43, 46] Immunohistochemical staining with monoclonal antihuman DAF and antihuman CD59 has been used to determine the presence of these proteins in tissues. Because expression of these transgenes is variable in different tissues and organs, histologic evaluation of protein expression in these transgenic animals is of importance if these animals are to be bred to become clinical organ donors.[47]

In vivo transplant studies have also been performed to evaluate the function and survival of these transgenic organs. White and Yannoutsos have shown that hearts from heterozygous offspring of transgenic founder animals expressing suprahuman levels of DAF did not undergo hyperacute rejection when transplanted heterotopically into nonimmunosuppressed cynomolgus monkeys. These transgenic hearts survived for a median of 5.1 days in untreated monkeys. Hearts from DAF transgenic pigs have been transplanted into immunosuppressed cynomolgus monkeys, and the median survival was 40 days. Hyperacute rejection occurred in less than 1 hour in immunosuppressed monkeys receiving nontransgenic pig hearts.[48]

TRANSGENIC TECHNOLOGY DIRECTED AT XENOREACTIVE ANTIBODY

Since identification of the Gal epitope as the main target of human xenoreactive antibody, strategies have focused on inhibiting the xenoantibody component of hyperacute rejection. Inactivating the gene responsible for the GalT enzyme has been suggested as a means of eliminating the Gal epitope. Tearle et al. reported the use of a GalT-targeting construct to inactivate one of the *GalT* alleles in murine embryonic stem cells via homologous recombination. To accomplish allele inactivation, mice chimeric for the embryonic stem cell genotype were first generated and subsequently bred to obtain mice homozygous for the inactivated *GalT* gene. Further studies showed limited binding of naturally occurring IgG and IgM xenoantibodies and reduced complement activation when normal human serum was reacted with murine cells lacking the Gal epitope.[49]

Sandrin et al. and Sharma et al. have shown that intracellular competition exists between the enzymes galactosyltransferase and α-1,2-fucosyltransferase (H-transferase) for the common substrate N-acetylgalactosamine.[50, 51] When both these enzymes are coexpressed in a porcine cell by transfection, the H-transferase is dominant over galactosyltransferase, the result being remodeling of the cell surface, with dominant expression of the H-epitope and poor expression of the highly antigenic Gal epitope. Introduction of human H-transferase into porcine cells has resulted in significantly reduced human IgG and IgM antibody binding and susceptibility to human serum–mediated lysis when compared with control porcine cells. Transgenic mice expressing H-transferase have been produced and demonstrate decreased expression of the Gal epitope and loss of human antibody binding. Sharma et al. were also able to show a reduction in galactosyltransferase enzyme levels in transgenic pigs by expression of the fucosyltransferase enzyme.[51]

Sandrin et al. developed another approach to the inhibition of natural antibody that involves constitutive in vivo expression of the galactose-cleaving enzyme α-galactosidase, which could decrease α-Gal epitope expression. Transgenic mice expressing the human α-galactosidase gene were produced; splenocytes from these transgenic mice showed a reduction in the binding of natural antibodies. However, the use of α-galactosidase alone did not completely eliminate expression of α-Gal epitope. Furthermore, this resulted in the exposure of new *N*-acetylgalactosamine residues and potential new xenoepitopes. However, the use of a combination of α-galactosidase and α-1,2-fucosyltransferase enzymes resulted in negligible cell surface expression of galactosyltransferase, and these cells were not susceptible to lysis mediated by human serum containing antibody and complement.[52]

In conclusion, these studies show that both xenoantibody and complement activation are decreased when human serum reacts with discordant cells lacking the Gal epitope; in addition, they suggest that strategies for elimination of the Gal epitope in the pig will probably prove to be clinically desirable.

TRANSGENIC TECHNOLOGY DIRECTED AT THE ENDOTHELIAL CELL

Attempts are also being made to introduce genes into endothelial cells that are involved in endothelial cell activation or the consequences of endothelial cell activation. The transcription factor NFκB has been found to be essential for the induction of genes that are upregulated via type II endothelial cell activation. Bach et al. have introduced IκB, a natural inhibitor of NFκB, into porcine endothelial cells by using a recombinant adenovirus. Significant inhibition of genes associated with type II activation occurred when these cells were confronted with an activating stimulus. Inhibition of NFκB in vivo may beneficially modulate many of the events resulting in delayed xenograft rejection.[53]

Thrombomodulin, which is present on the surface of normal resting endothelial cells, is lost with endothelial cell activation, and platelet aggregation is promoted. This process facilitates the development of a procoagulant state and results in microvascular thrombosis, which is a common pathologic event in the rejection of discordant xenografts. Possible therapeutic approaches to the problem of microvascular thrombosis include the systemic administration of antithrombotic agents. However, genetic engineering has provided an alternative approach to maintaining the natural anticoagulant state of the xenograft. Bach et al. transduced porcine endothelial cells with the gene for human thrombomodulin with transcriptional regulation that does not permit loss of thrombomodulin when endothelial cell activation occurs.[54] This high-level expression of thrombomodulin in an activated endothelial cell allows it to play a role in the generation of activated protein C, which is the most important natural anticoagulant. The advantage of this approach is achievement of a localized anticoagulant effect as opposed to a systemic effect. A similar approach could promote an anticoagulant rather than a procoagulant state in a xenotransplanted organ.

FUTURE IMPLICATIONS

The evidence is now sufficient to show the benefit of transgenic organs in xenotransplantation. However, clinically relevant prolonged xenograft survival has yet to be achieved. It is not known whether the development of transgenic animals that express multiple complement regulatory proteins would result in more complete inhibition of the complement system. It is likely that strategies to inhibit or block the antibody component of hyperacute rejection, as well as inhibit complement, will be necessary for the long-term survival of xenografts. Coexpression of genes that target complement inhibition and natural antibody reactivity have recently been developed. This approach led to the development of transgenic mice and pigs that express both human CD59 and α-1,2-fucosyltransferase. Splenocytes from animals expressing both transgenes showed complete protection from complement-mediated lysis with human serum as opposed to the partial protection from cell lysis seen in control animals expressing either one of the transgenes.[55]

Sandrin et al. have shown the additive effect of the enzymes α-galactosidase and α-1,2-fucosyltransferase in reducing the expression of α-Gal epitope on the cell surface.[52] In all probability, a combination of transgenes directed at the inhibition of complement, antigen expression, and endothelial cell activation will be required to achieve xenograft survival.

It is believed that the key to successful long-term xenograft survival will be the ability to induce tolerance to xenogeneic antigens. Sachs et al. have pioneered the approach of mixed hematopoietic chimerism to induce allogeneic and concordant xenogeneic transplantation tolerance.[56] Schumacher et al. reported the induction of antigen-specific B-cell tolerance to xenoantigens in mice reconstituted with autologous bone marrow cells into which foreign MHC genes have been introduced and expressed.[57] In time, gene therapy may be used to obtain antigen-specific transplantation tolerance, which could potentially decrease the requirement for potent immunosuppressive medication.

The development of cloned lambs such as Dolly and Polly have led to the speculation that nuclear transplantation from somatic cells could be used to produce clones of animals that have been selected for certain traits such as those that would not induce a xenogeneic immune response. These techniques could allow the development of animals with customized genomes, including genomes that have had genes added or removed. Despite the enormous ethical and scientific controversy that cloning has sparked, it is likely that cloning will become the method of choice for producing transgenic animals. When compared with current techniques, which are relatively laborious and inefficient, cloning would allow the rapid generation of large numbers of engineered animals.

Rapid advances in molecular biology have resulted in great excitement over pig organs that could be used for the treatment of end-stage organ failure. A combination of genetic engineering, immunosuppressive therapy, and continued insight into the pathobiology of xenotransplantation could bring this field from the distant future to the present.

REFERENCES

1. United Network for Organ Sharing Scientific Registry: *UNOS Facts and Statistics.* Richmond, Va, United Network for Organ Sharing, 1996.
2. Spital A: The shortage of organs for transplantation: Where do we go from here? *N Engl J Med* 325:1243–1246, 1991.

3. Evans RW, Oriens CE, Ascher NL: The potential supply of organ donors; an assessment of the efficiency of organ procurement efforts in the United States. *JAMA* 267:239–246, 1992.
4. Orriens CE, Evans RW, Ascher NL: Estimates of organ-specific donor availability for the United States. *Transplant Proc* 25:1541–1542, 1993.
5. Michler RE, Chen JM, Itescu S, et al: Two decades of transplantation at the Columbia Presbyterian Medical Center 1977–1997, in Terasaki PI, Cecka JM (eds): *Clinical Transplants 1997.* Los Angeles, UCLA Tissue Typing Laboratory, 1997.
6. Reemtsma K, McCracken BH, Schlegel JU, et al: Renal heterotransplantation in man. *Ann Surg* 160:384–410, 1964.
7. Nowak R: Xenotransplants set to resume. *Science* 266:1148–1151, 1994.
8. Starzl TE, Marchioro TL, Peters GN, et al: Renal heterotransplantation from baboon to man: Experience with 6 cases. *Transplantation* 2:384–410, 1964.
9. Hardy JD, Kurrus FE, Chavez CM, et al: Heart transplantation in man: Developmental studies and report of a case. *JAMA* 188:1132, 1964.
10. Cooley DA, Hallman GL, Bloodwell RD, et al: Human heart transplantation: Experience with 12 cases. *Am J Cardiol* 22:804–810, 1968.
11. Ross DN: In Shapiro H (ed): *Experience With Human Heart Transplantation.* Durban, South Africa, Butterworths, 1969, pp 227–228.
12. Bailey LL, Nehlsen-Cannerella SL, Concepcion W, et al: Baboon-to-human cardiac xenotransplantation in a neonate. *JAMA* 254:3321–3329, 1985.
13. Starzl TE, Fung JJ, Tzakis A, et al: Baboon-to-human liver transplantation. *Lancet* 341:65–71, 1993.
14. Starzl TE: Clinical xenotransplantation. *Xenotransplantation* 1:3–7, 1994.
15. Auchincloss H: Xenogeneic transplantation. *Transplantation* 46:1, 1988.
16. Platt JL, Vercelloti GM, Dalmasso AP, et al: Transplantation of discordant xenografts: A review of progress. *Immunol Today* 11:450, 1990.
17. Platt JL, Fischel RJ, Matas AJ, et al: Immunopathology of hyperacute xenograft rejection in a swine-to-primate model. *Transplantation* 52:214, 1991.
18. Leventhal JR, Dalmasso AP, Cromwell JW, et al: Prolongation of cardiac xenograft survival by depletion of complement. *Transplantation* 55:887, 1993.
19. Pruitt SK, Kirk AD, Bollinger RR, et al: The effect of soluble complement receptor type 1 on hyperacute rejection of porcine xenografts. *Transplantation* 57:363–370, 1994.
20. Leventhal JR, John R, Fryer JP, et al: Removal of babbon and human antiporcine IgG and IgM natural antibodies by immunoadsorption. *Transplantation* 59:294–300, 1995.

21. Cooper DKC, Good AH, Ye Y, et al: Specific intravenous carbohydrate therapy: A new approach to the inhibition of antibody-mediated rejection following ABO-incompatible allografting and discordant xenografting. *Transplant Proc* 25:377–378, 1993.
22. Jaenisch R: Transgenic animals. *Science* 240:1468–1473, 1988.
23. Mullins LJ, Mullins JJ: Transgenesis in the rat and larger mammals. *J Clin Invest* 97:1557–1560, 1996.
24. Niemann H, Reichelt B: Manipulating early pig embryos. *J Reprod Fertil Suppl* 48:75–94, 1994.
25. Langford GA, Yannoutsos N, Cozzi E, et al: Production of pigs transgenic for human decay accelerating factor. *Transplant Proc* 26:1400–1401, 1994.
26. Kroshus TJ, Bolman RM III, Dalmasso AP, et al: Expression of human CD59 in transgenic pig organs enhances organ survival in an ex vivo xenogeneic perfusion model. *Transplantation* 61:1513–1521, 1996.
27. Byrne GB, McCurry KR, Martin ML, et al: Transgenic pigs expressing human CD59 and decay accelerating factor produce an intrinsic barrier to complement-mediated damage. *Transplantation* 15:149–155, 1997.
28. Langford GA, Cozzi E, Yannoutsos N, et al: Production of pigs transgenic for human regulators of complement activation using YAC technology. *Transplant Proc* 28:862–863, 1996.
29. Pedersen RA: Studies of in vitro differentiation with embryonic stem cells. *Reprod Fertil Dev* 6:543–552, 1994.
30. Wigley P, Becker C, Beltrame J, et al: Site-specific transgene insertion: An approach. *Reprod Fertil Dev* 6:585–588, 1994.
31. Campbell KHS, McWhir J, Ritchie WA, et al: Sheep cloned by nuclear transfer from a cultured cell line. *Nature* 380:64–66, 1996.
32. Pennisi E, Williams N: Will Dolly send in the clones. *Science* 275:1415–1416, 1997.
33. Wilmut I, Schnieke AE, McWhir J, et al: Viable offspring derived from fetal and adult mammalian cells. *Nature* 385:810–813, 1997.
34. Pennisi E: Transgenic lambs from cloning lab. *Science* 277:631, 1997.
35. Lawson JH, Platt JL: Molecular barriers to xenotransplantation. *Transplantation* 62:303–310, 1996.
36. Xu H, Edwards NM, Chen JM, et al: Newborn baboon serum lacks natural anti-pig xenoantibody. *Transplantation* 59:1189–1194, 1995.
37. Kaplon RJ, Michler RE, Xu H, et al: Absence of hyperacute rejection in newborn pig-to-baboon cardiac xenografts. *Transplantation* 59:1–6, 1995.
38. Dalmasso AP: The complement system in xenotransplantation. *Immunopharmacology.* 24:149, 1992.
39. Zhow XJ, Niessen N, Pawlowski I, et al: Prolongation of survival of discordant kidney xenografts by C6 deficiency. *Transplantation* 50: 896–898, 1990.

40. Dalmasso AP, Vercellotti GM, Platt JL: Inhibition of complement-mediated endothelial cell cytotoxicity by decay accelerating factor. *Transplantation* 52:533, 1991.
41. Morgan BP: Complement regulatory molecules: Application to therapy and transplantation. *Immunol Today* 16:257–259, 1995.
42. Fodor WL, Williams BL, Matis LA, et al: Expression of a functional human complement inhibitor in a transgenic pig as a model for the prevention of xenogeneic hyperacute organ rejection. *Proc Natl Acad Sci USA* 91:11153–11157, 1994.
43. McCurry KR, Kooyman DL, Alvarado CG, et al: Human complement regulatory proteins protect swine-to-primate cardiac xenografts from humoral injury. *Nat Med* 1:423–427, 1995.
44. Mulder LCF, Mora M, Ciccopiedi E, et al: Mice transgenic for human CD46 and CD55 are protected from human complement attack. *Transplant Proc* 27:333–335, 1995.
45. Carrington CA, Richards AC, Cozzi E, et al: Expression of human DAF and MCP on pig endothelial cells protects from human complement. *Transplant Proc* 27:321–323, 1995.
46. Schmoeckel M, Nollert G, Shahmohammadi M, et al: Prevention of hyperacute rejection by human decay accelerating factor in xenogeneic perfused working hearts. *Transplantation* 62:729–734, 1996.
47. Rosengard AM, Cary NRB, Langford GA, et al: Tissue expression of human complement inhibitor, decay-accelerating factor, in transgenic pigs. *Transplantation* 9:1325–1333, 1995.
48. White DJG, Yannoutsos N: Production of pigs transgenic for human DAF to overcome complement mediated hyperacute xenograft rejection in man. *Res Immunol* 147:88–94, 1996.
49. Tearle RG, Tange MJ, Zannettino ZL, et al: The alpha-1,3-galactosyltransferase knockout mouse. *Transplantation* 61:13–19, 1996.
50. Sandrin MS, Fodor WL, Mouhtouris E, et al: Enzymatic remodelling of the carbohydrate surface of a xenogenic cell substantially reduces human antibody binding and complement-mediated cytolysis. *Nat Med* 1:1261–1267, 1995.
51. Sharma A, Okabe J, Birch P, et al: Reduction in the level of gal(alpha1,3) gal in transgenic mice and pigs by the expression of an alpha(1,2)fucosyltransferase. *Proc Natl Acad Sci USA* 93:7190–7195, 1996.
52. Osman N, McKenzie IFC, Ostenreid K, et al: Reduction in gal alpha(1,3) gal by expression of alpha-galactosidase DNA (abstract). Presented at the Fourth International Congress for Xenotransplantation, Nantes, France, 1997.
53. Bach FH, Robson SC, Winkler H, et al: Barriers to xenotransplantation. *Nat Med* 1:869–873, 1995.
54. Wrighton CJ, Kopp CW, McShea A, et al: High-level expression of functional human thrombomodulin cultured porcine aortic endothelial cells. *Transplant Proc* 27:288–289, 1995.

55. Costa C, Ebert KM, Squinto SP, et al: Transgenic cells expressing alpha 1,2-fucosyltransferase and h CD59 are completely protected from human serum cytolysis (abstract). Presented at the Fourth International Congress for Xenotransplantation, Nantes, France, 1997.
56. Sachs DH, Sykes M, Greenstein JL, et al: Tolerance and xenograft survival. *Nat Med* 1:969, 1995.
57. Schumacher I, Jeevarathnam S, Rubbocki, et al: Use of gene therapy to induce antigen-specific immunologic unresponsiveness to class I xenogeneic major histocompatibility complex antigens. *Transplant Proc* 27:313–314, 1995.

CHAPTER 11

Hypertrophic Obstructive Cardiomyopathy

Bruno J. Messmer, M.D.
Professor and Chief of Thoracic and Cardiovascular Surgery, University Hospital Aachen, Aachen, Germany

Heinrich G. Klues, M.D.
Associate Professor, Department of Cardiology, Medicine Clinic I, University Hospital Aachen, Aachen, Germany

Sebastian Reith, M.D.
Junior Fellow, Department of Cardiology, Medicine Clinic I, University Hospital Aachen, Aachen, Germany

Friedrich A. Schoendube, M.D., Ph.D.
Associate Professor, Department of Thoracic and Cardiovascular Surgery, University Hospital Aachen, Aachen, Germany

Peter Hanrath, M.D.
Professor and Chief of Cardiology, Medicine Clinic I, University Hospital Aachen, Aachen, Germany

Hypertrophic obstructive cardiomyopathy (HOCM) is one of the most controversially discussed cardiac diseases. The etiology, the exact pathophysiology of the obstruction, and the treatment are not clear, and the multitude of theories for each sector is the best proof of ignorance. The present report summarizes our 20 years' surgical experience with this disease, paying special attention to intraoperative pathology, surgical technique, and long-term follow-up. Furthermore, we have to describe and evaluate newer techniques such as DDD-pacing and catheter-induced localized septal infarction (The acronym TASH stands for transcoronary ablation of septal hypertrophy.)

ETIOLOGY OF HYPERTROPHIC OBSTRUCTIVE CARDIOMYOPATHY

For years the etiology of HOCM was thought to be idiopathic, which means unknown. Because of the idiopathic origin, Braunwald et al.[1] gave the disease the classical name of idiopathic hypertrophic subaortic stenosis, or IHSS. Nevertheless, an inherent genetically fixed component has been discussed ever since Davies[2] in 1952 first described an English family with five of nine siblings affected by the disease and three of them dying suddenly. New basic research has detected genetic mutations associated with HOCM predominantly at the β-myosin heavy chain, the myosin-binding protein C, and the troponin T and a-tropomyosin levels.[3, 4, 5]

The result of such mutations is a rather heterogenic entity of a bizarre hypertrophic myocardial structure defined by malaligned and disrupted muscle fibers, either diffuse or restricted to some areas, i.e., the basal septum. The variety of pathologic anatomical appearances is explained by the variety of possible genetic mutations, which result in similar changes of the sarcomere but with different expression. Diffuse hypertrophic cardiomyopathy reflects one end of the spectrum; predominant basal septum hypertrophy with left ventricular outflow tract (LVOT) obstruction represents the other.

PATHOPHYSIOLOGY OF OUTFLOW-TRACT OBSTRUCTION

The obstructive form of hypertrophic cardiomyopathy is defined by the presence of a pressure gradient across the LVOT. The gradient varies with the dynamic status of the left ventricle. It might be mild at rest but becomes always significant under stress.

Two basic anatomical structures are relevant for the obstruction:

1. Asymmetric hypertrophy of the ventricular septum, which can be confined to the basal part, the midventricular part, or the complete septum.
2. The structure of the whole mitral valve apparatus, including the papillary muscles.

Although asymmetric septal hypertrophy and especially a bulging of the basal part narrows directly the LVOT, the active part of the mitral valve apparatus is more complex. A systolic anterior motion of the septal leaflet of the mitral valve (SAM) has been recognized as an important factor of LVOT obstruction. However, this phenomenon was thought to be secondary to the muscular obstruction ever since Wigle et al.[6] explained the SAM to be induced by a Venturi effect resulting from high velocity flow across the obstructed LVOT. This on the Bernoulli equation basing and therefore convincing theory has been copied across the literature, but nobody has ever calculated the velocities necessary to create sufficient force to attract the mitral leaflet. Although other theories for the SAM were discussed long ago,[7, 8] it has not been until recently that the Venturi effect has seriously been questioned. Instead, a theory of flow deviation with understreaming of the mitral leaflets and therefore a flow-induced active anterior displacement of the mitral leaflet becomes more plausible. The theory of active displacement is further supported by anatomical features such as displacement and therefore malalignment of the papillary muscles—which in addition are not only hypertrophic but also heavily attached to the ventricular wall, either by broad fusion or by atypical trabeculae hindering their proper mobility. Interpapillary fusion or interpapillary trabeculae may further impede proper function of the mitral valve, enhancing the SAM phenomenon and mitral insufficiency, respectively. In addition, the mitral leaflets in HOCM are significantly larger and longer than in normal hearts,[9] which helps understreaming and displacement during early systole. Less common but significantly more frequent than in the normal population is a direct insertion of a papillary muscle at the free margin of the anterior leaflet.[10] Such an anomaly may interfere with free movement of the anterior leaflet and may give origin to mitral valve insufficiency.

Put it to the point, the bulge of the septum not only narrows directly the LVOT, but it also changes left ventricular geometry along its longitudinal axis to an extent that early systolic blood flow is deviated toward the posterio-basal wall and therefore underneath the mitral leaflets (Fig 1).

The relevant factors for obstruction and for the SAM phenomenon in hypertrophic cardiomyopathy can be summarized as follows:

- Anterior basal septal hypertrophy
- Narrowed LVOT
- Changes in left ventricular geometry
- Malposition and malattachment of papillary muscles
- Malalignment of mitral valve apparatus
- Increased size and length of septal mitral leaflet

Considering that both the muscular and the valvular part are equally important and responsible for the obstruction, a therapeutic approach to both of them seems rational.

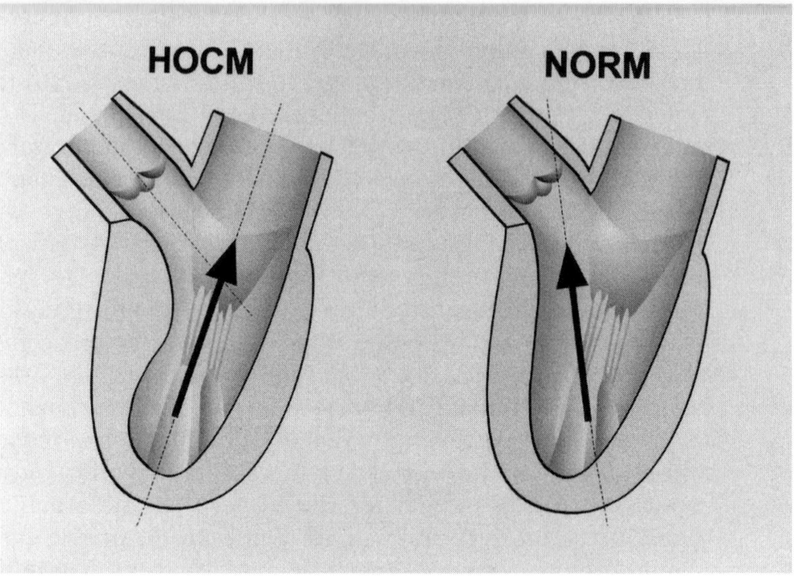

FIGURE 1.
Because of the subaortic septal hypertrophy, the apico-aortic longitudinal axis is angled, which results in early systolic flow deviation toward the posterior wall and underneath the mitral leaflets, respectively, which by this mechanism are moved in anterior position.

THERAPEUTIC OPTIONS FOR HYPERTROPHIC OBSTRUCTIVE CARDIOMYOPATHY

Today four basic therapeutical options are available for treatment of HOCM:

1. Medical therapy, mainly with Ca-antagonists and β-blocking agents
2. Surgical therapy with myectomy or procedures on the mitral valve apparatus or both
3. DDD-pacing
4. Catheter-induced local infarction of the basal septum (TASH).

MEDICAL THERAPY

The complexity of HOCM can only be understood by regarding the variable features contributing to the pathophysiology of this disease, such as obstruction, ischemia, diastolic dysfunction, and arrhythmias. The medical treatment of HOCM is largely empirical, mostly depending on the patient's subjective perception of symptomatic benefit. There are only a few drugs available and so far there are only a few randomized data. According to these data, the drug selection is frequently based on the experience and preference of individual investigators. There is a common use of β-blockers, which are especially effective in mild resting obstruction but have hardly any effect on high basal gradients. β-blockers achieve their symptomatic benefit by improving the left ventricular filling through reduction of the heart rate and the oxygen demand. The alternative standard drug used in HOCM is verapamil, a calcium antagonist, which usually reduces the outflow tract gradient through its negative inotropic properties.[11] The symptomatic benefit may be due to improved passive filling and a reduction of ischemia. However, some unpredictable verapamil-related side effects are still feared by some investigators.[12] The vasodilatating properties may increase the obstruction and lead to serious hemodynamic complications, including cardiogenic shock and pulmonary edema. Some investigators prefer the Ia antiarrhythmic drug disopyramide, especially when treating symptomatic HOCM.[13] The negative inotropic effect of this drug has evidently shown a significant reduction of outflow gradient followed by significant symptomatic benefit. Nevertheless, disopyramide should be used with caution because it may be proarrhythmic. Frequently, a combination with a β-blocker is recommended, particularly when the heart rate increases. There are still a few other drugs available for the treatment of HOCM, such as diltiazem, amiodarone (for the treatment of patients at high risk because of malignant arrhythmias), and angiotensin-converting enzyme inhibitors. Unfortunately, only a few data exist for the use of these drugs.

Generally, the management of medical treatment of HOCM should follow a certain pattern. In case of a completely asymptomatic patient, the prophylactic use of either verapamil or β-blockers is still questionable. Patients who have mild to moderate symptoms should receive verapamil or a β-blocker. If symptoms increase and must be classified as severe with signs of congestive heart failure, a diuretic agent can be added to the initial treatment. Diuretics, however, should be used with caution because of significant diastolic dysfunction often accompanying HOCM. In case of treatment failure at that stage, there are only a few medical alternatives, including disopyramide, diltiazem, and the combination of β-blockers and verapamil. In case of refractory severely symptomatic patients, nonmedical treatment should be considered, either surgical or, alternatively, a less invasive treatment with either induced septal infarction or DDD-pacing.

TABLE 1.
Surgical Techniques for Hypertrophic Obstructive Cardiomyopathy

Year	Author	Technique
1957	Brock[14]	Closed transventricular myotomy
1958	Cleland[15]	Transaortic myotomy
1961	Kirklin and Ellis[17]	Transaortic- + transventricular myectomy
1961	Morrow and Brockenbrough[18]	Transaortic myectomy
1963	Lillehei and Levy[19]	Transatrial myectomy
1967	Cooley et al.[20]	Rightventricular myectomy
1968	Binet et al.[21]	Extended ventriculo-aortic myotomy
1971	Cooley et al.[22]	Mitral valve replacement
1976	Rastan and Koncz[23]	Aortoventriculoplasty
1976	Dembitzky and Weldon[24]	Apico-aortic conduit
1992	McIntosh et al.[25]	Myectomy and mitral valve plication
1994	Messmer[26]	Extended myectomy

SURGICAL THERAPY

Indication for surgery remains with symptomatic patients refractory to medical therapy or intolerance of drugs. A variety of surgical techniques have been proposed and performed ever since Brock[14] made the first surgical attempt by closed transventricular myotomy in 1957. From the numerous techniques developed over the past 40 years, some are specially worth mentioning (Table 1). Cleland[15] reported in 1963 transaortic longitudinal myotomy of the bulging septum, which resulted in a gap, widening the LVOT (a technique he first performed in 1958).

Later, this method became better known as the Bigelow technique.[16] In 1961, Kirklin and Ellis[17] described the transaortic-transventricular approach with resection of parts of the hypertrophic septum, and in the same year Morrow and Brockenbrough[18] published the classical method of transaortic myectomy. A right ventricular approach in order to avoid the risk of atrioventricular (AV)-block was clinically introduced by Cooley et al.[20] All these operations dealt only with the septal hypertrophy, neglecting the important impact of the mitral valve and papillary muscles, respectively. It was Cooley et al.[22] who changed the operation to the mitral valve, neglecting vice versa the hypertrophic septum. Even though mitral valve replacement definitely eliminated the obstruction, the method did not gain acceptance because of its extremism and the negative impact of the artificial valve. For extremely severe stenoses and especially for tunnel-shape forms, Rastan and Koncz[23] proposed the aortoventriculoplasty, whereas Dembitzky and Weldon[24] used an apico-aortic conduit in these cases.

In 1992, McIntosh et al.[25] published a combined approach of septal myectomy and shortening of the elongated septal mitral leaflet by plication.

TECHNIQUE OF EXTENDED MYECTOMY AND PAPILLARY MUSCLE MOBILIZATION

Taking into account the double origin of obstruction, one of us (BJM), already in the 1970s, elaborated on an extended technique of myectomy and simultaneous mobilization of the papillary muscles. Since then, this operation has been performed in all patients, but it has not been published before 1994[26] to prove its superiority on the basis of long-term results.[27]

The operation consists of two parts: (1) transaortic resection of the septal bar, extending it to the basal lateral wall of the left ventricle; and (2) complete mobilization of the papillary muscles.

The operation is performed via a total sternotomy on cardiopulmonary bypass under moderate hypothermia and crystalloid cardioplegic arrest. A minimal invasive approach—as often propagated nowadays for aortic valve replacement—is not advisable because surgery is not restricted to the level of the aortic valve but reaches all the way down to the apex of the left ventricle. The aorta is incised in an oblique fashion, and the anterior wall of the distal aorta is transaortically fixed by a 4-0 stay suture to the posterior wall, thus keeping the free margin out of the surgeon's view. Stay sutures (2-0) are placed at all three commissures of the aortic valve, and the valve area is gently pulled upward. The aortic cusps are kept in open position by three 6-0 monofilament sutures placed at the noduli Arantii. These preliminary steps are important to gain optimal view and access across the valve to the obstructed subvalvular area.

While he is looking into the left ventricle, the surgeon's view is markedly reduced by the angle between the longitudinal axis of the left ventricle and the surgeon's axis of sight. Because the surgeon cannot look around the corner, he cannot recognize the deepest point of the septal bulge. To correct this inconvenience, Morrow[16] in his operation used pressure on the anterior wall of the right ventricle, pushing the septum down. In addition, he used an

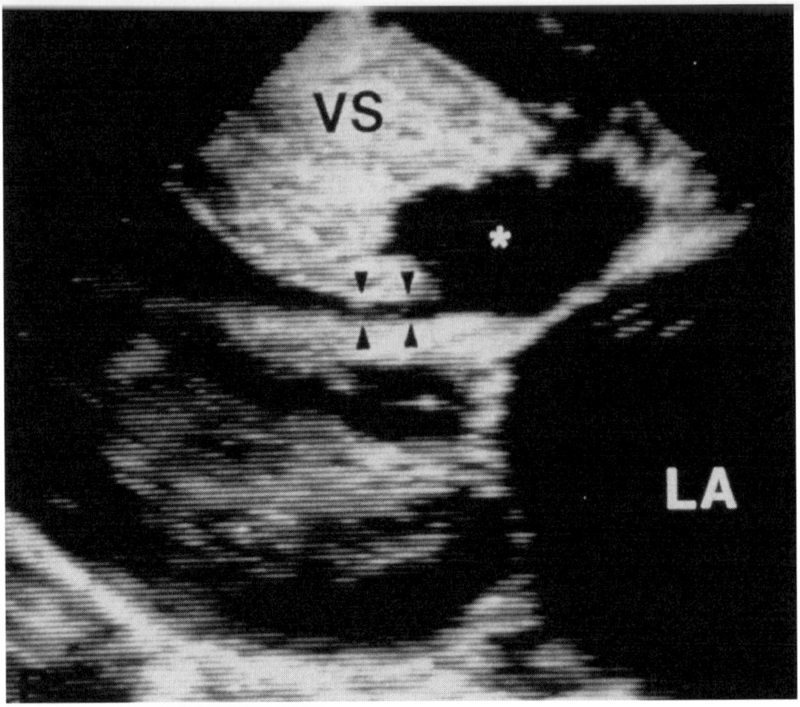

FIGURE 2.
Echocardiographic picture after septal myectomy *(asterisk)* by the classical Morrow technique. Note that the deepest point of the septum bulge has not been reached and residual obstruction *(arrows)* remains. *Abbreviations: VS,* ventricular septum; *LA,* left atrium.

angled handle for the knife. Despite these measurements, the muscle bar is rarely excised to its deepest point, and relief from obstruction remains often incomplete (Fig 2).

One of the secrets of our own modified technique is the use of a sharp triple-hook retractor (Fig 3) which, after exposure of the septal bulge, is gently inserted into the left ventricle and along the anterior septal wall toward the apex. The retractor is used as a lever with its prongs hooked into the septum at the deepest point of the muscle bar (Fig 4). Similarly to the classic Morrow procedure, a deep longitudinal incision is made with a blade 10 knife on a straight handle at the level of the right coronary artery and a second at the junction between the septum and the lateral wall. In between these two incisions the septum is excised, pushing the knife toward the points of the prongs of the triple hook, which guaran-

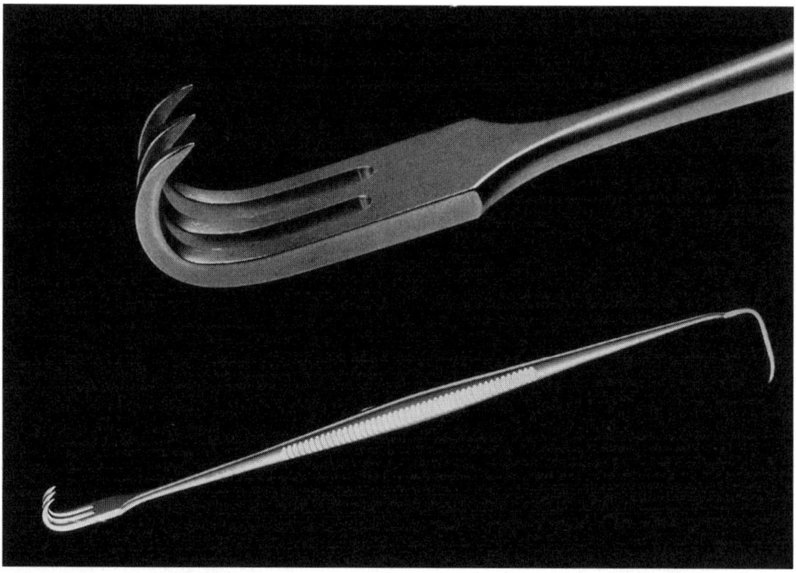

FIGURE 3.
Sharp triple-hook retractor for elevation of the deepest point of the hypertrophic septum.

tees complete excision to the deepest point. This technique also prevents septum perforation because the septal bulge is fixed between the aortic root and the prongs of the triple-hook retractor so that the direction of the excision is clearly defined.

It is important to leave a small ring of intact septum underneath the right coronary cusp of the aortic valve to prevent secondary aortic insufficiency. It is also important that this first excision is as extensive as possible because it must not only release primary obstruction but also give ample access to the depth of the left ventricle and the papillary muscles, respectively (Fig 5). Additional resection at the lower part of the septum is generally difficult because of often present trabecularization and the risk of a rough and chopped surface. Once the first big bite is excised, further resection is done toward the lateral wall well behind the mural leaflet of the mitral valve and in an oblique fashion in the midpart of the septum toward the posterior wall. Not touched, however, is the basal part of the muscular septum below its membranous part where the bundle of His is localized. The weight of the excised muscle mass may well exceed 10 g but is dependent on the preoperatively measured thickness of the basal septum.

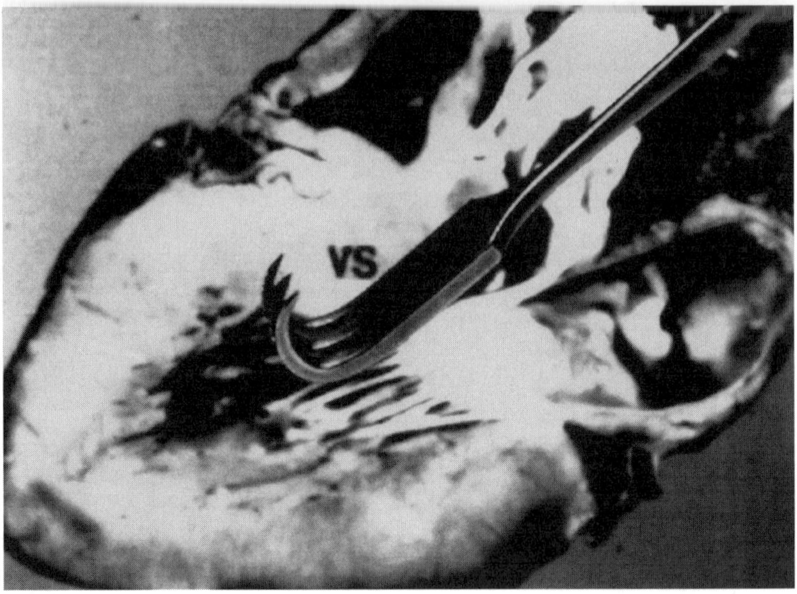

FIGURE 4.
Photomontage demonstrating the sharp triple hook inserted through the aorta into the left ventricular cavity and elevating the deepest point of the septal muscle bulge. *Abbreviation: VS,* ventricular septum.

Once septal excision is done, a right-angled retractor is inserted into the left ventricle to keep the slimed septum away. With a nerve hook the chordae to the anterolateral papillary muscle are grasped. Traction on the chordae gives view to the pathologic attachments of the muscle, which is then completely freed from the lateral wall and the neighboring posterior papillary muscle if necessary. In a further step, the latter is mobilized in the same manner. If necessary, the papillary muscles themselves are trimmed. By the end of the procedure, both papillary muscles should stay like slim columns inside the ventricle, fixed only at their basis, which guarantees free movement in the interplay with chordae and leaflets. Figure 6 demonstrates graphically the structures to be resected by this technique.

CLINICAL EXPERIENCE WITH THE EXTENDED MYECTOMY TECHNIQUE

Since 1979, a total of 74 patients underwent extended myectomy and reconstruction of the subvalvular mitral valve structures for severe forms of HOCM. There were 45 males and 29 females rang-

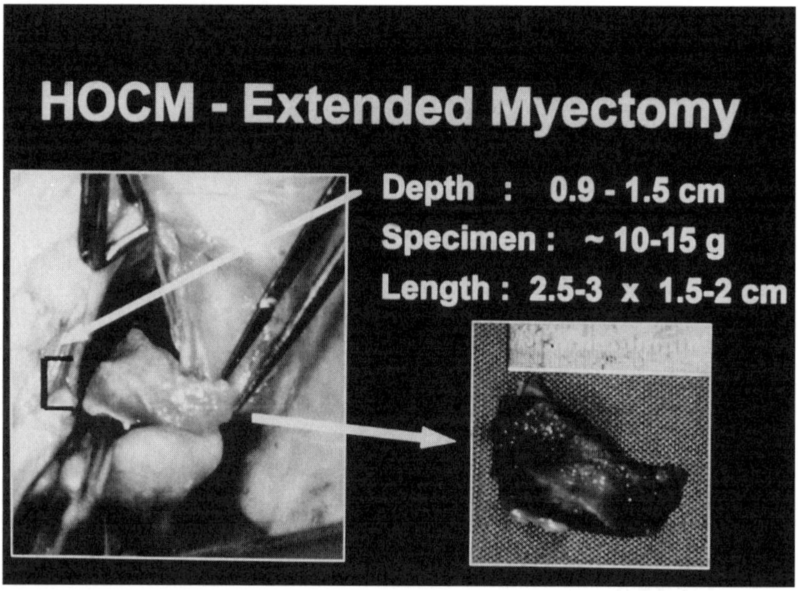

FIGURE 5.
Intraoperative view of transaortic excision of the septal bulge. The *black mark* indicates the site for further excision on the transitional zone to the basal part of the posterolateral wall.

ing in age between 8 and 73 years (mean age, 49 ± 12). In all patients medical therapy had failed. According to the New York Heart Association classification, 51 patients (69%) were in class III and 14 (19%) in class IV, respectively. Nine patients (12%) in class II underwent surgery either because of a high gradient or because of concomitant coronary artery disease (Fig 7).

All patients underwent preoperative cardiac catheterization. Most (80%) had additional echocardiography with Doppler evaluation of the pressure gradient across the LVOT. Transoesophageal echocardiography with direct visualization of the relevant anatomical structures became routine since 1986. Three-dimensional reconstruction allows for even better presentation.

Preoperatively, the peak systolic gradients across the LVOT at rest was 71 ± 36 mm Hg (range, 7–185 mm Hg). Provocation with the aid of amyl-nitrite inhalation, isoproterenol infusion, or the Valsalva maneuver resulted in gradients between 46 and 300 mm Hg with an average of 137 ± 46 mm Hg. In all patients, a significant SAM was present. Furthermore, mild to moderate mitral regurgitation (Sellers class I or II) was found in 20 patients (27%); 4

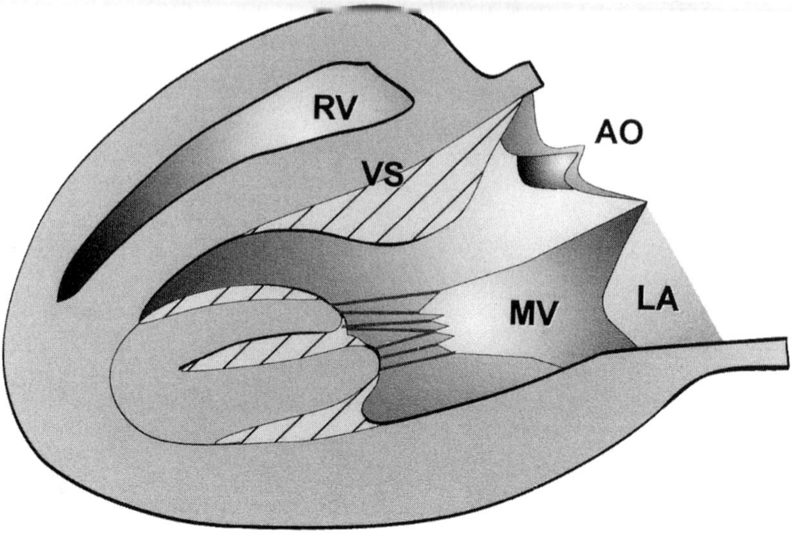

FIGURE 6.
Graphic design of muscular resection on the septum and mobilization of both papillary muscles by liberalization from the ventricular wall and from interpapillary hypertrophic trabeculae. Structures to be resected are marked by *hachures. Abbreviations: AO,* aorta; *LA,* left atrium; *VS,* ventricular septum; *MV,* mitral valve; *RV,* right ventricle.

patients (5%) had severe mitral insufficiency (Sellers class III). Significant coronary artery disease was detected in 10 patients (13.5%) and resulted in simultaneous coronary artery bypass grafting. Other concomitant procedures consisted of additional enlargement of the right ventricular outflow tract in 4 patients, anuloplasty (Kay-Wooler) for residual mitral insufficiency in 3 patients, and repair or replacement of the aortic valve as well as implantation of an internal cardiac defibrillator in 1 patient each.

Early postoperative implantation of a pacemaker was required in 3 patients (4%) for complete AV-block, but 2 of them had right bundle-branch block before surgery. Because creation of a left bundle-branch block is an inherent factor of adequate septal myectomy, a total AV-block is almost inevitable in these patients. During late follow-up, another 7 patients needed a pacemaker for various forms of bradycardia.

Statistics

For statistical analyses, the Kaplan-Meier[28] method was used for calculation of actuarial survival. Differences in survival were ana-

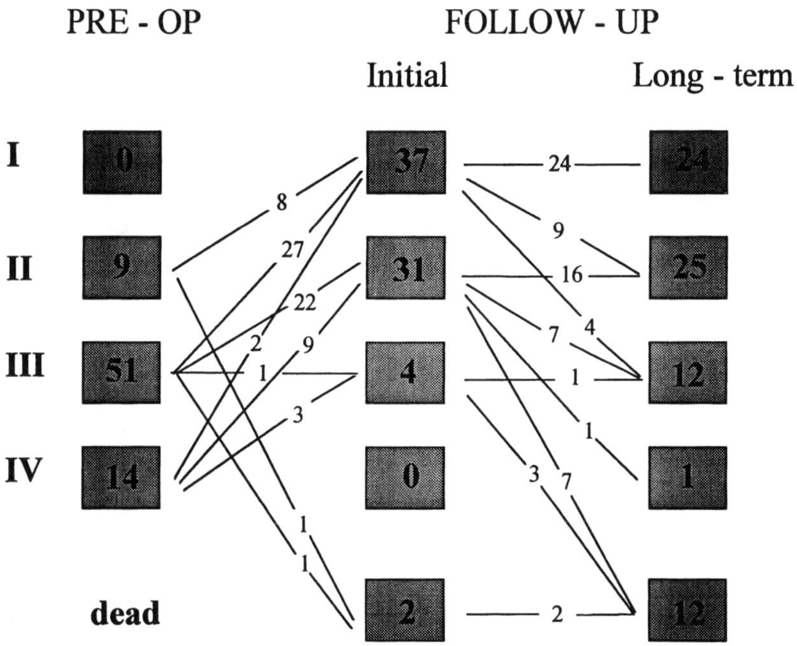

FIGURE 7.

Preoperative *(Pre-op)* and postoperative *(Post-op)* functional class in 74 patients. The initial follow-up was done at 6 months, the long-term at the last routine control. The *numbers in between the columns* indicate the number of patients who changed from one class to another.

lyzed by the log-rank test for dichotomy variables. The Wilcoxon test was used for unpaired parameters and the Cox regression mode for multivariate analyses. Calculations were done with the Statistical Analysis System software (SAS-Institute).

Mortality

Hospital mortality was 1.3% and was due to a patient who died at 7 weeks for multi-organ failure after a complicated postoperative course. One female with a preoperative high gradient and severe left ventricular impairment with an end-diastolic pressure of 40 mm Hg died—after an initially uneventful recovery—2 months later of multi-organ failure. During a long-term follow-up period (up to 17 years) and a mean follow-up time of 149 ± 5 months, another 10 patients died. Causes of late death were congestive heart failure in 6 and multi-organ failure, myocardial infarction, and malignancy in 1 patient each. In 1 patient, the cause of death could not be determined. It is noteworthy that half of the late deaths oc-

TABLE 2.
Data of the 12 Patients Who Died Early and During Late Follow-up

Patient	Age at Death (Yr)	Sex	Duration of Follow-up (Mo)	Preoperative LVOT gradient (mm Hg)	Preoperative LVEDP (mm Hg)	Preoperative NYHA (class)	Postoperative NYHA (class)	Type of Surgery	Cause of Death
1*	47	M	2	100	24	II	II	EM/IVR;MR	MOF
2	59	F	29	185	20	III	II	EM/IVR	CHF
3	62	M	128	75	15	IV	II	EM/IVR;MR	CHF
4	64	M	69	80	24	IV	II	EM/IVR;CABG	CHF
5	72	F	166	79	12	IV	III	EM/IVR	MOF
6	54	F	90	76	29	IV	III	EM/IVR	CHF
7	54	F	2	173	40	III	II	EM/IVR	MOF
8	69	M	118	95	20	III	II	EM/IVR;CABG	MI
9	71	M	122	110	23	III	II	EM/IVR;CABG	Malign
10	81	M	127	85	16	III	II	EM/IVR;CABG	CHF
11	73	M	121	140	20	III	II	EM/IVR	CHF
12	76	F	126	100	21	III	II	EMI/IVR	Unknown

Abbreviations: LVEDP, left ventricular end-diastolic pressure; *NYHA,* New York Heart Association; *EM/IVR,* extended myectomy/intraventricular repair; *MR,* mitral repair; *CABG,* coronary artery bypass graft; *CHF,* congestive heart failure; *MOF,* multi-organ failure; *MI,* myocardial infarction; *Malign,* malignancy.

curred in patients older than 70 years of age at 10 or more years after the operation. Furthermore, 4 of the late deaths were in patients with concomitant coronary bypass surgery (Table 2).

In the present series, the linearized mortality rate was 1.4% per patient year. The overall actuarial survival was 96 ± 2% at 5 years, 89 ± 5% at 10 years, and 71 ± 9% at 15 years (Fig 8). Although age at operation was not a risk factor for late survival, coronary artery disease when corrected did not seem to have a negative influence on late survival up to 10 years (Fig 9). When different risk factors were analyzed statistically the preoperative gradient at rest and as well as concomitant coronary bypass surgery demonstrated a significant risk for late survival but not the age at the time of surgery. By multivariate analysis, however, only the preoperative gradient at rest became an independent risk factor for late survival. Functional class has not been included in the analysis because classification in patients who have HOCM cannot be based on hard data but rather depends on the physician's impression (Table 3).

In the literature, hospital mortality varies between zero in newer series and up to 12% in older series (Table 4). It has been reported that concomitant coronary disease represents a risk factor for early mortality.[40] In the present series, early mortality was not influenced by concomitant coronary bypass surgery, and survival up to 10 years was practically identical for patients with and with-

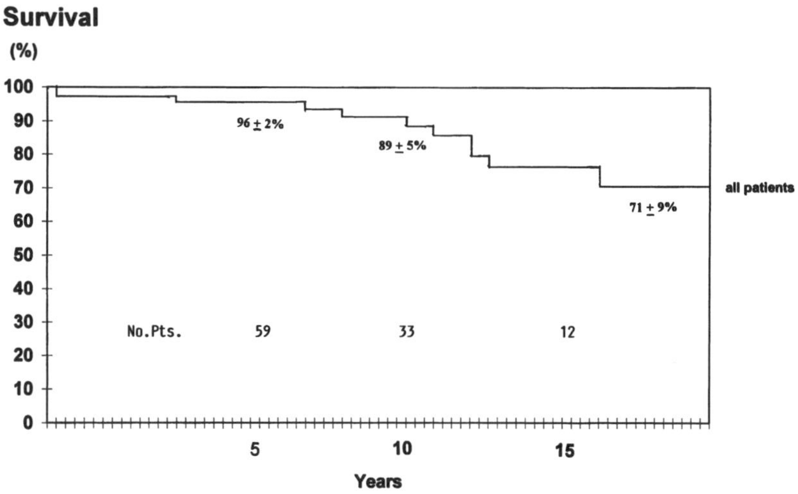

FIGURE 8.
Actuarial survival (Kaplan-Meier) for all 74 patients.

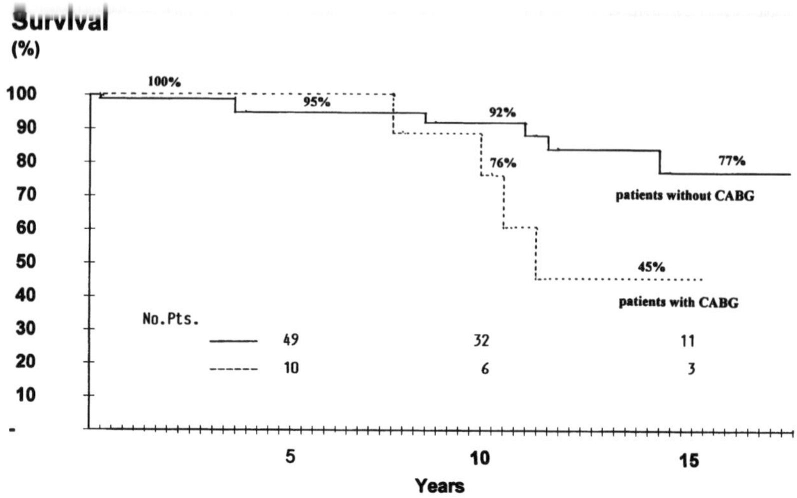

FIGURE 9.

Actuarial survival (Kaplan-Meier) for patients with and without coronary artery bypass graft *(CABG)*. Even though both curves are not different up to 10 years, statistical analysis yields a *P* value of 0.05 (log-rank test) over the whole period.

out coronary artery bypass graft. Nevertheless, statistically, coronary bypass surgery had a negative influence on late survival. Another important finding in the present series is that no patient was lost for sudden death, which is thought to be the most frequent cause of death in patients with HOCM.

The Late Clinical Status

The late clinical status was first evaluated in all patients at 6 months. At this time, 68 patients (92%) were in functional class I or II and only 4 (5%) were in class III; 2 patients were dead. At the most recent follow-up, still two thirds of the patients were in class I or II, whereas 12 (16%) had to be assigned to class III and 1 to class IV. Twelve patients had died. As shown in Figure 7, all but one of the survivors improved by at least one functional class shortly after the operation. During the late course, however, 31 patients either deteriorated or died.

Hemodynamics

In patients in whom comparable preoperative and postoperative measurements of the gradients across the LVOT were available, the gradient at rest decreased from an average of 85 ± 36 mm to 4.9 ± 7 mm Hg at follow-up. A similar drastic reduction was found for

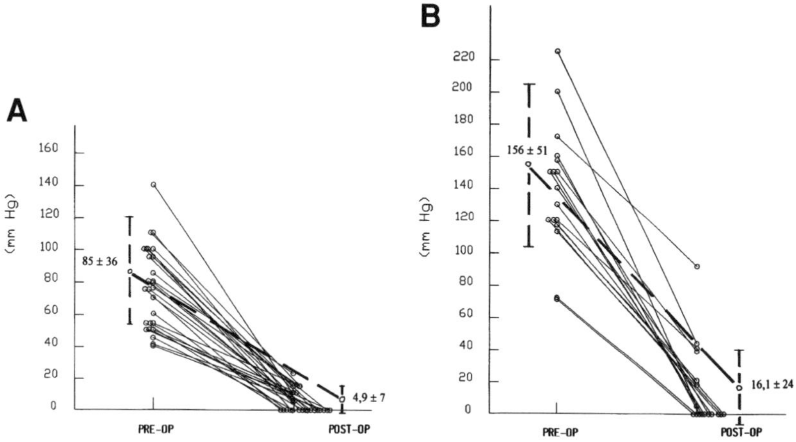

FIGURE 10.

Preoperative *(Pre-op)* and postoperative *(Post-op)* (6 months) pressure gradients at rest **(A)** and under stress **(B)** in patients who had comparable measurements of the hemodynamics.

TABLE 3.

Statistical Analysis of Risk Factors for Possible Influence on Long-term Results

Risk Factor	Log-rank Test (*P* values)	Multivariate Analysis (*P* values)
Age at operation	0.08	0.18
Gender	0.43	0.18
Year of operation	0.48	0.46
Pressure gradient at rest > 70 mm Hg	0.03	0.01
Coronary artery bypass graft	0.05	0.76

the gradient under stress, which fell from 156 ± 51 mm Hg preoperatively to 16.1 ± 24 mm Hg at follow-up (Fig 10).

Echocardiography

Echocardiography is probably the most important tool for evaluation of patients with HOCM, and especially for precise measurement of extension and thickness of the septal hypertrophy and for

TABLE 4.
Early and Late Linearized Mortality for Surgical Treatment of Hypertrophic Obstructive Cardiomyopathy in the Literature

Author	Year	Technique	*n*	Hospital Mortality	Late Mortality
Tajik et al.[29]	1974	MM	41	12%	—
Morrow et al.[30]	1975	MM	83	7.2%	—
Senning[31]	1976	MM	39	—	2.6%
Beahrs et al.[32]	1983	MM	36	10%	2.3%
Maron et al.[33]	1983	MM	240	8%	1.5%
Birks and Schulte[34]	1983	MM	137	6.6%	—
	1963–1973	MM	41	9.2%	—
	1977–1982	MM	96	3.1%	—
McIntosh and Maron[35]	1988	MM	123	8.1%	2.2%
	1988	MM	108	2.7%	—
		MVR	48	6.2%	—
Kraijcer et al.[36]	1989	MM	127	4.7%	0.7%
		MVR	58	6.9%	1.3%
Seiler et al.[37]	1991	MM	79	—	2.4%
Cohn et al.[38]	1992	MM	31	0%	1.4%
Ten Berg et al.[39]	1994	MM	38	0%	0.4%
Messmer (present series)	1997	ext.M	74	1.3%	1.4%

Abbreviations: MM, myotomy/myectomy; *MVR,* mitral valve replacement; *ext.M,* extended myectomy.

verification of the operative result in patients treated surgically. In the present series, septal thickness varied between 15 and 30 mm before the operation. At the latest follow-up it ranged from 8 to 22 mm. A significant decrease ($P < 0.001$) was found in those patients in whom comparable preoperative and postoperative measurements were available. It is also possible to measure directly the area of the LVOT before and after myectomy and to demonstrate the mobility of the papillary muscles after their operative liberalization (Fig 11). Until now we were able to determine the cross-section area of the LVOT in 11 patients preoperatively and postoperatively. The cross-section area increased from an average of 1.1 cm^2 before operation to 4.4 cm^2 late after surgery. It is therefore possible to

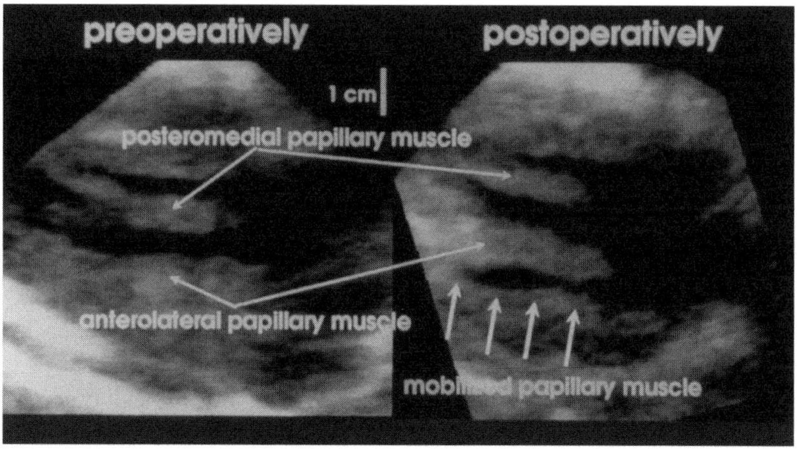

FIGURE 11.
Echocardiographic picture demonstrating the papillary muscles before and after complete mobilization.

achieve near-normal values (4.5–5.0 cm^2) with the method of extended myectomy presented here.

Although in all patients a significant SAM phenomenon was present before surgery, there was none at follow-up. Similarly, neither mild nor moderate or severe mitral insufficiency could be detected at follow-up. Complete resection of the septal muscle bulge realigns the longitudinal axis between the apex and the aortic valve, and early systolic flow deviation toward the inflow direction and the mitral valve leaflets, respectively, is successfully abolished.

TRANSCORONARY ABLATION OF SEPTAL HYPERTROPHY AND DDD-PACING

Recently, two newer techniques designed to decrease LVOT gradient have gained recognition. First, dual-chamber pacing was supposedly an alternative to the gold standard surgical treatment in patients with highly symptomatic HOCM. The exact mechanism by which dual-chamber pacing works is uncertain, but it may be related to a more favorable left ventricular excitation pattern, through a delayed timing of atrial contraction[41, 42] and a decreased left ventricular contractility.[43] In various studies, a significant reduction but not elimination of the basal outflow tract gradient could be shown, accompanied by a remarkable symptomatic improvement in most patients.[43, 44, 45] This effect is explained by a pre-excitation of the right ventricle that alters the synergy of ventricular contraction, especially the septum. The right ventricular pacing causes the interventricular septum to move paradoxically, with the consequence of an increase of the LVOT dimensions.[41, 43, 45–49] Consecutively, the LVOT gradient is markedly diminished, and a reduction of SAM-phenomenon is achieved.[44] Besides this short-term effect, however, there is presumably even a long-term effect of pacing in HOCM, described as remodeling of the left ventricle with a significant reduction of left ventricular wall thickness localized mainly locally around the pacing area.[45, 50, 51] According to those different studies, DDD-pacing can conclusively be regarded as an alternative treatment for class II–III patients who are refractory to maximal tolerated drug therapy and for whom surgical myectomy represents a too-high risk or is not available.[42, 44, 52] Furthermore, pacing offers the opportunity to optimize drug therapy without fearing bradycardia and does not exclude other available treatment options because it is a reversible method.[44] On the other hand, pacing in HOCM requires full ventricular capture. Therefore an optimized AV-delay is necessary.[41, 43, 52] Particularly, patients with a PR interval shorter than 120 ms need an extremely short AV delay (50 ms) to achieve complete ventricular capture. Thus in some cases, further support such as drug administration (β-blocker, calcium-antagonist) for PR-interval prolongation or AV nodal ablation is required.[42, 53] With regard to the short-term improvement, some investigators discussed the possibility of a placebo effect.[42, 54] Furthermore, the relatively high incidence of complications for pacemaker implantation—which is not different from the generally accepted standards—has to be considered.[44]

The latest alternative of treating symptomatic patients with HOCM is a catheter-based technique that induces a localized infarct in the septum through the instillation of an alcohol solution in a septal branch. This method was first described by Sigwart.[49] He based his concept on the observation that a transient occlusion of the first large septal branch of the left anterior descending coronary artery with a balloon catheter leads to a significant reduction of the LVOT obstruction in patients with HOCM.[55] Further development of this observation led to a permanent occlusion of this septal branch by the injection of alcohol into the vessel. Recently, this procedure has been successfully performed by several groups[56–59] in more patients than even expert surgeons have seen over years. This raises some questions about the indication for this procedure, and some critical remarks are certainly justified.[60]

The promising results seen in the short-time follow-up period of various studies were explained by a localized infarct of the proximal interventricular septum followed by a significant reduction of LVOT gradient, a reduction of wall thickness, and an enlargement of the left ventricular outflow area.[56, 58] Besides those hemodynamic benefits, a remarkable improvement of the clinical status could be seen in those patients who underwent an induced septal infarct during short-term follow-up.[56–58] Nevertheless, the relatively high incidence of complications—such as chest pain during the procedure, complete heart block with the necessity of pacemaker implantation, the occurrence of malignant arrhythmias, and even the fatal event of alcohol leakage down the left anterior descending coronary—limit this procedure to patients who are highly symptomatic despite maximal drug therapy and not considered to be candidates for surgery.

Conclusively, both methods represent possible alternatives to the standard treatment of HOCM with remarkable hemodynamic and symptomatic improvement. But further investigation and particularly long-term follow-up data are required and have to be compared with the excellent long-term results of surgical treatment and especially with the results of extended myectomy and mobilization of the subvalvular mitral valve structures.

CONCLUSIONS

Hypertrophic obstructive cardiomyopathy consists of a heterogeneous entity of gross and histopathologic changes of the cardiac musculature. Obstruction of the LVOT varies from mild to severe and is dependent on the form and expansion of asymmetric septum hypertrophy as well as on the degree of the SAM. Systolic anterior motion of the mitral valve is not the result of an attracting force caused by high flow velocity across the outflow tract but is due to active leaflet displacement as a result of early systolic understreaming in a geometrically altered left ventricle.

Initial treatment is medically with β-blocking agents, especially propanolol, verapamil, and disopyramide alone or in combination. Patients whose condition is resistant to medical therapy must be considered for surgery. For complete relief of the obstruction, both the septal and the mitral part must be approached, and the septal muscle bulge must be resected to its deepest point best reached by elevation with the aid of a sharp triple-hook retractor. The technique presented here of an extended myectomy with mobilization of the papillary muscles yielded low early and late mortality with no sudden death in this series. Hemodynamic and echocardiographic results up to 17 years are excellent. More recently, proposed alternative treatments such as DDD-pacing or transcoronary ablation of septal hypertrophy by alcohol instillation have shown to be effective, but the value of these methods can only be judged when long-term follow-up data are available. Furthermore, both DDD-pacing and TASH should be compared with extended surgical myectomy in randomized studies to be sure that truly symptomatic patients resistant to medical therapy are selected for these modes of treatment.

REFERENCES

1. Braunwald E, Morrow AG, Cornell WP, et al: Idiopathic hypertrophic subaortic stenosis: Clinical hemodynamic and angiographic manifestations. *Am J Med* 29:924–945, 1960.
2. Davies LG: A familial heart disease. *Br Heart J* 14:206–212, 1952.
3. Watkins H, Rosenzweig A, Hwang D-S, et al: Characteristics and prognostic implications of myosin missense mutations in familial hypertrophic cardiomyopathy. *N Engl J Med* 326:1108–1114, 1992.
4. Anan R, Greve G, Thierfelder L, et al: Prognostic implications of novel beta cardiac myosin heavy chain gene mutations that cause familial hypertrophic cardiomyopathy. *J Clin Invest* 93:280–285, 1994.
5. Watkins H, McKenna WJ, Thierfelder L, et al: Mutations in the genes for cardiac Troponin T and a-Tropomyosin in hypertrophic cardiomyopathy. *N Engl J Med* 332:1058–1064, 1995.
6. Wigle ED, Felderhof C, Silver MD, et al: Hypertrophic obstructive cardiomyopathy (muscular or hypertrophic subaortic stenosis), in Fowler NO (ed): *Myocardial Disease.* New York, Grune and Stratton, 1973, pp 297–318.
7. Reis RL, Bolton MR, King JF, et al: Anterior-superior displacement of papillary muscles producing obstruction and mitral regurgitation in idiopathic hypertrophic subaortic stenosis: Operative relief by posterior-superior realignment of papillary muscles following ventricular septal myectomy. *Circulation* 49/50 (Suppl II):181–188, 1974.
8. Henry WL, Clark CE, Griffith JM, et al: Mechanism of left ventricular outflow obstruction in patients with obstructive asymmetric septal hypertrophy (idiopathic hypertrophic subaortic stenosis). *Am J Cardiol* 35:337–345, 1975.
9. Klues HG, Maron BJ, Dollar AL, et al: Diversity of structural mitral valve alterations in hypertrophic cardiomyopathy. *Circulation* 85: 1651–1660, 1992.
10. Klues HG, Roberts WC, Maron BJ: Anomalous insertion of papillary muscle directly into anterior mitral leaflet in hypertrophic cardiomyopathy. *Circulation* 84:1188–1197, 1991.

11. Kaltenbach M, Hopf R, Kober G, et al: Treatment of hypertrophic obstructive cardiomyopathy with verapamil. *Br Heart J* 42:35–42, 1979.
12. Epstein SE, Rosing DR: Verapamil: Its potential for causing serious complications in patients with hypertrophc cardiomyopathy. *Circulation* 64:437–441, 1981.
13. Pollick C: Muscular subaortic stenosis: Hemodynamic and clinical improvement after disopyramide. *N Engl J Med* 307:997–999, 1982.
14. Brock R: Aortic subvalvular stenosis: Surgical treatment. *Guy's Hosp Rep* 108:126, 1959.
15. Cleland WP: The surgical management of obstructive cardiomyopathy. *J Cardiovasc Surg* 4:489–491, 1963.
16. Bigelow WG, Trimble AS, Auger P, et al: The ventriculomyotomy operation for muscular subaortic stenosis: A reappraisal. *J Thorac Cardiovasc Surg* 52:514–524, 1966.
17. Kirklin JW, Ellis FH Jr: Surgical relief of diffuse subvalvular aortic stenosis. *Circulation* 24:739–742, 1961.
18. Morrow AG, Brockenbrough EC: Surgical treatment of idiopathic hypertrophic subaortic stenosis: Technique and hemodynamic results of subaortic ventriculomyotomy. *Ann Surg* 154:181–189, 1961.
19. Lillehei CW, Levy MJ: Transatrial exposure for correction of subaortic stenosis: A new approach. *JAMA* 186:8–12, 1963.
20. Cooley DA, Bloodwell RD, Hallman G, et al: Surgical treatment of muscular subaortic stenosis: Results from septectomy in twenty-six patients. *Circulation* 35/36 (Suppl I):124–132, 1967.
21. Binet JP, Langlois J, Leiva-Semper A, et al: Ventriculomyotomy in hypertrophies of the left ventricle. *J Thorac Cardiovasc Surg* 56:469–476, 1968.
22. Cooley DA, Leachman RD: Hallmann GL: Idiopathic hypertrophic subaortic stenosis: Surgical treatment including mitral valve replacement. *Arch Surg* 103:606–612, 1971.
23. Rastan H, Koncz J: Aortoventriculoplasty: A new technique for the treatment of left ventricular outflow tract obstruction. *J Thorac Cardiovasc Surg* 71:920–927, 1976.
24. Dembitzky WP, Weldon CS: Clinical experience with the use of valve-bearing conduit to construct a second left ventricular outflow tract in cases of unresectable intra-ventricular obstruction. *Ann Surg* 184:317, 1976.
25. McIntosh CL, Maron BJ, Cannon RO, et al: Initial results of combined anterior mitral leaflet plication and ventricular septal myotomy-myectomy for relief of left ventricular outflow tract obstruction in patients with hypertrophic cardiomyopathy. *Circulation* 86 (Suppl II): 60–67, 1992.
26. Messmer BJ: Extended myectomy for hypertrophic obstructive cardiomyopathy. *Ann Thorac Surg* 58:575–577, 1994.
27. Schoendube FA, Klues HG, Reith S, et al: Long-term clinical and echocardiographic follow-up after surgical correction of hypertrophic ob-

structive cardiomyopathy with extended myectomy and reconstruction of the subvalvular mitral apparatus. *Circulation* 92 (Suppl II):122–127, 1995.
28. Kaplan E, Meier P: Nonparametric estimation for incomplete observations. *J Am Stat Assoc* 53:475–481, 1958.
29. Tajik AJ, Giuliani ER, Weidmann WH, et al: Idiopathic hypertrophic subaortic stenosis: Long-term surgical follow-up. *Am J Cardiol* 34:815–821, 1974.
30. Morrow AG, Reitz BA, Epstein SE, et al: Operative treatment in hypertrophic subaortic stenosis: Techniques and the results of pre and postoperative assessments in 83 patients. *Circulation* 52:88–102, 1975.
31. Senning A: Transventricular relief of idiopathic hypertrophic subaortic stenosis. *J Cardiovasc Surg* 17:371–375, 1976.
32. Beahrs MM, Tajik AJ, Seward JB, et al: Hypertrophic obstructive cardiomyopathy: Ten to 21-years follow-up after partial septal myectomy. *Am J Cardiol* 51:1160–1166, 1983.
33. Maron BJ, Harding AM, Spirito P, et al: Systolic anterior motion of the posterior mitral leaflet: A previously unrecognized cause of dynamic subaortic obstruction in patients with hypertrophic cardiomyopathy. *Circulation* 68:282–293, 1983.
34. Birks W, Schulte HD: Surgical treatment of hypertrophic obstructive cardiomyopathy with special reference to complications and to atypical hypertrophic obstructive cardiomyopathy. *Eur Heart J* 4 (Suppl F):187–190, 1983.
35. McIntosh CL, Maron BJ: Current operative treatment of obstructive hypertrophic cardiomyopathy. *Circulation* 78:487–495, 1988.
36. Kraijcer Z, Leachman RD, Cooley DA, et al: Septal myotomy-myectomy versus mitral valve replacement in hypertrophic cardiomyopathy. *Circulation* 80 (Suppl I):57–64, 1989.
37. Seiler C, Hess OM, Schoenbeck M, et al: Long-term follow-up of medical versus surgical therapy for hypertrophic cardiomyopathy: A retrospective study. *J Am Coll Cardiol* 17:634–642, 1991.
38. Cohn LA, Trehan H, Collins JJ: Long-term follow-up of patients undergoing myotomy/myectomy for obstructive hypertrophic cardiomyopathy. *Am J Cardiol* 70:657–660, 1992.
39. Ten Berg JM, Maarten JS, Knaepen PF, et al: Hypertrophic obstructive cardiomyopathy: Initial results and long-term follow-up after Morrow septal myectomy. *Circulation* 90:1781–1785, 1994.
40. Siegmann IL, Maron BJ, Permut LC, et al: Results of operation for coexistent obstructive cardiomyopathy and coronary artery disease. *J Am Coll Cardiol* 13:1527–1533, 1989.
41. Fananapazir L, Cannon RO, Tripodi D, et al: Impact of dual chamber pacing in patients with hypertrophic obstructive cardiomyopathy with symptoms refractory to verapamil and β-adrenergic blocker therapy. *Circulation* 85:2149–2161, 1992.

42. Wigle ED, Rakowski H, Kimball BP, et al: Hypertrophic cardiomyopathy: Clinical spectrum and treatment. *Circulation* 92:1680–1692, 1995.
43. Jeanrenaud X, Goy JJ, Kappenberger L: Effects of dual chamber pacing in hypertrophic obstructive cardiomyopathy. *Lancet* 339:1318–1323, 1992.
44. Kappenberger L, Linde C, Daubert C, et al: Pacing in hypertrophic obstructive cardiomyopathy. *Eur Heart J* 18:1249–1256, 1997.
45. Fananapazir L, Epstein ND, Curiel RV, et al: Long-term results of dual chamber (DDD) pacing in obstructive cardiomyopathy: Evidence for progressive symptomatic and hemodynamic improvement and reduction of left ventricular hypertrophy. *Circulation* 90:2731–2742, 1994.
46. Duck HJ, Hutschenreiter W, Pankau H, et al: Vorhofsynchrone Ventrikelstimulation mit verkürzter av-Verzögerungszeit als Therapieprinzip der hypertrophen obstruktiven Kardiomyopathie. *Z Gesamte Innere Med Ihre Grenzgebiete* 39:437–447, 1984.
47. McDonald K, McWilliams E, O'Keeffe B, et al: Functional assessment of patients treated with permanent dual chamber pacing as a primary treatment for hypertrophic obstructive cardiomyopathy. *Eur Heart J* 9:893–898, 1988.
48. Spirito P, Seidman CE, McKenna W, et al: The management of hypertrophic cardiomyopathy. *N Engl J Med* 336:775–785, 1997.
49. Sigwart U: Non-surgical reduction for hypertrophic obstructive cardiomyopathy. *Lancet* 346:211–214, 1995.
50. Reneman RS, Prinzen FW, Cherieux EC, et al: Asymmetrical changes in left ventricular diastolic wall thickness induced by chronic asynchronous electrical activation in man and dogs. *FASEB J* 7:752A, 1993.
51. Delhaas T, Arts T, Prinzen FW, et al: Relation between regional electrical activation time and subepicardial fiber strain in the canine left ventricle. *Pflugers Arch (Eur J Physiol)* 423:78–87, 1993.
52. Nishimura RA, Danielson GK: Dual chamber pacing for hypertrophic obstructive cardiomyopathy: Has its time come? *Br Heart J* 70:301–303, 1993.
53. Gras D, De Place C, Leclerq C, et al: Key importance to individually optimize atrioventricular synchrony in obstructive hypertrophic cardiomyopathy treated by DDD-pacing. *Eur Heart J* 15 (Suppl):552A, 1994.
54. Nishimura RA, Trusty JM, Hayes DL, et al: Dual chamber pacing for hypertrophic cardiomyopathy: A randomized, double-blind, crossover trial. *J Am Coll Cardiol* 29:435–441, 1997.
55. Sigwart U, Gerbic M, Essinger A, et al: L'effet aigu d'une occlusion coronarienne par ballonet de la dilatation transluminale. *Schweiz Med Wochenschr* 45:1631A, 1982.
56. Knight C, Kurbaan AS, Seggewiss H, et al: Non-surgical septal reduction for hypertrophic obstructive cardiomyopathy: Outcome in the first series of patients. *Circulation* 95:2075–2081, 1997.

57. Lakkis N, Kleiman N, Killip D, et al: Hypertrophic obstructive cardiomyopathy: Alternative therapeutic options. *Clin Cardiol* 20: 417–418, 1997.
58. Kuhn H, Gietzen F, Leunen CH, et al: Induction of subaortic septal ischemia to reduce obstruction in hypertrophic obstructive cardiomyopathy: Studies to develop a new catheter-based concept of treatment. *Eur Heart J* 18:846–851, 1997.
59. Seggewiss H, Gleichmann U, Faßender D, et al: Catheter treatment of hypertrophic cardiomyopathy: Acute hemodynamic and clinical results. *Circulation* 94 (Suppl I):617, 1996.
60. Braunwald E: Induced septal infarction: A new therapeutic strategy for hypertrophic obstructive cardiomyopathy. *Circulation* 95:1981–1982, 1997.

CHAPTER 12

Traumatic Rupture of the Thoracic Aorta

Kenneth L. Mattox, M.D.
Professor and Vice Chair of Surgery, Baylor College of Medicine; Chief of Staff and Chief of Surgery, Ben Taub General Hospital, Houston, Texas

Blunt injury to the thoracic aorta continues to be the sine qua non example of severe thoracic injury. This injury taxes all elements of a trauma system, from societal prevention and educational programs to complex rehabilitation and medical activities. Furthermore, numerous and often conflicting opinions have resulted from educational bias and polarized interpretation of limited data. Many of the data available on aortic injury are Class 3 evidence-based information. Finally, available transportation, imaging, and operative technology make adaptability of historical control information extremely difficult. Changing opinions, comfort levels with managing this injury, the overall complex nature of traumatic injuries, limited numbers of cases an individual surgeon or team of surgeons will perform, operative options, and individual skill variability make this a very complex surgical problem.

Knowledge of thoracic aortic injury is basically limited to the past 50 years of this century. The first successful repair of a chronic blunt thoracic injury occurred in 1953, and the first acute injury repair occurred in 1959.[1, 2] During each decade since 1960, new technical advances have been made in emergency medical services, resuscitation, imaging, monitoring, cardiopulmonary bypass technology, drugs, and surgical critical care. There are many, often conflicting, data in each of these categories, creating tremendous polarization and confusion. Nevertheless, the data are often cited in a courtroom when an undesirable result occurs. If these opposing views are analyzed in light of the year of the report, institutional preferences, and changing/emerging technology, the differences are not so much at variance. This chapter attempts to focus on the most practical and applicable standards of practice. Even as this chapter is being written, paradigms of resuscitation, operative decision making, timing of operation, and technology are undergoing significant change.

INCIDENCE

Between 2% and 10% of patients with blunt chest injury have an injury to the thoracic great vessels, including the aorta.[3, 4] In a review by Oller et al. in 1992,[5] 26,617 trauma patients from North Carolina were entered into a single trauma registry over a 39-month period. From this population-based registry, 1,148 vascular injuries were recorded in 908 patients. Fifty-eight had injury to the thoracic aorta. This database did not include patients who died before arrival at a hospital. By some estimates, up to 85% of the patients with this injury die before any chance of clinical diagnosis or therapeutic intervention.[6] North Carolina has relatively few trauma centers and much rural geography. Extrapolations from this database should take into consideration these epidemiologic factors.

PITFALLS IN AORTIC INJURY

When one approaches a patient with a potential aortic injury, especially to the thoracic aorta, many potential pitfalls exist:

EXCESSIVELY AGGRESSIVE RESUSCITATION

Aggressive resuscitation and its attempts to elevate blood pressure create several undesirable side effects for the patient with an aortic injury. With less than 1,000 mL of crystalloid fluid, a statistically significant elevation in the PTT, PT, and platelet count occurs, compared with patients with no or limited resuscitation with crystalloid fluid.[7] Elevation of blood pressure in a patient with an aortic injury, as in the patient with a leaking abdominal aortic aneurysm, has a greater potential to cause excessive additional blood loss and a secondary fatal hemorrhage. Limited resuscitation, maintaining the blood pressure under 120/-, therefore, is more desirable than aggressive fluid resuscitation.

FAILURE TO APPRECIATE OR RECORD PHYSICAL FINDINGS

Patients with multi-organ or complex trauma require a systematic approach to evaluation and treatment. Review of original medical records of patients discovered hours or days after an event to have a secondary injury often reveals incomplete record keeping. Distal pulses and neurologic status—as well as all other aspects of the primary and secondary survey—must be evaluated and recorded.

EXCESSIVE EXPECTATIONS

A patient with aortic trauma has a life-threatening injury. Despite a surgeon's best efforts, the patient's condition may not improve, complications may develop, and death may occur. Society has come to expect a good outcome if a trauma patient reaches a trauma center. This perception is unrealistic and poses pitfalls for the patient, the patient's family, and the medical team, especially in patients with aortic injury.

VARIATION IN THE PRESENTATION SYMPTOMS

Up to 50% of patients subsequently found to have aortic injury have no initial sign of external trauma. Up to 8% have relatively normal-appearing initial chest x-ray scans. Other patients with aortic injury are seen in extremis—with unstable vital signs, including hypertension—and may also have diverting abdominal, head, or extremity injury.

VARIATION IN SUGGESTIVE FINDINGS ON THE INITIAL CHEST X-RAY SCAN

At least 20 suggestive signs associated with thoracic aortic injury have been described on a plain anteroposterior or lateral chest x-ray scan. Each may occur in the *absence* of an aortic injury, just as an aortic injury may be present with *no* suggestive radiologic signs present.

VARIATION IN LOCATION OF THE AORTIC INJURY

Although the descending thoracic aorta just distal to the subclavian artery is the most common site of injury, the thoracic aorta can be injured at the aortic root, the ascending aorta, the transverse aortic arch, and the distal thoracic aorta at the diaphragm. Between 2% and 5% of patients have more than one injury of the aortic site.

VARIATION IN AVAILABILITY OF IMAGING TECHNOLOGIES

Although aortography remains the "gold" standard for precisely diagnosing an aortic injury and any thoracic arterial anomalies (occurring in up to 30% of patients), some trauma centers use CT scanning and transesophageal echocardiography (TEE) to evaluate the condition of a patient with a mediastinal hematoma. Both CT and TEE currently yield false negative, false positive, and misleading readings.

VARIATIONS IN DIAGNOSTIC AND TREATMENT PHILOSOPHIES WITHIN A GIVEN HOSPITAL, WITHIN A REGION, AND AROUND THE COUNTRY

At least three (or more) standard and acceptable perioperative approaches exist for the management of aortic injury. Both good and undesirable results have been reported with use of *each* of the techniques. Regardless of the technique used, a good outcome results in praise, and an unfavorable outcome is usually met with criticism.

TIME OF DAY WHEN PATIENTS ARE SEEN WITH THIS INJURY

More than 60% of thoracic aortic injuries are seen at the hospital between 11 PM and 7 AM. Over 50% of these patients have elevated blood alcohol levels. Most hospitals are not staffed with as many experienced personnel during these hours as they are during daylight hours.

EXTENT OF ASSOCIATED INJURIES

In some patients, the aortic injury is an isolated injury; others have extensive head, chest, orthopedic, abdominal, and vascular injuries, creating a diagnostic and logistic problem in management.

POSSIBILITY OF A CONCOMITANT COAGULOPATHY

A dilutional or hypothermia coagulopathy is common in trauma patients, especially if aggressive prehospital and emergency center crystalloid resuscitation has occurred. Such coagulopathies create problems in the timing and safety of any surgery.

TIMING OF OPERATIONS

Some surgeons mandate that an operation be performed immediately after a diagnosis has been established, whereas other surgeons prefer to delay surgery for hours, or even days and weeks.

CHOICE OF ADJUNCTIVE TECHNOLOGY

Tremendous variations exist in the literature regarding use of adjunctive techniques to achieve perfusion distal to any aortic clamps. For aortic root and ascending aortic injury, cardiopulmonary bypass is almost always required, but in aortic arch and descending thoracic aortic injuries, other techniques—such as clamp/repair without shunts, use of passive shunts, use of active shunts without heparinization, and use of routine cardiopulmonary bypass with heparinization—are available. With the addition of each technology, the complexity of the surgery and the possibility for technology-associated complications increase.

VARIATIONS IN TECHNICAL ADJUNCTS AVAILABLE IN A HOSPITAL

Tremendous variability exists in the type and complexity of adjunctive equipment available among hospitals. Autotransfusion devices, automated anesthesia records, cardiopulmonary bypass, active/passive shunting techniques, and other items may or may not be available. Availability is often a function of managed care philosophies and determined by nonphysicians. Furthermore, the age, functionality, and availability of technicians varies considerably, depending on budget allocations. This variation often forces surgeons, especially in a rural setting, to use a technique or a piece of equipment that they would not have normally used in a large urban hospital.

VARIATIONS IN THE AVAILABILITY OF IMAGING TECHNIQUES

Not only is there variability in imaging technologies and equipment, but there also is tremendous variability in the availability of a radiologist to both perform angiography and interpret any CT, TEE, or even angiographic findings. The surgeon is often the only professional available to interpret subtle findings and make appropriate decisions.

VARIABILITY IN EXPERIENCE OF BOTH THE SURGICAL AND THE NURSING STAFF

A surgeon's familiarity and experience with aortic trauma—as well as that of the surgical team—varies considerably among trauma centers and nontrauma centers around the world. Most hospitals seeing trauma patients see two aortic injury cases per year. This low number does not allow the surgeon to gain much experience with this injury. Nonetheless, when this injury is encountered, the surgeon is often required to operate.

VARIABILITY OF AVAILABILITY AND DISTRIBUTION OF TRAUMA SYSTEMS AND TRAUMA CENTERS

Trauma center distribution is spotty and trauma center policies vary greatly. Emergency physicians often do not involve the surgeon in the case of a patient with an aortic injury until after an aortogram is done.

POSSIBILITY OF CONCOMITANT CNS INJURY

Central nervous system injury, including spinal cord contusion, might be present but not manifest until up to several days after the injury. Furthermore, concomitant head injury creates logistic pitfalls for the surgeon.

ANATOMICAL ANOMALIES

Vascular rings, anomalous origin of the right subclavian artery, ductus diverticulum, situs inversus, common origin of the innominate and left carotid arteries, among others, are not uncommon anatomical anomalies that may be encountered. These are precisely diagnosed only by aortography, and if their presence is discovered during an operation, problems could result intraoperatively.

NATURAL HISTORY AND PATTERNS OF PRESENTATION

Aortic root injury is probably a result of lateral deceleration, whereas all of blunt thoracic aortic injury at other locations is secondary to an osseous pinch.[8] An automobile passenger has a 50% greater chance of sustaining aortic injury if ejected from the automobile on impact. Seventy percent to 85% of patients with aortic injury die before arriving at a hospital; 2% to 5% of patients have an unstable condition during transport. During the first 4 hours at a hospital, the latter group has a 90% to 98% mortality, often from both aortic and nonaortic causes, especially concomitant head injury. Fifteen percent to 25% of patients with aortic injury are hemodynamically stable during transport and during the 4–8 hours of evaluation for their multiple traumatic injuries. Among this group, a 25% mortality is seen, with most dying of concomitant abdominal or head injury or both. In up to 5% of patients with aortic injury, the condition is initially undiagnosed, and chronic pseudoaneurysms of the thoracic aorta develop in them. Among this group, 22% are symptomatic at 1 year, 42% are symptomatic at 5 years, 58% at 10 years, and 85% at 20 years. The mortality for chronic traumatic aneurysms is higher in symptomatic patients.

MAKING THE DIAGNOSIS—CONSENSUS AND CONTROVERSY

HISTORICAL AND CLINICAL INDICATORS

Aortography is often obtained because of historical or clinical indicators suggesting thoracic aortic injury. In the stable patient, this practice is both indicated and effective. Historical clues that should cause the surgeon to consider an aortic injury include:

- Evidence of excessive decelerative forces in an automobile accident, including deformity of the steering wheel
- Survivors of an aircraft crash
- Falls from heights
- Automobile-pedestrian accidents
- History of being ejected from an automobile during a crash

- History of postinjury paralysis
- History of lateral deceleration (for aortic root injury)

Physical examination clues that should cause the surgeon to consider aortography include:

- Upper extremity hypertension
- Evidence of postinjury lower extremity paralysis or paresis
- Intrascapular murmur
- Steering wheel imprint on the anterior chest wall
- Major chest wall fractures, including sternum, flail chest, scapula, and bilateral clavicles after blunt trauma

RADIOGRAPHIC INDICATORS

Suggestive findings on emergency center chest x-ray scans are the most common reason imaging studies are obtained. At least 20 different suggestive clues seen on AP or lateral chest x-ray scans should lead to secondary imaging. These clues all are a function of the presence of a mediastinal hematoma and its effect on secondary structures, such as the trachea or the esophagus. These clues are present whether the chest x-ray scan is a 36-inch AP projection or a 72-inch posterior-anterior projection. In some hospitals where the availability of aortography is delayed because of nonavailability of either an angiographic technologist or an interventional radiologist, the next recommended imaging study has been a CT scan, adding delays and expenses. Most often, the CT scan merely confirms the presence of a mediastinal hematoma. Newer, spiral-enhanced CT scanners might document the site of an aortic tear but fail to clearly document any anomalies in the thoracic vasculature. In virtually every trauma center, a positive CT scan result is followed by a delayed formal aortogram, with its duplicative expenses. Transesophageal echocardiography has also been recommended as an imaging technique of choice, but its sensitivity produces false positive readings, is user dependent, and also does not document aortic anomalies. In many hospitals, a TEE is also followed by an aortogram. As the aortogram remains the only definitive examination to demonstrate both aortic pathology and anomalies, it is recommended that this test be initially performed in patients with historical examination or radiologic clues consistent with thoracic injury.

WHEN AORTOGRAPHY IS NOT POSSIBLE

Some patients either have such extensive associated injuries or are so hemodynamically unstable that transport to an interventional radiology suite is impossible or impractical. In some such instances, the surgeon may wish to know whether a strong probability of aortic injury exists, for overall logistic and planning purposes. In these cases, a screening TEE can be helpful, performed in the emergency center, operating room, or ICU.

In the hemodynamically unstable patient, a surgeon may be forced to perform an operation without benefit of an aortogram. In such instances, if the incision choice is incorrect, the subsequent control, exposure, and attempted repair can be catastrophic. An ascending aortic injury cannot be repaired easily through a posterolateral thoracotomy, and a descending thoracic aortic injury cannot be repaired via a median sternotomy. In such instances, if the hematoma is seen toward the right side of the chest or is in the thoracic outlet, the surgeon should perform an emergent median sternotomy. Should the mediastinal hematoma be seen in the left side of the chest and be centered at the aortic isthmus, a left fourth posterolateral thoracotomy is the incision of choice.

CONCOMITANT ABDOMINAL, BRAIN, AND THORACIC AORTIC INJURY

Many patients with thoracic aortic injury also have life-threatening intracranial or abdominal injury or both. Except in the patient who has chest tube drainage suggesting an exsanguinating hemorrhage from the chest, a craniotomy or a laparotomy should be performed before a thoracotomy. In some instances, an abdominal damage control tactic can be applied and the patient can be taken for an aortogram if one had not been obtained earlier. On rare occasions, a thoracotomy may be required (without benefit of an aortogram, after a craniotomy or laparotomy).

OPERATIVE APPROACHES

POSITION AND INCISIONS

Patients with injuries to the aortic root, the ascending aorta, and the aortic arch, including blunt injury to the innominate artery, are placed supine on the operating table and the injury is approached via a median sternotomy. For all but the innominate artery injuries, cardiopulmonary pump bypass is usually required. For patients with injury to the descending thoracic aorta, a left posterolateral incision, usually through the fourth interspace, is indicated. Anterolateral incisions do not provide the best exposure and only are used as part of a transsternal bilateral resuscitative thoracotomy.

OPERATIVE ADJUNCTS

Communication among all members of the operative team is essential. Many adjunctive maneuvers and equipment are favored by various surgeons and include:

- Swan-Ganz pulmonary catheters
- Intra-arterial pressure monitoring, sometimes in both the right arm and a femoral artery
- Autotransfusion
- Ability to perform single-lung anesthesia with collapse of the left lung
- Consideration for CSF drainage (not yet reported in patients with acute aortic injury)
- Devices for active and passive shunting, if these are the surgeon's preference

REPAIR/CLAMPING AND PERFUSION PHILOSOPHIES

Aortic injuries may be deliberately treated nonoperatively (at least acutely) or treated with attempted repair or exclusion. More than 10 different approaches have been used; at least 5 are standard in some localities. The reason for the variety of approach philosophies relates to complexity and difficulty of reconstruction; medical, legal, and managed care sanctions; and a desire to prevent (as much as possible) a significant mortality rate as well as a frustrating (and continuing to occur) complication rate, particularly for paraplegia.

Historically, thoracic aneurysms, including posttraumatic ones, were *not* directly reconstructed. Wrapping with cellophane, insertion of piano wire, and other tactics to retard a potential rupture were attempted. In some high-risk patients, permanent exclusion by a permanent clamp proximal and distal to the aneurysm, with an extra-anatomical bypass routing, was used. Direct repair—whether in the 15% of cases that can be repaired primarily or the majority that require graft interposition, clamping above and below the injury, with subsequent repair—has been termed a clamp/repair approach.

The segmental arteries and the adjacent spinal cord between these clamps are at risk if there is unfavorable anatomy or a spinal compartment syndrome, regardless of additional adjuncts. At least three standard adjuncts to clamp/repair are in current use. None should be condemned nor championed, and the surgeon operating on a blunt thoracic aortic injury must be familiar and adept with each and understand the advantages and disadvantages of each. Use of a passive shunt, use of an active shunt, use of routine cardiopulmonary bypass, and a dependence on collateral circulation are standard adjuncts to clamp/repair. Passive shunts have unpredictable flow rates and currently are rarely used. The pump and shunt adjuncts add a degree of complexity and potential additional complications relating to the cannula, tube sites, and pump circuit, which are not present in the simple nonshunted clamp/repair approach.

Deliberate nonoperative approaches will be discussed later in this chapter.

DISTAL PERFUSION

Perfusion distal to the aortic clamps has been a subject of considerable debate. For many years, passive shunts were claimed to provide "adequate" distal protection and provide an element of "protection" to the spinal cord between the two aortic clamps. It is now recognized that this "practice guideline" of the 1980s did not result in a reproducible distal flow rate and, at times, had virtually no flow through the passive shunt. Some surgeons who used such passive shunting in the past have now progressed to use of "active" shunts because they claim that the distal perfusion is more reproducible. Three methods of standard distal perfusion are in use:

1. routine cardiopulmonary bypass, usually with nonpulsatile flow and with routine total body heparinization;
2. shunting, using either a passive (Gott shunt) or an active (centrifugal pump) shunt, and usually not total body heparinization;
3. and reliance on the body's collateral circulation to the distal body circulation.

Even with the last method, profuse retrograde bleeding occurs when the distal clamp is released for flushing purposes at the completion of the distal suture line. Regardless of the philosophy for distal perfusion, the spinal cord circulation between the clamps is at risk for underperfusion should the spinal cord circulation be unfavorable. The first two methods add a degree of complexity to the procedure, and each cannulation site has a potential for additional complications and problems.

FACTORS CONTRIBUTING TO TIMING OF SURGERY

Although cross-clamp times less than 15 minutes have been reported, the average reported cross-clamp times are in the range of 35–45 minutes. The length of the cross-clamp time is most often determined by extent of injury, rather than an individual surgeon's technical prowess. The minority of patients have cross-clamp times in excess of 50–60 minutes, and in most of these instances, very complex lesions were encountered. Considerable debate centers on cross-clamp times, a "magical" 30-minute "safe" time, and the contribution that the various approaches might have on the incidence of the dreaded complication of paraplegia. Such statements have more emotion than scientific supportive data.[9] stated that the mortality from thoracic aortic injury after trauma has remained constant over time, despite improvements in EMS, resuscitation, and operative techniques; and cross-clamp time does not predict the occurrence of postoperative paraplegia.

PURPOSEFUL DELAY IN OPERATIVE MANAGEMENT

A number of interesting anomalies that occurred during the past 15 years suggest that delay in operation for deciding thoracic aortic injury might be considered in selected patients. When concomitant thoracic aorta and abdominal injury exists, virtually all authors recommend laparotomy before thoracotomy in "stable" patients. Chronic traumatic thoracic aneurysms are seen more commonly. Healed arterial injuries that have not undergone previous operation are increasingly described in the aorta and in peripheral vascular surgery. Purposeful surgical delays on traumatic thoracic aortic tears are increasingly being reported, with more than 300 currently appearing in the literature.

Early surgery on the thoracic aorta is contraindicated in selected patients, such as in the patient with a Glasgow Coma Scale score of less than 6. When CT of the head demonstrates extensive hemorrhage and when the PT and the PTT are 1½ times normal or greater, early operation is contraindicated. A patient requiring inotropic support or one whose left lung cannot be collapsed should have operative repair delayed for hours, days, weeks, and sometimes months.

Currently, over 300 patients with descending thoracic aortic injury have had reported delay in surgery for hours, days, weeks, and sometimes months. Delays have been either for the reasons previously stipulated or because of other extensive injuries. Of these 300, only the 5 patients who had an aorta-related mortality had uncontrolled hypertension. Virtually all 300 patients were stable for the first 6 hours after injury, with no sign of expansion of the periaortic hematoma, and most received afterload reduction agents.[10] In 1995, Pate indicated that aortography is performed 2.7–71 hours after injury in most institutions, with operation occurring an average of 9 hours after injury (range, 4.2–68.3 hours). In his review of cases, all but 1 of 89 patients who had delay in surgery did well and did not sustain aortic rupture during the delay period. The one patient who had aortic rupture while awaiting surgery had uncontrolled hypertension. Increasingly, in stable patients with descending thoracic aortic injury in combination with multiple injuries (especially head injury), initial nonoperative management is being recommended by trauma and thoracic surgeons. Afterload reduction is recommended in the patient without hypotension, and the decision for "conservative" vs. immediate operative management should always be an informed decision, with informed consent from the patient and the patient's family. This final decision must always rest with the patient's surgeon. In considering initial nonoperative repair, there are a number of caveats:

1. the patient must be hemodynamically stable;
2. the mediastinal hematoma must not be expanding;
3. the patient should probably be receiving β blockade, although a prospective randomized study has not been conducted to substantiate this recommendation;
4. and the blood pressure should be controlled so that systolic pressure does not exceed 120 mm Hg.

FUTURE PROJECTIONS

Technological and logistic paradigm shifts continue to dominate thoracic aortic injury. The areas for current and future developments will include:

- Training, qualifications, and credentialing of surgeons who evaluate, diagnose, and treat thoracic aortic injury
- Purposeful delay and surgery using controlled blood pressure in patients hemodynamically stable 4–6 hours after injury
- Better understanding and treatment of potential spinal compartment syndrome
- Endovascular imaging, including US
- Endovascular stented grafts
- Advanced monitoring technology
- Integrated relational database artificial intelligence to assist in decision making
- Teleconsultation and teletreatment across political jurisdictions

REFERENCES

1. Stranahan A, Alley RD, Sewell WH, et al: Aortic arch resection and grafting for aneurysm employing an external shunt. *J Thor Surg* 29:54–65, 1955.
2. Klausner JM, Rozin RR: Late abdominal complications in war wounded. *J Trauma* 38:313–317, 1995.
3. Glinz W: Priorities in diagnosis and treatment of blunt chest injuries. *Injury* 17:318–321, 1986.
4. Kemmerer WT: Patterns of thoracic injuries in fatal traffic accidents. *J Trauma* 1:595, 1961.
5. Oller DW, Rutledge R, Clancy T, et al: Vascular injuries in a rural state: A review of 978 patients from a state trauma registry. *J Trauma* 32:740–746, 1992.
6. Parmley LF, Mattingly TW, Marion WC, et al: Nonpenetrating traumatic injury to the aorta. *Circulation* 17:1086–1101, 1958.
7. Bickell WH, Wall MJ Jr, Pepe PE, et al: Immediate versus delayed fluid resuscitation for hypotensive patients with penetrating torso injuries. *N Engl J Med* 331:1105–1109, 1994.
8. Cohen AM, Crass JR, Thomas HA, et al: CT evidence for the "Osseous Pinch" mechanism for traumatic aortic injury. *AJR* 159:271–274, 1992.
9. Duhaylongsod FG, Glower DD, Wolfe WG: Acute traumatic aortic aneurysm: The Duke experience from 1970 to 1990. *J Vasc Surg* 15:331–343, 1992.
10. Pate JW: Imaging of traumatic rupture of the aorta (letter). *J Thorac Cardiovasc Surg* 109:190–191, 1995.

Index

A

B

D

E

F

G

H

I

K

L

S

T

U

V

W

X

Y